DATE DUE

Countertransference
in the
Treatment of PTSD

Countertransference in the Treatment of PTSD

Edited by
JOHN P. WILSON
JACOB D. LINDY

Foreword by Bessel A. van der Kolk

THE GUILFORD PRESS
New York   London

Last digit is print number: 9 8 7 6 5 4 3 2 1

Library of Congress Cataloging-in-Publication Data

Countertransference in the treatment of PTSD / edited by
    John P. Wilson, Jacob D. Lindy: foreword by Bessel A. van der Kolk.
        p.   cm.
    Includes bibliographical references and index.
    ISBN 0-89862-369-3
    1. Post-traumatic stress disorder—Treatment.
    2. Countertransference (Psychology) 3. Psychotherapist and patient.
    I. Wilson, John P. (John Preston) II. Lindy, Jacob D., 1937–
    [DNLM: 1. Stress Disorders, Post-Traumatic—therapy.
    2. Countertransference (Psychology) 3. Professional–Patient
    Relations. WM 170 C855 1994]
    RC552.P67C68 1994
    616.85′21—dc20
    DNLM/DLC
    for Library of Congress   93-43029
                                                                       CIP

Contributors

Petra G. H. Aarts, PhD, National Institute for Victims of War, Utrecht, the Netherlands

Inger Agger, PhD, Liaison Officer, EC-Task Force, Zagreb, Croatia, and Licensed Psychologist, Aalborg, Denmark

Joseph Colletti, MA, Department of Clinical Psychology, University of Kansas, Lawrence, Kansas

Yael Danieli, PhD, Private practice, New York, New York, and Director, Group Project for Holocaust Survivors and Their Children, New York, New York

Christine Dunning, PhD, Department of Governmental Affairs, Division of Outreach and Continuing Education, University of Wisconsin–Milwaukee, Milwaukee, Wisconsin

Carol R. Hartmen, RN, DNSc, Department of Psychiatric Nursing, Boston College, Chestnut Hill, Massachusetts

Helene Jackson, PhD, Columbia University School of Social Work, New York, New York

Søren Buus Jensen, MD, PhD, Chief Psychiatrist, Aalborg Psychiatric Hospital, Aalborg, Denmark, and Director, Center for Psychosocial and Traumatic Stress, Aalborg, Denmark

J. David Kinzie, MD, Department of Psychiatry, Oregon Health Sciences University, Portland, Oregon

Richard P. Kluft, MD, Director, Dissociative Disorders Programs, The Institute of Pennsylvania Hospital, Philadelphia, Pennsylvania, and Clinical Professor of Psychiatry, Temple University School of Medicine, Philadelphia, Pennsylvania

G. Frank Koerselman, MD, Department of Psychiatry, St. Lucas Hospital, Amsterdam, the Netherlands

Jacob D. Lindy, MD, Center for Psychoanalysis, Cincinnati, Ohio

Michael J. Maxwell, MS, Department of Veterans Affairs Medical Center, Portland, Oregon.

I. Lisa McCann, PhD, Women's Trauma Recovery Services, Kansas City, Missouri

Kathleen Nader, DSW, Director of Evaluations, UCLA Trauma, Violence and Sudden Bereavement Program, UCLA Neuropsychiatric Institute, Laguna Hills, California

Wybrand Op den Velde, MD, Department of Psychiatry, St. Lucas Hospital, Amsterdam, the Netherlands

Erwin Randolph Parson, PhD, Clinical Psychologist and Consultant to the Perry Point Post-Traumatic Stress Disorder Clinical Team, Department of Veterans Affairs Medical Center, Perry Point, Maryland

Beverley Raphael, MD, Royal Brisbane Hospital, University of Queensland, Herston, Australia

Cynthia Sturm, PhD, Private practice, Portland, Oregon

Bessel A. van der Kolk, PhD, Chief, Massachusetts General Hospital Trauma Clinic, Boston, Massachusetts, and Associate Professor of Psychiatry, Harvard Medical School, Boston, Massachusetts

John P. Wilson, PhD, Professor of Psychology, Cleveland State University, Cleveland, Ohio, and Chairperson, Disaster Services, The American Red Cross

Foreword

Our patients are our teachers, but psychologists and psychiatrists have been very slow in learning our patients' lessons about the impact of trauma on their lives. It has taken us a long time to recognize the extent to which people, with all their innate resilience, can actually be wounded by external injuries. This book explores the obstacles to learning the lessons from our traumatized patients and the various ways in which we avoid listening and "being there" for them. Often, the same issues that cause victims to become fixated on the trauma (numbing, dissociation, fascination, revulsion, rescuing, and blaming) obstruct therapists in their attempts to undo the effects of that trauma. We must understand and tame these inevitable aspects of taking on the task of accompanying people on their journey to integrate the effects of overwhelming experiences into their lives. This book tries to help therapists be aware of their counter-transference, so it can be used in the service of that task, rather than becoming an obstacle that leads to the re-creation of the trauma in the therapy.

Lessons learned under conditions of intense emotional arousal have a lasting impact. Working with people who have been traumatized confronts all participants with intense emotional experiences and requires them to explore the darkest corners of the mind and face the entire spectrum of human glory and degradation. Sooner or later, those experiences are bound to overwhelm; the repeated exposure to our own vulnerability becomes too intense, the display of man's infinite capacity for cruelty too unbearable, the enactment of the trauma within the therapeutic relationship too terrifying.

There always have been therapists who have understood the role of trauma in the therapist–patient relationship and struggled with it. Sandor

Ferenczi wrote a paper in 1929 about the "Confusion of Tongues between the Adult and the Child: The Language of Tenderness and the Language of Passion," in which he described the incompatibility between a child's need for tenderness and care and an adult's use of these needs to discharge sexual and aggressive tensions. His courageous description of the resulting confusion about the boundaries of sexuality, aggression, and tenderness, and the reenactment of this confusion within the therapy relationship, eventually contributed to his professional isolation. John Bowlby started his studies on the vital role of secure attachments while a resident in Melanie Klein's clinic in London, where he was taught to apply drive theory to explain the behavior of sexually and physically abused children. During and after World War II, innumerable psychoanalysts had close encounters with the consequences of Nazi concentration camps, but only a handful called attention to the ways in which devastating realities could deform the psyche. Leo Eitinger, Jan Bastiaans, Shamai Davidson, William Niederland, Henry Krystal, Robert J. Lifton, and a few others were lone voices until the 1970s, when the reality of violence became central to our culture. Judith Herman has emphasized how acknowledgment of the true impact of trauma can only occur in the context of a favorable political climate. The simultaneous emergence of the women's movement and the recognition of the psychological effects of the Vietnam War created the unlikely alliance necessary to recognize the central role of trauma in creating long-lasting individual suffering and societal malfunction.

Despite the fact that between 40 and 60% of psychiatric patients have histories of significant trauma, a straightforward evaluation of the role of trauma in the creation of psychological malfunction is extremely difficult. Little is known about the various paths that people take to cope with traumatic experiences, what contributes to and constitutes resilience, and to what degree trauma can spawn creative transformations that lead to new personal and cultural values. The wide variety of adaptations to traumatic life experiences makes it impossible to resort to facile constructs. Simply ascribing the entirety of a person's psychological functioning to the trauma, or proposing that our patients "really" suffer from a biological disorder that can be fixed with drugs, constitutes a countertransference reaction aimed at avoiding the complexity and harshness of our patients' lives. The devastating effects of trauma on affect modulation, attention, perception, and the giving and taking of pleasure bring us face to face with the full destructive impact of people's urges to dominate, use, and control others. And those urges are shared by ourselves and by our patients.

After years of neglecting and denying the reality of trauma, we have almost come to glorify it. In recent years, much of human suffering and human cruelty has been recast as the result of victimization, sometimes at the expense of attention to other factors that contribute to these immemorial issues. In a simplistic psychological world, victims provide us with heroes and heroines, and perpetrators provide us with villains. Facing trauma tempts us to split the world into uncomplicated realms of good and evil. But such simple distinctions can only be maintained if we ignore the complex issues of attachment, dominance, and competition, and the universal tendency to split the world into dichotomies of us versus them, good versus evil. These issues are even more complicated in people who have been traumatized, where bizarre attachments may have developed between victims and perpetrators, victims and their helpers, and victims and the people they are supposed to care for—all of whom may play roles in a compulsive repetition of the trauma. There is a constant pressure on the people in victims' lives to help reenact, rather than to remember, the trauma, to give in to the frustration of being unable to help victims engage and experiment with new challenges, and to get fed up with having to continuously earn their fragile trust. How does someone deal with the issue of taking responsibility for one's life after having experienced that it is futile to take action? How does one agree to abide by the rules when the rules were made solely to gratify the whims of others?

Trauma confronts people with the futility of putting up resistance, the impossibility of being able to affect the outcome of events. This book explores how the shattering of assumptions about predictability and mastery inflicts a "narcissistic wound to the fabric of the self." This recognition forces us to deal with the cardinal, twin issues of control and safety in our patients' lives—and therapy becomes the arena in which the battle to regain control and a sense of safety needs to be waged. The successful negotiation of these pivotal issues determines whether therapy will, in fact, prove to be therapeutic and lead to a resolution of the trauma, whether patients will experience current life as a challenge and opportunity, or whether they will sink into the "black hole of the trauma."

Thus, the therapist must become what Lindy has called "the trauma membrane," the person who personifies predictability and safety, as well as the person with whom the dimensions of control and ambivalence can be worked through. Idealization is a necessary component of these transactions, but so is the space to experience and explore disappointment, autonomy, and disagreement. As Kohut has pointed out, idealization of a caregiver is necessary as long as a person is not capable of restoring internal homeostasis after being upset. Ideally, children gradually gain a feeling of control and autonomy as they gain mastery over their internal and external world. An increased sense of mastery allows for an increasingly realistic assessment of caregivers and the development of ambivalence. Trauma destroys this sense of mastery and throws people back into a state where external sources are vitally needed to regulate internal emotional states. When the trauma is inflicted by a human agent, particularly by a familiar person, the conflict between the need for external reassurance and the fear of revictimization becomes the central issue in the transference.

It is important for therapists to accept the fact that this need for idealization is not founded on their real attributes (which, through the anxiety of trying to stay in control, patients often barely perceive), but that patients idealize in order to provide them with the anchor that was destroyed by the trauma. This need for security in the patient is echoed in the therapists' own needs—to be effective, to be good caregivers in contrast with evil perpetrators, whose help is accepted, appreciated, and understood. The patients' passive dependence or stubborn inability to trust is mirrored in the therapists' feelings of being powerless and incompetent. The patients' fragility and vulnerability is reflected in the therapists' attempts to be perfect and in control. It is a tremendous strain on therapists to keep an honest appraisal of their own capacities while tolerating their patients' intense need for rescue and constant scanning for imperfections. Only when both patients and therapists understand the etiology of these interactions (the traumatic past) can ambivalence and humor enter into the therapeutic relationship. If the origins of this tenacious clinging and intolerance of flaws remain unaddressed, therapy is likely to evolve into what Kohut called "transference bondage," in which the patient trades in autonomy for safety.

Thus, idealization is a double-edged sword: It provides an illusory sense of safety while immobilizing people from taking autonomous action. A patient's energies are focused on watching the therapist like a hawk and keeping the situation under control. These patients have problems with being still, and they are unable to establish an autonomous sense of security without resorting to withdrawal, sensation seeking, or substance abuse. All of this places tremendous demands on the therapist, who becomes the patient's lifeline. As early as possible, therapist and patient need to have an understanding of how trauma-induced vulnerability sets the stage for an exquisite sensitivity to specific actions and aspects of the therapist. Setting limits and creating clear therapeutic contracts are essential to ensure the safety of the therapeutic dyad. The challenge is to set limits while keeping open the exploration and expression of aggression. Although therapists also need to feel safe, they need to be wary of their own needs to be comforted by their patients. After all, abusers often attempt to find solace in their victims as well, and when they do, it is at the victim's expense. Safety does not consist of coming up with answers to the incomprehensible. The therapy of traumatized people does not allow for giving patients sage advice about how to live their lives. They are the survivors—therapists can only imagine how they might have been affected by similar experiences.

When the safety of relationships is threatened, people resort to the emergency responses of fight or flight. With traumatized patients it often does not take much to trigger these reactions, which may have been appropriate for a helpless child or a traumatized adult, but which are not very helpful in the context of current reality. The threatened loss of a powerful protector will activate very primitive responses. At times, traumatized patients may see death as their only means of escape from an intolerable threat. In our studies of traumatized borderline patients, many subjects identified their therapists' reaction to their suicide attempts and self-destructive actions as a critical point in helping them gain a sense of autonomy: "Good therapists were the ones who helped me figure out how to control my behavior, rather than attempting to control me."

Various chapters in this book explore the shame, powerlessness, and longing for revenge that suicidal and self-destructive episodes elicit in the therapist. Yet, often these crises will provide new building blocks for the capacity to tolerate ambivalence, which is essential for the restoration of a sense of autonomy. Only when patients (and therapists) learn to tolerate ambivalence will they become less clinging, and their self-esteem, long sapped in the service of self-protection, can be liberated and mobilized for action.

Clinicians have long noticed that before autonomy can occur, the safety of the relationship needs to be internalized. Our own research has confirmed that when there is no prior idealized person, as occurs in chronically neglected people, it is virtually impossible to mobilize the trust necessary for eventual internalization and growth.

Psychotherapy is a business that tries one's patience, and the psychotherapy of frightened, paralyzed, angry, and secretive survivors of trauma requires the patience of a saint. Because the schooling of psychotherapists rarely includes religious training, we are personally ill prepared for this enterprise. Patience is quite incompatible with the intense feelings of helplessness, rage, rescue, and sadism that these patients evoke in us. Victims invite us to violate the basic tenets of psychotherapy—to suspend value judgments, moralizing, and therapeutic activism. The desire to take a moral stance, to actively side with positive action, interpersonal connections, and empowerment, puts a great strain on our capacity to take a passive, listening stance from which we can help our patients figure out how the trauma has affected their inner world and outer expressions. The less one is in a position to address and explore the effect of trauma on patients' perceptions and decision-making processes, the more one is tempted to do something to take over control or to pass control on to other outside parties. Therapeutic activism implies accepting the helplessness of the patient as at times inevitable. Taking over control at times when patients need to learn to establish control for themselves may result in passivity and failure: The price for trying to run our patients' lives usually is abandonment.

Whether the therapist has a behavioral or a psychodynamic approach, the work of therapy basically consists of helping the patient acknowledge the facts, bear the feelings associated with them, and find ways of going on with his or her life. The need to make thought, not action, the currency of the therapeutic process is extremely difficult to accomplish in view of the fact that trauma-related thoughts and feelings bring back the intolerable affects that patients so carefully avoid, which, if countenanced to their full extent, may prove to be well-nigh unbearable for the therapist.

This book emphasizes the need for empathy and thought over action. Yet, at the same time, the contributors, without exception, understand the deeply political nature of traumatization and the need for social action to prevent trauma, or at least to alert the world to the psychological cost of traumatic experiences. One step in that direction was their coming together, as all therapists dealing with victims must, to scrutinize their own personal experiences and reactions in their therapies. We all agree that the regular and open communication about our own feelings and actions in the therapeutic setting is essential in harnessing the intense countertransference responses elicited by this work.

BESSEL A. VAN DER KOLK

BIBLIOGRAPHY

Herman, J. L. (1992). *Trauma and recovery*. New York: Basic Books.

Kohut, H. (1977). *The restoration of the self*. New York: International Universities Press.

Lindy, J. (1988). *Vietnam: A casebook*. New York: Brunner/Mazel.

McCann, I. L., & Pearlman, L. A. (1990). *Psychological trama and the adult survivor*. New York: Brunner/Mazel.

van der Kolk, B. A. (1987). *Psychological trauma*. Washington, DC: American Psychiatric Press.

van der Kolk, B. A. (1989). The compulsion to repeat trauma: Revictimization, attachment and masochism. *Psychiatric Clinics of North America*, *12*, 389–411.

Acknowledgments

In the 3 years that we spent working with the contributors to this book, many persons labored with dedication behind the scenes to bring it to fruition. As its past presidents we wish to acknowledge the International Society of Traumatic Stress Studies for its cooperation and for the support of our colleagues there in the field of trauma studies. We remember especially the late Sarah Haley and Robert Laufer for their contributions, courage, and personal character of great integrity. A very special thank you to Lynn Viola of the Department of Psychology at Cleveland State University (CSU), who oversaw the production process on a daily basis. Without her efforts and willingness to go beyond the call of duty, the publication would have been significantly delayed. We also extend our thanks to Jennifer Kling, graduate assistant at CSU, who typed and retyped the manuscripts. At the Center for Psychoanalysis in Cincinnati, Jo Gerth and Melinda Russell merit special appreciation for their hard work throughout the editing process. Finally, a special thank you to Søren Buus Jensen and Inger Agger of the Center for Psychosocial and Traumatic Stress in Aalborg, Denmark, for allowing me (JPW) to be the Guest Professor of the Year for 1992–1993 and to present many of the ideas in this book at the Center and its conference.

Preface

Much of this book is about what we, as clinicians, wish were not true of us and our limitations as therapists. Much of it is about what we, as survivors, wish were not true about the world. And in the sanctuary of our office, the two realities meet face to face in the psychotherapy of trauma survivors.

This is a book about what we go through as we listen to and work with our trauma patients and how our own experience may help or hinder the recovery process. It is also about how awareness of our human reactions to patients' trauma is indispensable in keeping these powerful treatments on track. It is a book about how we must apply this awareness judiciously, functioning not outside but within the boundaries of our professional relationships with survivors. In this way we strive to help our clients regain a sense of continuity and meaning in life, and to enhanced our own function as clinicians.

When we began to share our work in trauma research and therapy over a decade ago, one of us (JDL) was a psychiatric teacher and advanced candidate in psychoanalytic training, anxious to apply a psychoanalytic language, which he felt was uniquely prepared to assist in dealing with issues of trauma. The other (JPW) was a university faculty member in psychology, who was deeply moved by the tragic stories of Vietnam veterans (then our forgotten warriors), and who argued for new and creative approaches to help trauma survivors. JDL was distressed to find a generally negative attitude toward the work of psychoanalysts among many of our colleagues working with post-traumatic stress disorder (PTSD). Although some of their objections were based on theoretical concerns, at that time we were more interested in the objections based on personal experiences. Our colleagues, in their clinical efforts to assist victims of trauma (from such sources as incest, war, and the Holocaust), had sought help from senior psychoanalysts. They found to their dismay that people whom they had respected as teachers and therapists, some of whom they had experienced as being empathic with other intimate details of their lives and through supervision, were simply unable to tolerate the content of trauma-related issues and their personal and professional impact. Frequently, these analysts would try to explain away the emotions the trauma elicited by subsuming them under previously discussed early childhood dynamics, or, more damagingly, they concluded, as did Freud (1917) long ago, that memories of such events were primarily the product of fantasy, not reality. The supervising therapists gave clues, subtly or grossly, that the trauma was too much for them to tolerate. Our colleagues felt dismay and turned away in disillusionment, thinking, "Above all, *this person* could not hear me." We felt chagrined by these stories of additional pain to already traumatized friends, and we sought to learn how and why these events had occurred.

It was these experiences that first to drew JDL's attention to the powerful role of countertransference in the process of the psychotherapy of PTSD. For JPW, a second set of stories from trauma survivors about unsuccessful treatment efforts elicited special attention. These were stories that emerged after innovative, storefront outreach programs with survivor therapists had been established. Survivors of warfare revealed that therapists and their groups in the storefront programs had over-responded on the basis of their own unresolved war trauma experiences. Whereas the "scholarly" analysts had been too rigid and disbelieving, these fellow survivor counselors had drowned out the uniqueness of the client's trauma experiences, often inhibiting the unfolding of the story and preventing its being resolved in an individualized way. (In Chapter 1, we call the former "avoidant," or Type I, countertransference, and the latter "overidentification," or Type II, countertransference.)

Our colleagues who themselves were victims and survivors were forthright in what they expected of their therapists (and theirs were not small expectations). These survivors had gone through the unthinkable and, in Des Pres's (1980) language, felt a great drive to bear witness to the injustices that had befallen them. They had selected therapists who they hoped would have the psychological strength to be able to understand and cope with the tragedies that overwhelmed them, and when these therapists failed, the disillusionment was overwhelming. In time, we both came to see the psychotherapy of PTSD in a contextual basis, perhaps best expressed in the first-person singular, as in Martin Buber's "I–thou" relationship. It is a special communication between the "I" who survived and the "thou" with whom the survivor chooses to bear witness. The fracture of this relationship through countertransference seemed a worthy subject of exploration.

In the psychotherapy of trauma survivors, the "I" and the "thou" are not simply points on a graph or another piece of data; inevitably, these treatments are intimate matters and must, therefore, seek a disciplined professional language of trauma and intimacy in order to convey what happens in the treatment setting. These considerations have consistently drawn our attention in recent years to the specifics of transference and countertransference interactions as they occur in the psychotherapy of PTSD.

The idea for a book on countertransference and trauma grew out of an earlier, encyclopedic task of compiling as complete a picture as possible of the current state of knowledge of trauma, in the form of the 1993 publication *The International Handbook of Traumatic Stress Syndromes* (Wilson & Raphael, 1993). In this publication, numerous leaders in the field, particularly those involved in the clinical care of trauma survivors, alluded to the problems and burdens therapists experience from managing the emotional consequences of their work with trauma survivors. They seemed jointly to identify the powerful role of irrational forces within the therapist as the major interference with successful treatment. This consensus crossed the lines of the various schools of psychotherapy. Therapists working in different countries with different trauma survivors were grappling with similar countertransference issues and beginning to discuss their importance in the treatment process.

The contributors to this volume are recognized leaders in the psychotherapy of trauma, with expertise in dealing with specific survivor populations. They share the view that countertransference is an obstacle to successful work in this field.

Their participation in this project, to a person, involved much more than the usual contribution to an edited volume, that is, a review of the literature and a statement with regard to currently recommended practices. Instead it involved individual soul searching as each of us examined carefully, and at times painfully, difficult survivor–therapist interactions. The contributors in this volume are not only supervisors and consultants, but they are also on the spot as clinicians facing difficult moments, some of which evoked memories of their own victimization or survivorhood.

For the two of us, reading and revising these manuscripts was both an introspective and an expositional activity. The contributors in fact acted as consultants to one another, offering, as it were, one more trauma membrane within which we could support and encourage each other.

In addition to their own clinical work, it is no accident that the contributors to this volume are also steeped in strong advocacy and leadership positions in the area of trauma and trauma research. Individual experience with the therapist's disequilibrium evoked by intensive work with trauma survivors has motivated five of the contributors to serve as presidents of the International Society for Traumatic Stress Studies.

Traditionally, traumatic experiences have been divided into human-made and natural phenomena and into large-scale group catastrophes as opposed to individual traumatic events. Traumas occurring in war are contrasted with those in civilian life; traumas occurring to those who choose high-risk roles such as firemen, policemen, and soldiers are compared to those upon whom victimhood seems to fall in a random manner; there are traumas that occur primarily to children and those that occur in adulthood; traumas that violate sexual boundaries such as rape and incest and other violent crimes that threaten bodily security and life itself in other ways. There are traumas that destroy community and values and those that leave these elements intact.

Traumas may also be distinguished in terms of the role expected of the clinician and the chronology of the interaction after trauma. For example, in the actual response to disaster, mental health workers, like other rescue workers, are part of the landscape of the trauma event itself. Clinicians working within or consulting to businesses and industry are caring for the immediate support network involved in the recovery process. Rape crisis counseling may occur chiefly at the time of the event or alternatively may not take place until years later. Survivors of political oppression and torture finally meet up with a clinician either after they have escaped the territory of persecution or when shifts in political leadership have made it safe to acknowledge the past terror. In most situations, the survivor seeks the clinician's help with protracted symptoms that persist beyond the experience of the traumatic events. However, on other occasions, it is during the survivor's efforts to seek restitution that the encounter with the clinician occurs. For Holocaust survivors, resistance fighters, and Vietnam War veterans the first encounter with clinicians may not be in their roles as healers but when the therapists are making assessments and judgments with regard to restitution to the victim. Thus, clinicians take on many roles such as on-site comforters and consultants, or as professionals helping to reduce symptoms of acute stress years later, or in assessing survivor pathology in a restitution process. Each role has considerable bearing on the nature and quality of countertransference reaction (CTRs) that may be expected.

The impact of a survivor on a helping professional can be conceptualized in many ways. In Figure P.1, we have illustrated that regardless of the type of traumatic event that adversely affects the survivor/victim and his or her circle of loved ones, the resulting state of traumatization may lead to trauma-specific transference reactions at any point along a chronological timeline, from immediately after the event to years later, in

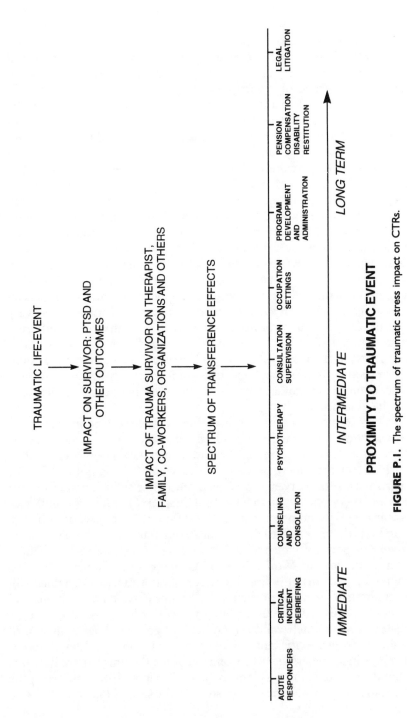

FIGURE P.I. The spectrum of traumatic stress impact on CTRs.

such activities as litigation, compensation evaluations, or disability determinations. However, those who work with trauma survivors are never immune from CTRs. From our perspective, those professionals identified as helpers will benefit by understanding the ubiquitous nature of countertransference, especially in work with PTSD.

We have elected in this book to organize the chapters along the following lines: Part I (Chapters 1–3) is a theoretical and practical introduction to the book, outlining the general issues raised historically and currently in the area of countertransference and trauma. In Chapter 1 we provide a schema for trauma therapy, clarifying where countertransference can lead to breaks in empathy and can fracture and derail recovery. We also introduce two major categories of empathic strain that may lead to such CTRs: Type I (avoidance) and Type II (overidentification). Chapter 2 presents a schema integrating patterns of affective reactions to the client's trauma story with defensive and cognitive modes. Here we also suggest that the understanding and acknowledgment of empathic strain and countertransference may ultimately help build a new psychological containing structure within the treatment, in which trauma survivors can find emotional safety. In such a safe, containing environment, recovery can occur. Chapter 3 uses specific cases of work with survivors of different trauma populations to illustrate how such empathic breaks occur at different points in the treatment process. Chapter 3 further illustrates signs and symptoms of CTRs and illustrates how such tendencies, through introspection and insight, can actually build a new therapeutic structure in which healing occurs.

In Part II, we examine the special forces at work in countertransference when helping women and children who have witnessed, or been the victims of, violent and/or sexual assault. The clinical interaction may be immediate (Chapters 6–8), or it may be years later (Chapters 4 and 5). The clinician most often serves as therapist, but may also be a consultant for others on the scene or in the family (Chapter 6). Many examples of avoidant (Type I) and overidentification (Type II) responses are offered.

In Part III, we examine countertransference arising in those who treat survivors of political violence and war. These survivors include Dutch resistance fighters in World War II (Chapter 12), Vietnam veterans, (Chapter 11), victims of political torture in South America (Chapter 10), and Cambodian survivors of the Pol Pot camps (Chapter 9). Trauma and recovery here tends to occur within a network of survivors. Therapists struggle to find uniquely valid ways to address groups whose trauma must be understood in specific cultural and historical contexts. Again, there is wide range in acuteness versus chronicity: Some therapists share the same current dangers of trauma as their patients (Chapter 10), some are in the first decade of survival (Chapter 9), some in the second (Chapter 11), and some are in the fourth decade after the events (Chapter 12). Because of the wide and creative modes of outreach and treatment, clinicians are in a range of roles: group leaders, counselors, consultants, medical physicians, and triage managers, as well as therapists. Additionally, clinicians are asked to make judgments about restitution, raising further countertransference (Chapter 12).

In Part IV, we expand our discussion of trauma and countertransference to indirect trauma survivors as well as direct ones. During natural disasters, for example, many types of rescue workers are exposed both to the threat of the disaster and to the plights of those they attempt to help (Chapter 13). Their reactions are both to the event itself *and* to the CTR-like, role-specific situations they experience. In individual accidents (Chapter 14), managers and coworkers have strong CTR-like responses to their traumatized employees and coworkers. The training of professionals to recognize and manage CTRs is discussed in Chapter 15. Finally, Chapter 16 presents a summary of the advances made in our knowledge of CTRs in work with trauma survivors and outlines tasks for future research.

Thus, each chapter highlights certain special features of the trauma experience, of the trauma recovery process, and the roles through which clinicians engage survivors.

The tables and illustrations in Chapter 1 of this volume outline many of the variables discussed above. Further graphics function like computer windows to clarify subcomponents that bear on the trauma experience and the countertransference of the particular event. The use of these graphs, like all of the information contained in the chapters, is heuristic in nature and designed to stimulate thinking, thereby advancing the capacity of clinicians to more adequately assist victims of trauma suffering from PTSD.

REFERENCES

Des Pres, T. (1980). *The survivor: An anatomy of life in the death camps.* New York: Oxford University Press.

Freud, S. (1917). Introductory lectures on psycho-analysis. *Standard Edition, 16,* 241–478.

Wilson, J. P., & Raphael, B. (Eds.). (1993) *The international handbook of traumatic stress syndromes.* New York: Plenum Press.

Contents

PART I

Theoretical and Conceptual Foundations of Countertransference in Post-Traumatic Therapies

Part I contains three interrelated chapters that attempt to build a theoretical scaffold by which to understand the nature, dynamics, and subtypes of countertransference processes in the treatment of post-traumatic stress disorder (PTSD). The overall focus of these chapters is to present the common pathways of countertransference processes faced by clinicians, researchers, and others who work and live with the victims of trauma. Central to our discussion of the interpersonal dynamics in therapy, and indigenous to this intense work, are the twin concepts of sustained empathic inquiry and empathic strain.

Traumatized clients present many challenges to those who attempt to work with them in clinical settings. Their personal trauma stories frequently contain painful accounts of events that altered their inner sense of self, creating psychic scars and unhealed wounds to the core of their personality. To recover from the various emotional injuries caused by trauma, the victim requires a therapeutic sanctuary that is experienced as a safe and constantly secure place where the work of therapy, the *integration and resolution* of the trauma experience, can occur. In this regard, the therapist's task of creating a safe therapeutic structure is never an easy one. The clinician not only confronts the pain and personal struggle of the client but must do so with a capacity for sustained empathy. However, as the trauma story of the client unfolds and deepens with treatment, empathic strain occurs, making it difficult to stay closely attuned to the dynamics of the client. As the therapeutic alliance strengthens, the client

1

tends to project *trauma-specific transferences,* which have the potential to elicit very complex countertransference reactions (CTRs) and unique role enactments in the therapist.

In Chapter 1, we introduce two poles of a countertransference continuum—Type I (avoidance, counterphobia, distancing, detachment) and Type II (overidentification, overidealization, enmeshment, excessive advocacy) processes. We consider these forms of countertransference to be expectable, indigenous, reactive processes in post-traumatic therapy. Moreover, when the continuum of Type I and Type II CTRs are considered in conjunction with *objective* (normative) reactions to the client's trauma story or *subjective* (personalized) reactions, those reflecting unresolved conflicts from the therapist's life, it is possible to derive four distinct modes of empathic strain. In Chapter 1, we have identified these modes as *empathic withdrawal, empathic repression, empathic enmeshment,* and *empathic disequilibrium.* We believe it is important to identify different modes of empathic strain because they (1) identify differences in therapists' reactive styles, (2) manifest at different times during treatment, (3) are not static processes but dynamic ones that reflect information about trauma-specific transference projections, (4) enable thematic material to emerge as the process unfolds and elaborates in greater detail and meaning, and (5) direct the therapist's attention to the locus of work necessary to move beyond the strain.

The relation of empathic strain to Type I and Type II CTRs has important implications for the process of therapy. In Chapter 1, we present a schema that demonstrates how countertransference can impact on the *stress recovery process,* the phases of treatment from the event to integration in the self-structure of the survivor. A highlight is the fact that if a rupture of empathy occurs, producing a form of empathic strain, a potentially pathological consequence may result. More specifically, a loss of the therapeutic stance may be associated with any or all of five categories of deleterious disruptions to the therapeutic relationship: (1) cessation of treatment, (2) fixation within a phase of recovery, (3) intensification of trauma-specific transference, (4) regression, and/or (5) acting-out behaviors. Thus, the identification of empathic strain and countertransference implies the necessity for therapists to recognize within themselves signs and symptoms of defensiveness and, perhaps, the subtle movement into specific types of roles (e.g., failed protector, fellow survivor). Chapter 1 concludes with a discussion of the need to properly manage countertransference in order to maintain a "safe–holding" environment in the context of post-traumatic therapy.

In Chapter 2, we expand the discussion of the various subtypes of Type I and Type II countertransference to illustrate the very complex ways in which they affect post-traumatic therapy. As an integral part of this analysis, we examine how the therapists' affective responses to traumatized clients are associated with defensive efforts to contain and bind their own distress as a manifestation of empathic strain.

In examining the subtypes of Type I and Type II CTRs, we were able to delineate a continuum of responses that characterize each tendency. In Type I, this continuum includes six specific modes or subtypes that encompass (1) forms of denial, (2) minimization, (3) distortion, (4) avoidance, (5) detachment, and (6) withdrawal. Likewise, Type II reactions include five modes or subtypes: (1) codependent relations, (2) enmeshment, (3) overcommitment and overidentification, (4) rescuer activities, and (5) overemphasis on the role of the traumatic event in the life of the client. Furthermore, our analysis of the *psychological structure* of Type I and Type II CTRs revealed five factors that can combine in different ways to determine the specific configuration of the countertransference.

The five factors underlying the structure and configuration of subtypes of Type I and Type II responses include (1) *affect*—the types of affect and impulses felt by the therapist during therapy sessions, (2) *defense*—efforts to contain distress and empathic strain, (3) *coping modes*—behaviors by the therapist to cope with the trauma-specific transferences of the client, (4) *impaired role boundaries*—the effects that empathic strain exerts on the management of effective role boundaries between therapist and client, and (5) *theoretical rationale*—cognitive attributions or rationalizations by the therapist about the aforementioned processes.

The recognition and identification of specific types of Type I and Type II constellations are important because, to a large extent, CTRs reflect how the therapist attempts to understand, interpret, and utilize information that emanates from the transference projections of the suffering client. In this regard, transference projections of traumatic material have differential *affect arousal potential* in the CTR, as well as the capacity to effect specific role enactments in a therapist (e.g., failed protector, collaborator, comforter, conspirator, fellow survivor). Thus, in the dual unfolding process of post-traumatic therapy, the analysis of the transference–countertransference dynamics becomes central to creating critical therapeutic role structures, which allow the work to proceed with sustained empathy, and to effectively managing potentially disruptive countertransference processes. Chapter 2 concludes with a discussion of *empathic growth,* a term that denotes positive integrative outcomes for both the client and the therapist.

In Chapter 3, the issue of countertransference is further elaborated within a modified psychoanalytic perspective that incorporates the conceptual ideas presented in the first two chapters. Consistent with the wisdom accumulated from psychoanalytic studies from Freud to the present, post-traumatic therapy that utilizes a psychoanalytic orientation places emphasis on unconscious manifestations of trauma-specific transferences, as well as their counterparts in CTRs.

In Chapter 3, we illustrate the concepts developed in Chapters 1 and 2, and we present nine case studies of trauma survivors. These case histories involve survivors of the Holocaust, the Vietnam War, and childhood sexual abuse, as well as other traumatic events. Each of the case histories is told from the therapist's vantage point and illustrates how specific affects, defenses, and empathic strain (Type I and Type II CTRs) can impact adversely or positively on the treatment process or emotional stability of the client. For example, in Case Example Two ("Dismembered Torso"), the therapist's personal traumas evoked in the treatment led to a dissociative countertransference state and resulted in reproducing the client's trauma, leading to decompensation and the need for hospitalization. In contrast, however, Case Example Five ("It's Your Turn") illustrates how sustained empathic inquiry in the face of severe empathic strain enabled conflicted material to break through in a Vietnam War veteran. Between these polar examples of the results of countertransference is Case Example Four ("Forgetting the Children") in which a therapist's anger at the idiosyncratic actions of a client represented a role enactment (countertransference) of the client's unconscious feelings about the death of her child.

Chapter 3 concludes with a discussion of the nature of countertransference and how trauma-specific role enactments are manifested during the course of treatment. This analysis attempts to weave together the central concepts presented in Part I of this book to establish a framework, or common conceptual ground, so that each of the subsequent chapters can be considered within these paradigms. Our hope and intent was to develop a theoretical scaffold that would be heuristic in nature so as to stimulate future research and clinical studies of the role of countertransference in work with victims of trauma and disaster. To date, our investigation has proved productive beyond expectation. Clearly, however, future work is needed to expand and refine the initial insights achieved at this writing.

I

Empathic Strain
and Countertransference

JOHN P. WILSON
JACOB D. LINDY

In recent years the study and treatment of post-traumatic stress disorder (PTSD) has grown at an exponential rate, reflecting not only the accumulation of scientific data and clinical knowledge but the worldwide pervasiveness of the events that cause PTSD and associated psychological conditions (Wilson & Raphael, 1993). Simultaneously, mental health professionals have attempted to assist victims of trauma and disaster through the use of modern techniques of psychotherapy, counseling, psychopharmacology, and behaviorally oriented approaches to treatment (Figley, 1985; Lindy, 1989, 1992; McCann & Pearlman, 1990; Ochberg, 1988). At present, however, there are only a few empirical studies that have been designed to evaluate psychotherapy outcome and to determine which modalities of treatment are most effective with different types of clients (Foa, Rathbaum, Riggs, & Mardock, 1991). The availability of such studies in the future will enable more systematic clinical programs to be developed in regard to training psychotherapists. Recently, a growing awareness has emerged of the importance of therapists' reactions and countertransference processes in the treatment of PTSD (Danieli, 1988; Lindy, 1985, 1989; McCann & Pearlman, 1990; Wilson, 1989). It is the purpose of this chapter to focus on issues that affect empathy and the treatment outcome of PTSD.

THERAPIST'S CONFRONTATION WITH TRAUMATIZED CLIENTS

Clinical work with trauma victims brings the clinician close to the "soul" of the pain and injury. Although the nature and severity of the specific issues that a trauma survivor with PTSD faces in the task of healing and psychologically integrating a traumatic experience varies from person to person (Ochberg, 1988, 1992; Wilson, 1989), survivors and victims who seek help often suffer from painful memories of the events and distressing affective states that may alter the structure of the self. As observed by Lifton (1988), traumatic events may cause a disequilibrium in psychoformative processes and lead to defensive attempts (e.g., withdrawal, aggressive compensation, psychic numbing) to protect the injured self-structure and personal sense of vitality and wholeness. Moreover, although there are alternative pathways of post-traumatic adaptation in the course of life cycle development, *the traumatized individual seeks a safe environment, a therapeutic sanctuary, in which to engage in an interpersonal relationship that facilitates recovery and movement toward integrating the stressful experience within the ego-structure in ways that are no longer distressing or disruptive of adaptive functioning* (see Herman, 1992, for a discussion).

Empathy and Empathic Strain in PTSD[1]

Although the client suffering from PTSD initially presents in a variety of ways, ranging from extreme psychic numbing and avoidance of self-disclosure to being psychically overloaded and feeling emotionally distraught and unable to modulate distressing affects (McCann & Pearlman, 1990), the treatment of this disorder usually follows a predictable path. In the early phase of treatment, the "trauma story" is explored and the therapist attempts to establish trust, rapport, and openness (Lindy, 1993; Wilson, 1989). Therapists listen in an empathic and nonjudgmental way to clients' descriptions and interpretations of what happened to them in the trauma (Ochberg, 1993). The creation of a "safe–holding" environment (Winnicott, 1960) is crucial to the establishment of mutual trust in the therapeutic process. We believe that the capacity for sustained empathy is pivotal for the recovery process—as the trauma unfolds, as new affect and imagery develops, and as trauma is placed in a newer meaning system. In our opinion, the clinician's capacity for genuine empathy is the *sine qua non* for laying the groundwork that enables the patient to perceive that

---

[1]Table 1.3 at the end of this chapter contains a glossary of terms and their definitions for this chapter and throughout the book.

the therapeutic context is a situation of security and protection, and a proper place to express anxiety and feelings of vulnerability. A similar position has been espoused by Maroda (1991), who states:

> Essentially, the first year [of treatment] is devoted to developing the relationship and setting the stage for the expression of the transference. Basic trust and empathy are the primary concerns—the patient wants to know that his therapist understands, is reliable and trustworthy, and is genuine in his desire to help him. In this initial stage, the self-psychological approach to treatment is very effective. Sustained empathic inquiry is ideal because the patient is telling his story and is seeking some symptom relief for the pain or crisis that brought him to treatment in the first place. (p. 67)

Achieving empathy requires the ability to project oneself into the phenomenological world being experienced by another person. While empathy is an integral part of any therapy, in the treatment of PTSD and allied conditions *sustained empathic inquiry* is both more necessary and more difficult to maintain. This empathic stance enables the therapist to help the client through traumatization to the point where its aftereffects can be successfully integrated into the individual's self-structure. Sustained empathic inquiry is also vital to the creation of a safe–holding environment, a milieu in which the client's reactions to victimization can be normalized and one that offers reassurance that what the client is experiencing is a human reaction to abnormally stressful life events. Yet it is no simple matter to maintain empathy when the treatment setting itself becomes a crucible into which aspects of the trauma became transferred. Rather, empathy is a complex enterprise in which the therapist must also be aware of his or her own partial identification with the client's phenomenological framework—in other words, therapists working with these patients *must* take into account the processes of countertransference.

Slatker's (1987) review of the literature on countertransference (which is consistent with our view) indicates that a rupture of empathy results in the loss of an effective therapeutic role, that is, one that permits sustained empathic inquiry into the patient's processing of traumatic memories and the undermodulated affect associated with cognitive processes, which operate on all levels of consciousness in the trauma patient. The factors that cause *empathic strain* in the therapeutic relationship are potential determinants of *affective reactions* (ARs) in the therapist. Although ARs are common in treatment, intense ARs can lead to negative countertransferential reactions (CTRs) by diminishing the capacity for sustained empathic inquiry and thereby producing a temporary rupture in the therapeutic role stance. Therapy-rupturing CTRs diminish the ability of the therapist to maintain the safe–holding environment necessary for recovery from PTSD. Yet, given the enormity of the therapist's task in containing intense trauma affect, which by definition is the human response to conditions outside the range of usual life experiences, countertransference tendencies should be anticipated. It is for this reason that we seek to understand the place of CTRs in the psychotherapy of trauma survivors.

Clearly, empathy, identification, and countertransference are interrelated processes. Slatker (1987), for example, has argued that the relation between empathy and countertransference depends on what he terms *counteridentification,* as well as on identification with the client's inner world of affect and psychological being. Here Slatker suggests that through the process of counteridentification "the analyst both identifies with the patient and at the same time pulls back from that identification so as to view the patient's conflict with objectivity" (p. 203). From this viewpoint, "empathy is based on counter-identification; indeed it is counter-identification that permits our empathy to be therapeutically useful. But counter-identification is also a component of countertransference, and if it operates imperfectly, whereby objectivity is not achieved, then the analyst's negative countertransferential reactions can cause empathy to diminish or to vanish altogether" (p. 203).

Affective Reactions, Sources of Empathic Strain, and Countertransference

The concept of countertransference as a clinical construct originates in Freud's essays on the technique of psychoanalysis (1910). The most thorough early monograph (Racker, 1968) distinguishes countertransference along several lines and introduces projective identification as a central mechanism. Many subsequent clarifications, refinements, and revisions have been proposed by analysts and other psychodynamically oriented therapists (see Slatker, 1987, for a review). Unfortunately, definitions vary, as do the prominent intrapsychic model (Isaacharoff & Hunt, 1978). The focus of this book does not permit us to discuss these variations, other than to note that (1) authors now employ an object relations intrapsychic model more often than a classical structural model; (2) authors define CTR more inclusively, as opposed to the earlier view of CTR as subjective and idiosyncratic; and (3) authors tend to advise therapists to work with countertransference insights through supervision and to disclose them rather than to seek their elimination as the treatment goal. Depending upon author and definition, the concept of countertransference has been regarded variously as controversial, important, irrelevant, or central to the outcome of psychotherapy.

Transference and Countertransference in the Treatment of PTSD: Trauma-Specific Transference

The terms *transference* and *countertransference* traditionally refer to the reciprocal impact that the patient and the therapist have on each other during the course of psychotherapy. In the treatment of PTSD and co-morbid states, transference processes may be *trauma specific* (Brandell, 1992; Danieli, 1988; Lindy, 1985, 1988; McCann & Pearlman, 1990; Wilson, 1988, 1989) and/or generic in nature, originating from pre-traumatic, life course development as well as from traumatic events.

Trauma-specific transference (TST) reactions are those in which the patient unconsciously relates to the therapist in ways that concern un-resolved, unassimilated, and ego-alien aspects of the traumatic event. These reactions include affective states, behavioral tendencies, and sym-bolic role relationships. In the context of a safe–holding environment, the TST reaction includes the tendency of the client to focus on the particular dynamics of the traumatic life event. The client casts the therapist into one or more trauma-specific roles through the transference process.

The therapist, in a complementary manner, may feel as though he or she has entered one of these particular roles as part of the countertrans-ference process. Countertransference positions (role enactments) range from positive (the therapist becomes a fellow survivor or a helpful sup-porter, rescuer, or comforter near the trauma) to negative (the therapist becomes a "turncoat" collaborator or hostile judge). In the worst case (most often following empathic error), the therapist may be seen as the perpetrator during a reenactment in the therapy.

The shape of the therapy is likely to arise from the ambivalence and paradoxes of these various positions and the capacity of the therapist to recognize their nuances and complexities. For example, some Holocaust survivors may be clear in their hatred for Nazi perpetrators but more mixed in their disdain for collaborators (e.g., Nazi *Kapos*). Some Vietnam veterans may think of themselves as perpetrators as well as survivors; they may even respect the enemy and identify faulty American political policy as the perpetrator. Rape victims have no fellow survivors, and they dis-cover that judges may recapitulate the perpetrator's role. Hostages may see their perpetrators as rescuers (e.g., Stockholm syndrome). Incest survi-vors may have had to turn for comfort to their perpetrators, while having no fellow victim or true comforter at all. In fact, small children who are repeatedly exposed to terrifying trauma and molestation may have no choice but to invent out of their imagination new personalities to fulfill the roles, such as protector and avenger, left vacant by adults during their trauma (e.g., multiple personality disorder and dissociative tendencies).

Trauma situations combine the emotional terror of each of these roles differently. Later, as dynamic relations play out in treatment, failures in therapist empathy are likely to evoke both negative transference reactions, in which the therapist is seen as a negative trauma figure, and negative CTRs, in which the therapist begins to feel as if he or she were in one of these roles vis-à-vis the client. These are critically important moments in the treatment and must be understood in order for the treatment to survive.

Sophie's Choice: A Historical–Fictional Example of Trauma-Specific Unconscious Reenactment from World War II Nazi Germany

One of the classic literary illustrations of unconscious reenactment processes and TST is found in William Styron's (1979) novel *Sophie's Choice*, in which the Nazi Holocaust survivor, Sophie, developed a sadomasochistic relationship after the war with her lover, Nathan. Delusional and obsessed with the glory and power of Nazi Germany, the psychotic Nathan brutally acts out against Sophie his grandiose and paranoid vision of Nazi omnipotence. His actions further victimize Sophie, whose psychic condition is fragile and depressed. Intertwined in their self-destructive relationship, as portrayed in the novel and motion picture, they reenact the traumatic choice forced on Sophie by the Nazi SS officer at the death camp's receiving platform: She had to determine which of her two young children would live. As portrayed by Styron (1979), Sophie's helplessness, confusion, terror, and indecision over having to choose which of her children would live or die form the nucleus of her post-traumatic symptomatology. In the pathology of their relationship, Nathan symbolically becomes many objects for Sophie, such as the revived child who had been sacrificed to the Nazis. An affair with him captures a carefree, spontaneous life of which both of them had been deprived. In another reenactment, Nathan becomes the Nazi who had rejected Sophie's brief attempt at seduction to save her children on the exit ramp. Through Nathan, she finally seduces him, then murders them both for their "crimes." Tragically, she symbolically reunites with her lost child by her dual suicide with Nathan. Viewed from the perspective of PTSD, Sophie's relationship with Nathan is a symbolic form of reenactment, driven by powerful, undermodulated affect, grief, and self-recrimination, all of which are highly trauma specific. The readers and audience of *Sophie's Choice* are cast in the role of overwhelmed witnesses to the Nazi atrocity. As the story unfolds we may be drawn in feeling the guilt of the surviving child, despair for the dead child, rage at the Nazi, or turmoil at Sophie's frantic yet empty life, finally explained by her impossible choice. Each of these positions ultimately confronts us with existential shame. Were we to be her therapists, each of these positions would be a potential point for empathic strain and powerful CTRs.

THE ELEMENTS OF COUNTERTRANSFERENCE AND THEIR RELATION TO PTSD

As the complement to transference, countertransference has been defined as a process that "denotes all those reactions of the analyst to the patient that may help or hinder treatment" (Slatker, 1987, p. 3). This brief definition calls attention to several elements of central significance to our understanding of the process of countertransference.

First, there are reactions of the therapist to the patient, which are *indigenous* to the context in which therapy occurs. Second, these reactions may enhance or disrupt therapeutic engagement. Third, they may be *complementary* or *concordant*. Racker (1968) distinguished concordant countertransference from complementary countertransference. In the first instance, therapists respond to the dilemma of their patients by identifying with some aspect of their plight, such as a wish (to survive), a defense (denial), or an ideal (courage). In a complementary countertransference, the therapist identifies with role or intrapsychic vantage point that captures that plight from another perspective than the survivor's intrapsychic search for understanding. For example, in a trauma case the therapist may temporarily feel like the perpetrator victimizing the patient rather than empathizing, or like the patient's own harsh superego that is criticizing the patient rather than empathizing with his plight.

Fourth, the transference–countertransference sequence is an *interactive* process and may stimulate reactions (e.g., emotional states, memories, fantasies, creative insights) in *both* the patient and the therapist. As noted initially by Winnicott (1949), the interactive processes of treatment make countertransference inevitable, including *objective* and *subjective* forms of reaction. Gorkin (1987) has reviewed this distinction between objective and subjective reactions. "What is of primary interest to me," he writes, "is that type of response which is the counterpart, or expectable, response to the patient's personality and behavior—objective countertransference. I distinguish this type of countertransference from the kind of response that is due to the analyst's personal conflict or idiosyncrasies—subjective countertransference" (pp. 34–35). Maroda (1991) has revived Racker's (1968) seminal concept of *dual unfolding*: "transference unfolds in conjunction with the countertransference. . . . From an interpersonal perspective, the countertransference can be as important as the transference, and the person of the therapist can be almost as important as the person of the patient" (Maroda, 1991, pp. 69–70).

Slatker's (1987) careful study of the psychoanalytic literature on countertransference reveals a wealth of insight about this complex phenomenon that is applicable to the treatment of PTSD. The concept of dual unfolding further informs us that countertransference is a *multidimensional phenomenon* that includes (1) ARs (e.g., guilt, shame, anxiety, tension), which are part of a psychobiological capacity for empathy; (2) cognitive reactions (e.g., fantasies, mental associations); and (3) dispositions to act in idiosyncratic or need-based ways toward the client as part of an ongoing interpersonal process (e.g., prosocial advocacy, rescuer reactions).

In the treatment of PTSD and allied conditions, the potential for developing both objective and subjective CTRs is quite significant because of the intensity of the transference process presented by a trauma survivor (McCann & Pearlman, 1990; Mollica, 1988; Wilson, 1989). Survivors of extremely stressful life events disclose trauma stories that are laden with affective intensity and descriptions of human experiences that so often and so far exceed the boundaries of a "just, equitable, and fair world" that they cause the therapist to be taken aback and temporarily dislodged from an empathic, objective, and nurturing professional role. Consider the following case example:

> Teresa, a woman in her 20s, disclosed to her counselor the following trauma story regarding her internment in a South American prison for political dissenters. Her captors demeaned and abused her sexually, using rape in all its human forms. Next, they unleashed specially conditioned Alsatian dogs that intimidated, threatened, and bit her, drawing blood from her breasts. The dogs then had sexual intercourse with her. During these events the captors watched, laughed, and made humiliating and disparaging remarks. Next, her captors beheaded her two young children while forcing her to watch. They kicked her children's decapitated heads as "soccer balls." Finally they placed her in an isolation cell and carried out a mock execution.

The counselor who was helping this client was badly shaken during the session when the trauma story was told and sought relief from the tension she experienced throughout the hour of treatment. Her AR was such that she was overwhelmed by the content of the trauma story, which raised personal issues for her, as she was herself a woman in prime childbearing years.

As the consultant, I (JPW), too, was powerfully affected by the counselor's intense, emotionally charged need to sort our her personal reactions to the torture victim who was her client. As I listened intently, I visualized the scenes the counselor described, a technique that not only assisted me in recognizing the counselor's feelings of helplessness, terror, anger, fear, and uncertainty, but also generated in me feelings of anger and the need to "set things right."

The powerful emotions evoked in this case are not uncommon in work with victims of trauma and disaster who suffer from PTSD, depression, anxiety, and injuries that "bruise the soul" (Simpson, 1993). The traumatized individual seeks help to let go of pain, confusion, and feelings of vulnerability. Yet, in order to do so, the survivor must find a safe–holding milieu in which the therapist can maintain an empathic stance with firm interpersonal boundaries, a milieu in which the dual unfolding process will enable the client to successfully work through the phases of recovery (Horowitz, 1986). Because the power of affect is so intense, the therapist must attend to countertransference processes in the treatment of PTSD. In these cases, countertransference can lead to empathic strain which, if unmanaged, will cause a rupture of empathy and a loss of therapeutic role.

The Groundwork of the Forbidden

It is now presumed that the psychotherapy of trauma survivors presents the therapist with uniquely intense encounters with trauma clients because of the types of events that cause PTSD. As Lifton (1967) observed many years ago in his pioneering work with Hiroshima survivors of the atomic bomb, the encounter with death and massive destruction, the perceived threat to the bases of human existence, and the need to generate meaning result in the difficult task of reformulating the significance of the event for the survivor. For most victims who suffer the personally painful damage to their well-being, it is their ongoing attempt to put the experience to rest with new meaning and insight brings them into treatment.

The patient's trauma story may reveal an overwhelming tragedy, a situation of coercive vulnerability, involvement as a victim in sinister activities of depravity, or a description of torment, pain, suffering, and loss. In listening to such stories, the therapist reels with the enormity of the trauma as it affects the patient. At the same time, the traumatized patient's attitudes, demeanor, and affect can also activate forbidden impulses and fantasies in the therapist, responses occurring in addition to the common range of Type I (avoidance) and Type II (overidentification) CTRs.

One of us (JPW) has presented the vignette of Teresa to hundreds of trauma counselors as a point of departure for discussion. Common responses among professionals are disgust, anger, sadness, denial, revulsion, and fear. Universally, counselors find the trauma story horrendous, and they are powerfully struck, if not immediately overwhelmed, by the image of a mother watching torturers kicking her children's decapitated heads. They sense a profound discomfort and disequilibrium as they consider what Danieli (1988) refers to as "existential shame." Moreover, these reactions occur within the safe and sterile environment of ongoing education and training. What if they had encountered Teresa themselves?

It should be noted that the therapist in this horrible case was able to hear the whole story, a story that began with sexual degradation and ended with mock execution. The torturers deliberately set out to degrade their prisoner sexually, to equate her political position with a feeling of disgust about herself, to punish her as though she were a criminal, and finally to leave her with the memory of anticipating a randomly timed, imminent execution as though she deserved it.

Countertransference to the first phase of the torture, while also evoking disgust and horror, might additionally elicit hints of forbidden feelings—such as arousal, voyeurism, erotic sadistic or masochistic impulses, identification with the aggressor—that might frighten the counselor by casting him or her in the perpetrator's role. Although the therapists' reactions might be quickly hidden from view, such countertransference phenomena could have interrupted the trauma story. From a more traditional point of view, one could also suggest that such fleeting fantasies or ARs should have been condemned as idiosyncratic, or at least disregarded as shameful and pathological. However, it could alternatively be argued that the therapist who was aware of such forbidden fantasies might discover a hidden organizing feature of the trauma experience, namely that, subjectively speaking, the torture survivor may still be confused or disoriented by the (invalid) fear that her action or inaction provoked the abusers' excesses and set the whole tragedy in motion. By seeing herself in an interactional context with her torturers, she might reveal the horrible "reality" that she continues to feel ashamed that these despicable actions were carried out even though she was helpless to stop them, or worse, that she believes that somehow she deserved the abuse.

In the psychotherapy of PTSD, *the groundwork of the forbidden* must be acknowledged as part of the domain of CTRs that occur as the dual unfolding process evolves during the course of treatment. The activation of *forbidden impulses,* like less extreme CTRs, contains information that can assist in the successful treatment of a patient by illuminating trauma-specific themes of transference. In fact, because these reactions are expectable, we must work to create the proper psychological and physical space for them to be acknowledged and shared with colleagues.

MODES OF EMPATHIC STRAIN: THERAPISTS' REACTIVE STYLES

Empathic strain results from those interpersonal events in psychotherapy that weaken, injure, or force beyond reasonable limits a salutary therapeutic response to the client. Countertransference processes are only one source of empathic strain, yet we believe that in the treatment of PTSD, CTRs are perhaps the primary cause of treatment failure.

Building on the seminal works of Slatker (1987), Danieli (1988), Lindy (1988), Parson (1988), Wilson (1989), Maroda (1991), and Scurfield (1993), it is possible to construct a schema for understanding modalities of empathic strain in the treatment of PTSD. Figure 1.1 illustrates these forms of empathic strain in a two-dimensional representation, based on Type I and Type II modes of CTRs divided by objective and subjective countertransferences processes. As noted earlier, objective CTRs are expectable affective and cognitive reactions experienced by the therapist in response to the personality, behavior, and trauma story of the

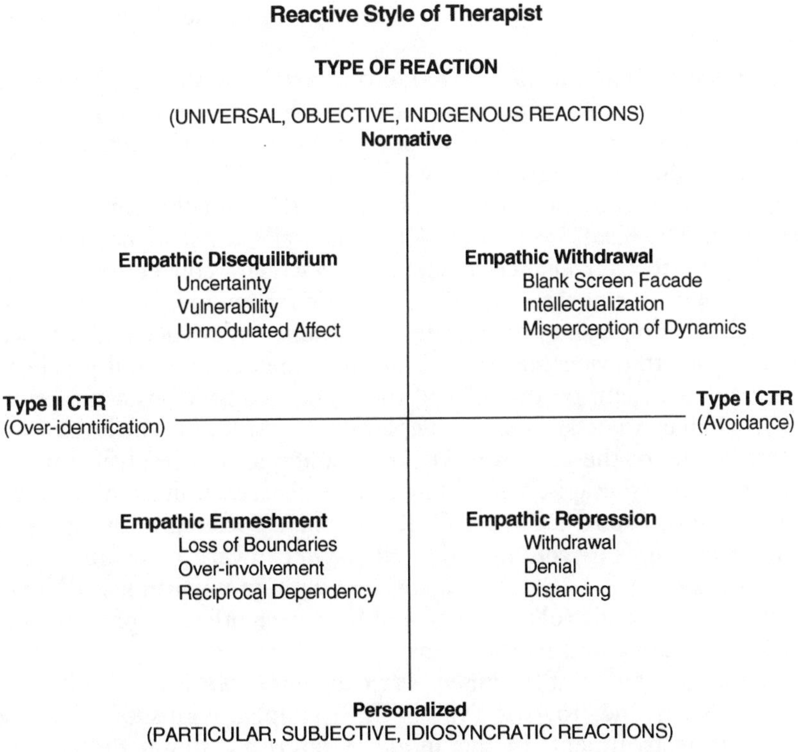

Reactive Style of Therapist

TYPE OF REACTION

(UNIVERSAL, OBJECTIVE, INDIGENOUS REACTIONS)
Normative

Empathic Disequilibrium	**Empathic Withdrawal**
Uncertainty	Blank Screen Facade
Vulnerability	Intellectualization
Unmodulated Affect	Misperception of Dynamics

Type II CTR   **Type I CTR**
(Over-identification)   (Avoidance)

Empathic Enmeshment	**Empathic Repression**
Loss of Boundaries	Withdrawal
Over-involvement	Denial
Reciprocal Dependency	Distancing

Personalized
(PARTICULAR, SUBJECTIVE, IDIOSYNCRATIC REACTIONS)

FIGURE 1.1. Modes of empathic strain in countertransference reactions (CTRs).

client, whereas subjective CTRs are personal reactions that originate from the therapist's personal conflicts, idiosyncracies, or unresolved issues from life course development.

Type I and Type II modes of countertransference refer respectively to the primary tendencies of counterphobic avoidance, distancing, and detachment reactions as opposed to tendencies to overidentify and become enmeshed with the client (see Chapter 2 for a discussion). Type I CTRs typically include forms of denial, minimization, distortion, counterphobic reactions, avoidance, detachment, and withdrawal from an empathic stance toward the client. Type II CTRs, in contrast, involve forms of overidentification, overidealization, enmeshment, and excessive advocacy for the client, as well as behaviors that elicit guilt reactions.

As Figure 1.1 illustrates, the combination of the two axes of countertransference processes produces four distinct modes or styles of empathic strain, which we have identified as (1) empathic withdrawal, (2) empathic repression, (3) empathic enmeshment, and (4) empathic disequilibrium. Although a therapist may experience one style or reaction pattern more than another, it is possible to experience any or all of the modes of empathic strain during the course of treatment with a traumatized client.

Empathic withdrawal is a mode of countertransference strain that occurs when the therapist experiences expected affective and cognitive reactions during treatment, and he or she is predisposed by defensive style and personality characteristics towards Type I avoidance and detachment responses. In this mode, a rupture occurs in the empathic stance toward the client. The result is often the loss of capacity for sustained empathic inquiry due to overreliance on the "blank-screen" conventional, or recently taught (for new therapist) therapeutic techniques. These reactions block the painful task of integrating the trauma experience and may lead the therapist to misperceive or misinterpret the behavior and psychodynamics of the client on the basis of the therapist's previous assumptions.

A similar process occurs in *empathic repression,* in which the transference issues of the patient reactivate conflicts and unresolved personal concerns in the therapist's life. Thus, a subjective reaction, combined with a disposition toward a Type I CTR, may be associated with repressive counter measures by the therapist. His or her inward focus on areas of personal conflict is likely to be associated with an unwitting withdrawal from the therapeutic role and denial of the full significance of the clinical issues being presented by the client.

The third mode of strain, *empathic enmeshment,* is the result of the therapist's tendency toward Type II CTRs coupled with subjective reactions during treatment. In this mode of empathic strain, the clinician leaves the therapeutic role by becoming overinvolved and overidentified with the client. The most common consequence is pathological enmeshment and a loss of role boundaries in the context of treatment. In the treatment of PTSD, therapists with a personal history of trauma and victimization are especially vulnerable to this mode of empathic strain and may unconsciously attempt to rescue traumatized clients as an indirect way of dealing with their own unintegrated personal conflicts. Perhaps the greatest danger that occurs within this mode of empathic strain is the potential for the therapist to unconsciously reenact personal problems through pathological enmeshment. When this occurs it not only causes an abandonment of the empathic stance toward the person seeking help but may lead to secondary victimization or intensification of the transference themes that the patient brought to treatment in the first place.

Empathic disequilibrium, as Figure 1.1 indicates, is characterized by a disposition to Type II CTRs and the experience of objective reactions during treatment, especially in work with patients suffering from PTSD and comorbid conditions. This mode of strain is characterized by somatic discomfort, feelings of insecurity and uncertainty as to how to deal with the client, and more. It occurs commonly in therapists who experience either Type I or Type II CTRs. In the case example described earlier in this chapter, the therapist indicated that she felt overwhelmed, tense, vulnerable, and uncertain of her own capacity to bind anxiety, and she experienced increased physiological arousal. She stated that she felt somewhat insecure in regard to her ability to adequately treat the torture victim, despite having worked quite successfully with other torture victims in the past. In particular, her objective CTR included vivid images of seeing the heads of the murdered children on the ground being sadistically abused by the victim's captors. These visual images and her natural identification with the woman as a mother and brutalized person were associated with an extreme state of autonomic nervous system arousal. Her concern following the session was that if she could not more effectively modulate her affect she would not be successful in her clinical efforts. An associated concern centered around her fear that the torture victim might become further isolated from sources of help or even worse, commit suicide.

This case illustration also indicates that empathic overarousal is associated with powerful ARs (e.g., anxiety, motor tension) and cognitive processes (e.g., images of sadistic torture) that extend beyond the therapy hour in distressing ways and are associated with self-doubt, feelings of vulnerability, and a need to discharge the therapist's hyperaroused state.[2]

To some degree the type of countertransference a given clinical

---

[2]It is interesting to note that one consequence of empathy is that the therapist may experience degrees of hyperarousal that are proportional to the level of hyperarousal the patient manifests as part of their PTSD. Clearly, this is a type of dual unfolding in the dynamics of transference and countertransference.

encounter will evoke is a function of the role of helper. In this volume clinicians and practitioners occupy many roles, such as rescue workers on the scene of a disaster, consultants to primary caregivers immediately after industrial and school trauma, or advisors to survivors during litigation proceedings (as with rape victims and children who witness murder). They are also experts in financial restitution proceedings regarding disability and compensation, and in legal proceedings regarding criminal charges.

Within psychotherapy, clinicians are called on to take trauma histories and to elicit the trauma story. Clients call on clinicians to protest and rescue, to judge and to accept, to constrain and to advocate, to comfort, and to endow with meaning. Each of these roles may reflect some unresolved aspects of the trauma experience and become the fulcrum around which the countertransference of withdrawal and enmeshment occurs.

Later in work of this nature, the client may begin to reexperience trauma-related feelings that he or she feels are activated in the here and now of the therapy. The former torture survivor, for example, may feel that the therapist is failing to protect her from harsh, current political forces that are blocking immigration and thereby persecuting her anew. She may feel that the therapist is judging her for sacrificing her children to her political cause, irreverently dismissing her attachment to her dead children, or failing to hear her sadness and pain at now feeling inhibited sexually (thereby disrespecting her sexuality). As each of these elements in the trauma situation is partially reenacted and transferred onto the treatment, new trauma-based countertransferences may appear, impairing empathy by rupture, repression, enmeshment, or overarousal, until these processes are understood as part of the dual unfolding of the treatment.

Individual Variations in Modes of Empathic Strain

We realize that elaborating a two-dimensional model for a topology of countertransference has its limitations as well as its value, and we do not mean to say that *all* relevant CTRs to PTSD fit neatly into one of the four quadrants. For example, CTRs may also need to be categorized in terms of affect range and intensity, trauma role reenacted, defense cluster mobilized, symptom experienced by therapist, or segment of the treatment frame distorted (see Chapter 3, this volume). Neither do we wish to imply a static mode, one that confines CTR in a given treatment to one quadrant. Indeed, there is more likely a dynamic interplay among quadrants over time in a single case. Nevertheless, this model provides an important starting point, one that includes rather than excludes other descriptive dimensions and, for purposes of clinical use, establishes an important point of orientation.

THE IMPACT OF EMPATHIC STRAIN AND COUNTERTRANSFERENCE ON THE PSYCHOTHERAPY OF TRAUMA SURVIVORS

Next we turn to an analysis of the factors that determine CTRs and how CTRs, in turn, affect the phases of stress recovery and potentially cause pathological results to the client.

Figure 1.2 presents a conceptual schema of countertransference effects in the treatment of trauma survivors. This schema is a general model that attempts to illustrate how CTRs cause a rupture of empathy and lead to a loss of the therapeutic role stance essential for sustained empathic inquiry. Of particular importance are the potential pathological consequences caused by an empathic break between the therapist and the client suffering from PTSD (see Chapter 3 for case illustrations).

Factors Associated with CTRs

We believe that there are at least four major categories that contain determinants of CTRs: (1) the nature of stressor dimensions present in the trauma and the trauma story, (2) personal factors in the therapist/helper, (3) institutional organizational factors affecting the therapist and the therapeutic process, and (4) specific characteristics in the client.

As Figure 1.2 indicates, each of these four categories of CTRs has the potential to affect the specific phases of the stress recovery process and cause a rupture of empathy. Further, when an empathic break does occur, it may cause a pathological outcome such as (1) cessation of the recovery process, (2) fixation within a phase, (3) regression, (4) intensification of transference, and (5) forms of acting-out behavior.

The Nature of Stressor Dimensions Present in the Trauma and in the Trauma Story

Table 1.1 summarizes the key elements that comprise the four categories of determinants of CTRs. The first set of factors common to work with trauma survivors concerns the therapist's reactions to the trauma story as presented by the client. With refugee torture victims, for example, the trauma story typically contains accounts of extremely stressful life ex-

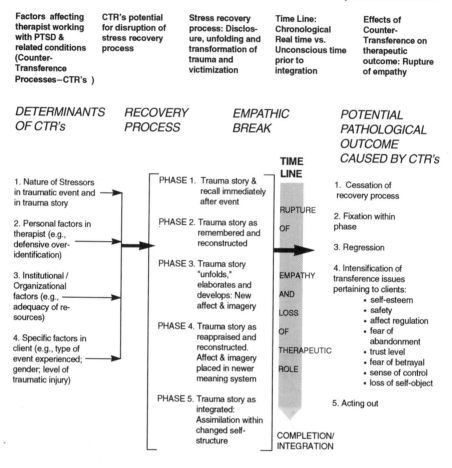

| Factors affecting therapist working with PTSD & related conditions (Counter-Transference Processes–CTR's) | CTR's potential for disruption of stress recovery process | Stress recovery process: Disclosure, unfolding and transformation of trauma and victimization | Time Line: Chronological Real time vs. Unconscious time prior to integration | Effects of Counter-Transference on therapeutic outcome: Rupture of empathy |

DETERMINANTS OF CTR's

RECOVERY PROCESS

EMPATHIC BREAK

POTENTIAL PATHOLOGICAL OUTCOME CAUSED BY CTR's

TIME LINE

1. Nature of Stressors in traumatic event and in trauma story

2. Personal factors in therapist (e.g., defensive over-identification)

3. Institutional / Organizational factors (e.g., adequacy of re-sources)

4. Specific factors in client (e.g., type of event experienced; gender; level of traumatic injury)

PHASE 1. Trauma story & recall immediately after event

PHASE 2. Trauma story as remembered and reconstructed

PHASE 3. Trauma story "unfolds," elaborates and develops: New affect & imagery

PHASE 4. Trauma story as reappraised and reconstructed. Affect & imagery placed in newer meaning system

PHASE 5. Trauma story as integrated: Assimilation within changed self-structure

RUPTURE OF EMPATHY AND LOSS OF THERAPEUTIC ROLE

COMPLETION/ INTEGRATION

1. Cessation of recovery process

2. Fixation within phase

3. Regression

4. Intensification of transference issues pertaining to clients:
 • self-esteem
 • safety
 • affect regulation
 • fear of abandonment
 • trust level
 • fear of betrayal
 • sense of control
 • loss of self-object

5. Acting out

COUNTER-TRANSFERENCES MAY CAUSE "RUPTURE OF EMPATHY" AND LOSS OF THERAPEUTIC ROLE WITH NEGATIVE IMPACT ON RECOVERY

FIGURE 1.2. Countertransference effects on recovery from trauma and victimization.

perience that involves injury, threat, mutilation, bereavement, humiliation, degradation, defilement, the confrontation of moral dilemmas, and exposure to death, dying, destruction, and chaos. During treatment, the therapist typically experiences strong ARs to the client's account and reliving of the traumatic event. Beyond that, of course, therapists react to their own images and understanding of the traumatic event through the mechanism of partial identification and counteridentification (Slatker, 1987). Thus, the complexity of countertransference can be seen in the multileveled way in which the therapist reacts to a particular client in the transference–countertransference, dual unfolding process. Countertrans-

TABLE 1.1. Factors That Interact in Determining the Nature, Quality, and Dynamics in CTRs in Work with Survivors of Trauma/Victimization

I. The Nature of Stressor Dimensions Present in the Trauma and the Trauma Story
    Complexity and type of stressor (natural vs. human origin)
    Grotesqueness, death, injury, mutilation, abuse
    Stage in life cycle at exposure
    Role(s) in event
    Moral dilemmas during event
    Degree of psychological ensnarement by perpetrator or events
    Duration, severity, frequency of exposure or victimization
    Personal role relations in event
    Degree of community involvement

II. Personal Factors in Therapist/Helper
    Personal beliefs, religious values, ideological systems, and preconceptions
    Defensive styles and dispositions
    Personal "historical" data from own life experiences
    Degree of training and experience with trauma and victimization
    Motivation to work in trauma field
    Theoretical assumptions about personality and life cycle development

III. Factors in the Client Relevant to Understanding CTRs
    Age, race, gender, ethnicity, and cultural dimensions
    Role in traumatic event (e.g., perpetrator, victim, witness)
    Personality characteristics
    Defensive and coping styles
    Level of traumatization and injuries
    Cultural differences affecting the cognitive process of trauma
    Pre-trauma ego strength or pre-morbidity
    Type of traumatic event experienced
    Family dynamics and background factors

IV. Institutional/Organizational Factors Relevant to Therapeutic Process
    Political context: Supportive versus oppositional
    Attitudes toward client population
    Adequacy of resources that help or hinder treatment
    Availability of "network" affiliations and resources to aid in treatment
    Internal or external mechanisms to provide necessary support for
      helpers
    Flexibility versus rigidity to change in existing organizational health
      care structures

ference includes reactions to the traumatic event (e.g., torture), the reliving of the trauma story by the distressed client (e.g., anguish, pain, bereavement), the social status characteristics (e.g., age, gender), and the role relations of the survivor (e.g., mother of murdered children).

Historical Events and Personality Characteristics in the Therapist

It is a truism to say that the therapist brings his or her own personality characteristics and idiosyncracies to the treatment situation. These include personal beliefs and ideological systems, defensive styles and personality traits, education, and personal "historical" data from life experiences relevant to the trauma circumstance (see Op den Velde et al., Chapter 12, this volume).

In work with persons suffering from PTSD, the degree of training and education for work in the field of traumatic stress can significantly influence the disposition to Type I and Type II CTRs. Therapists with little training or preparation to work with trauma survivors often report being overwhelmed by the self-disclosure of a profoundly disturbing life experience by a client with a history of trauma or abuse. If unmanaged by supervision or peer consultation, a Type I or Type II CTR may cause a rupture of empathy and disrupt progress in treatment. It is also important to critically examine the therapist's motivation to work with trauma survivors. A personal history of trauma or abuse in childhood, for example, can affect the type of CTR experienced. Moreover, it can create additional difficulty in the dual unfolding process because the client's personal struggle to integrate his or her own trauma experience can stimulate conscious or unconscious reenactment and reliving processes in the therapist as well.

Personality Characteristics of the Client

A broad range of factors in clients with PTSD can influence countertransference processes. Included in this list are demographic characteristics (e.g., race, gender, age, cultural attributes), personality characteristics and defensive styles, the type and degree of traumatization and immediate trauma-related support, pre-trauma ego-strength, and the psychosocial history of the client. These factors may facilitate or hinder the process of dual unfolding and the therapist's partial identification or counteridentification with a particular trauma survivor.

In our case example of the refugee victim of torture, the counselor, herself a young woman, identified with the gender, age, and role status of the client (i.e., a mother of two children). She identified with the victim as a woman raped by male captors and dogs. She also had a special appreciation of the victim's struggle to start life over again after fleeing her native culture.

The client was a survivor with PTSD, but she was also an indigent, single woman living alone in one of the most populated cities in the world. She was poor, lonely, and suicidal. The counselor, dedicated and compassionate, was strongly affected by the sheer emotional intensity of the trauma story as it unfolded in their work together and by the current life circumstances of the torture survivor as they added secondary stressors to her life. In her effort to maintain an empathic stance, the counselor shared the woman's sadness and desolation.

By imagining various different therapists working on Teresa's case, we see that there could be many combinations of forces affecting her interaction with them and the nature of their empathic strains and countertransferences. For example, would a male therapist's countertransference be the same as a female's? Would an older woman's resemble a younger woman's? Or, in another variation, would a male torture survivor evoke similar or different emotions? In discussing this case in training workshops, we have found that many male therapists who hear the story of the torture victim and her children experience degrees of anger and rage, and they often have fantasies of killing the captors. Yet, other male therapists describe their reactions as avoidance, distancing, or revulsion. Race, ethnicity, culture, and political orientation affect Type I and Type II reactions as well. All of this points to the need for systematic, controlled, empirical studies of the complex interactive processes affecting countertransference mechanisms in the psychotherapy of trauma survivors.

Institutional/Organizational Factors Relevant to CTRs

Although many mental health professionals work in organizations that have policies, procedures, methods, and rules that affect the care of clients, the impact of these institutional variables is neither well understood nor often studied empirically. One notable voice in this wilderness has been Arthur Blank (1985, 1993) in his studies of the irrational reactions to work with Vietnam veterans. Blank noted that until the U.S. Department of Veterans Affairs agreed to provide quality care to Vietnam-era veterans, that organization had institutionalized many obstacles to the development of needed health care programs, especially for the treatment of PTSD. These obstacles ranged from negative, stereotypic attitudes toward Vietnam veterans to the lack of recognition of PTSD as a clinical entity and the absence of adequate facilities to carry out readjustment counseling.

The example of the U.S. Department of Veterans Affairs and the difficulties faced by many of its professional health workers undoubtedly applies to other mental health agencies and the parent bureaucratic bodies that fund them. From our perspective, the concern is that institutions may be *supportive* of or *oppositional* to the efforts made by mental health care providers; *flexible* or *rigid* in responding to innovation, change, and improvement of services; *self-contained* or *collaborative* in efforts at networking with allied agencies for the benefit of the client with PTSD; and *nurturing* or *indifferent* in providing adequate mechanisms of support for the service providers themselves. What is clear, however, is that when institutions fail to create an environment in which the service provider feels that he or she is part of a cooperative team with shared values and a commitment to aid victims of trauma, the impact on that service provider is likely to be a negative one, which creates a dual form of countertransference: one toward the institution and one toward the client who accesses that agency for help.

In summary, it is possible to discern that the four categories of countertransference we have listed in Table 1.1 all interact with each other, at least in a logical way, if not empirically. Survivors of trauma with symptoms, reactions, or a diagnosis of PTSD tell their trauma stories through the filter of their unique personality styles, cultures, and life experiences. Similarly, the therapist helping the trauma survivor is a person with distinct personality attributes, a professional role, and a psychosocial history as well. Together they meet in a common psychological space for purposes of working to facilitate healing, recovery, and psychological integration from a traumatic past life event. The context of this task occurs in a private practice or within an organization that employs the helping professional. What then ensues is a joint relationship, a psychological and spiritual encounter, where together they try to understand events and profoundly disturbing experiences that alter the course of people's lives, so that they can attempt to understand the meaning of why the trauma occurred.

If this process goes well, the helper will be able, in a metaphorical sense, to "dance" delicately and gracefully with the survivor in a safe space that enables the survivor to feel his or her human vulnerability and to grow from it, and thus to overcome victimization, with a new sense of meaning and personal well-being. This metaphorical dance will not be easy for either participant, and they will encounter crises, impasses, and moments during which the whole enterprise will be at risk of fracture and a premature ending.

MANAGEMENT OF THERAPIST DISEQUILIBRIUM
IN THE TREATMENT OF PTSD

Given the ubiquity of empathic strain in working with trauma survivors and the consequent tendency toward CTRs, the question of management of the resultant disequilibrium in the therapist is a matter of utmost importance for treatment outcome. Among the memories likely to be activated are those of the therapist's own traumatic past. Among the affects likely to be stirred are the therapist's own reactions had he or she been in the trauma situation. Managing and working through these dysphoric affects and memories is an awesome, at times overwhelming, task, and the pressure to disclose unresolved affect prematurely to the client as a means of discharge can be intense. As a corollary, a need to avail oneself of peer support and supervision/consultation may even be an absolute, as in the case example. However, the private working through is both necessary to the therapist's self-understanding and an essential ingredient in communicating understanding to the survivor.

On the other hand, in treating PTSD the therapist cannot maintain a "blank screen" and fail to validate legitimate feelings. Before some trauma survivors are able to tell their stories or unconsciously permit partial reenactment in treatment, they may need to know the trauma credentials of the therapist. They may also need to test the therapist to ascertain that the hearer of the trauma story will be humane, sensitive, and compassionate. These are the nutrients in the "soil" that permit recovery work to grow. In fact, one essential difference between treating trauma survivors and other clients is the therapist's stance: What in another context is termed "disclosure," and considered counterproductive, may in this context define essential elements in the working alliance.

SIGNS OF DEFENSIVENESS AND COUNTERTRANSFERENCE IN
THE PSYCHOTHERAPY OF TRAUMA SURVIVORS

Defensive behavior by the therapist is typically counterproductive to the successful treatment of PTSD. Maroda (1991) suggests that defensiveness is in itself a sign of a countertransference problem, regardless of the factors that led to the use of defenses. She suggests that signs of defensiveness include attitudes of derision, condescension, criticalness, judgmental postures, passive repetition of past interpretations that were rejected, and problems around scheduling appointments. The latter includes forgetting appointments, double-scheduling, rescheduling, or canceling appointments. Other clues to defensiveness include a fear of being out of control with a patient or a narcissistic belief in one's special talents in working with trauma survivors (see Op den Velde et al., Chapter 12, this volume).

Table 1.2 summarizes four sets of indicators of CTRs in the psychotherapy of trauma survivors: (1) physiological and physical reactions, (2) affective reactions, (3) psychological reactions, and (4) behavioral symptoms. These four categories were derived by talking extensively with our colleagues in the field who work with trauma survivors (i.e., members of

---

TABLE 1.2. Factors Indicative of CTRs in Therapist/Helper

I.   Physiological and Physical Reactions
     Symptoms of increased ANS arousal
     Somatic reactions to trauma story or therapy as a contextual process
     Sleep disturbances
     Agitation
     Inattention, drowsiness, or avoidance reactions
     Uncontrolled and unintended displays of emotion

II. Emotional Reactions
     Irritability, annoyance, or disdain toward client
     Anxiety and fear reactions
     Depression and sadness reactions
     Anger, rage, hostility reactions
     Detachment, denial, avoidance, or numbing reactions
     Sadistic/masochistic reactions
     Voyeuristic and sexualized reactions
     Horror, disgust, dread, or loathing reactions
     Confusion, psychic overload, overwhelmed reactions
     Guilt, shame, embarrassment reactions

III. Psychological Reactions
     Detachment reactions based on defenses of intellectualization,
         rationalization, isolation, denial, minimization, fantasy
     Overidentification based on defenses of projection, introjection, denial

IV. Signs and Behavioral Symptoms of CTRs That May Be Conscious or
     Unconscious
     Forgetting, lapse of attention, parapraxes
     Leave therapeutic role stance of empathy
     Hostility, anger toward client
     Relief when client misses appointment or wish that client not show for
         session
     Denial of feelings and/or denial of need for supervision/consultation
     Narcissistic belief in role of being gifted specialist in PTSD
     Excessive concern/identification with client
     Psychic numbing or emotional constriction
     Self-medication as numbing
     Loss of boundaries during therapy
     Totalistic, concordant, complementary reactions

TABLE 1.3. Glossary of Terms Relevant to Countertransference Processes

AFFECTIVE REACTION (AR)	The experience of affect by the therapist in response to transference reaction by the client
COUNTERIDENTIFICATION	The process by which the therapist attempts to maintain objectivity in treatment by examining his or her identification with the client in an empathic role stance
COUNTERTRANSFERENCE REACTIONS (CTRs)	The affective, somatic, cognitive, and interpersonal reactions (including defensive) of the therapist toward the client's story and behaviors
DUAL COUNTERTRANSFERENCE	CTRs toward two or more objects at the same time (e.g., a client and an institution where therapist is employed)
DUAL UNFOLDING PROCESS	The evolving nature of the transference–countertransference process in the course of treatment
EMPATHY	The psychobiological capacity to experience another person's state of being and phenomenological perspective at a given moment in time
EMPATHIC STRAIN	Interpersonal events in psychotherapy that weaken, injure, or force beyond due limits a salutary response to a client
OBJECTIVE CTRs	Expectable and indigenous ARs by the therapist during the course of treatment
SAFE–HOLDING ENVIRONMENT	D. W. Winnicott's term for a therapeutic context that is perceived by the client as a safe, protective environment that can successfully contain or hold the emotional difficulties of the client that led to treatment
SUBJECTIVE CTRs	ARs manifested by the therapist to the transference that are idiosyncratic and particular and may involve personal conflicts that are unresolved
SUSTAINED EMPATHIC INQUIRY	The capacity of the therapist to remain in an empathic role stance toward the client throughout the course of treatment
TRANSFERENCE	The process and behaviors by which a client relates to the therapist in a manner similar to that in past relationships with significant others
TRAUMA-SPECIFIC TRANSFERENCE (TST)	Transference reactions that are specifically associated with unmetabolized elements of the traumatic event and which usually involve symbolic and other forms of reenactment with the therapist
TRAUMA STORY	The account of the trauma survivor of his or her experience in a traumatic event
TYPE I CTRs	CTRs that involve forms of denial, detachment, distancing, or withdrawal from the client
TYPE II CTRs	CTRs that involve forms of overidentification, enmeshment, or overidealization of the client

the International Society for Traumatic Stress Studies). For example, nearly all stated that physical reactions were common (e.g., headaches, increased motor tension, flushing, sleeplessness, increased autonomic nervous system [ANS] arousal), and were a salient clue that countertransference was at work.

The range of emotional reactions that are part of CTRs spans the continuum of human emotions and varies from one therapist to another, depending on the attributes of the client and the nature of his or her traumatic experience. Many therapists stated that increased tension, somatic reactions, irritability, and numbing were common reactions, especially if there was not adequate supervision, peer consultation, or other opportunities to defuse their personal reactions after prolonged contact with trauma survivors. Table 1.2 also indicates that therapists may develop behavioral symptoms indicative of CTRs, such as lapses of attention, relief when a client misses an appointment, or hostility toward the client who is vulnerable and dependent for help. Parapraxes, excessive identification with the client's experiences, or increased drug or alcohol use as self-medication are also employed to reduce states of arousal, tension, or fatigue.

The importance of recognizing and properly managing CTRs in the treatment of PTSD is critical to the maintenance of sustained empathic inquiry. Maroda (1991) states that "failure to express or analyze the counter-transference, particularly at critical moments in the treatment process, can result in long impasses, untimely terminations, and treatments that run their course dominated not by the transference, but by the countertransference" (p. 156). Given the therapeutic objective—to help survivors heal—the importance of countertransference in this population is pivotal to the successful transformation of trauma and the restoration of human integrity.

REFERENCES

Blank, A. S. (1985). Irrational reactions to PTSD and Vietnam Veterans. In I. Sonnenberg, A. S. Blank, & J. A. Talbott (Eds.), *The trauma of war* (pp. 69–99). Washington, DC. American Psychiatric Press.

Blank, A. S. (1993). Vet centers: A new paradigm in delivery services for victims and survivors of traumatic stress. In J. P. Wilson & B. Raphael (Eds.), *The international handbook of traumatic stress syndromes* (pp. 915–925). New York: Plenum Press.

Brandell, J. (1992). *Countertransference in psychotherapy with children and adolescents.* Northvale, NJ: Jason Aronson.

Danieli, Y. (1988). Confronting the unimaginable: Psychotherapists' reactions to victims of the Nazi Holocaust. In J. P. Wilson, Z. Harel, & B. Kahana (Eds.),

Human adaptation to extreme stress (pp. 219–237). New York: Plenum Press.

Figley, C. R. (Ed.). (1985). *Trauma and its wake* (Vol. I). New York: Brunner/Mazel.

Foa, E. B., Rathbaum, B. O., Riggs, D. S., & Mardock, T. B. (1991). Treatment of post-traumatic stress disorder in rape victims: A comparison between cognitive-behavioral procedures and counseling. *Journal of Consulting and Clinical Psychology, 59*(5), 715–723.

Freud, S. (1910). Future prospects for psycho-analytic therapy. *Standard Edition, 11*, 141–142. London: Hogarth Press, 1962.

Gorkin, M. (1987). *The uses of countertransference.* Northvale, NJ: Jason Aronson.

Herman, J. (1992). *Trauma and recovery.* New York: Basic Books.

Horowitz, M. (1986). *Stress response syndromes.* Northvale, NJ: Jason Aronson.

Isaacharoff, A., & Hunt, W. (1978). Beyond countertransference. *Contemporary Psychoanalysis, 14*, 291–310.

Lifton, R. J. (1967). *Death in life: The survivors of Hiroshima.* New York: Touchstone.

Lifton, R. J. (1988). Understanding the traumatized self: Imagery, symbolization, and transformation. In J. P. Wilson, Z. Harel, & B. Kahana (Eds.), *Human adaptation to extreme stress* (pp. 7–32). New York: Plenum Press.

Lindy, J.D. (1985). The trauma membrane and other clinical concepts derived from psychotherapeutic work with survivors of natural disaster. *Psychiatric Annals, 15*(3), 153–160.

Lindy, J. D. (1988). *Vietnam: A casebook.* New York: Brunner/Mazel.

Lindy, J. D. (1989). Transference and post-traumatic stress disorder. *Journal of American Academy of Psychoanalysis, 17*, 397–403.

Lindy, J. (1993). Focal psychoanalytic psychotherapy of posttraumatic stress disorder. In J. P. Wilson & B. Raphael (Eds.), *The international handbook of traumatic stress syndromes* (pp. 803–811). New York: Plenum Press.

Maroda, K. J. (1991). *The power of countertransference.* New York: Wiley.

McCann, I. L., & Pearlman, L. (1990). *Psychological trauma and the adult survivor.* New York: Brunner/Mazel.

Mollica, R. (1988). The trauma story: The psychiatric care of refugee survivors of violence and torture. In F. Ochberg (Ed.), *Post-traumatic therapy and victims of violence* (pp. 295–315). New York: Brunner/Mazel.

Ochberg, F. (Ed.). (1988). *Post-traumatic therapy and victims of violence.* New York: Brunner/Mazel.

Ochberg, F. (1993). Post-traumatic therapy. In J. P. Wilson & B. Raphael (Eds.), *The international handbook of traumatic stress syndrome* (pp. 773–785). New York: Plenum Press.

Parson, E. (1988). Post-traumatic self-disorder: Theoretical and practical considerations for psychotherapy of Vietnam War veterans. In J. P. Wilson, Z. Harel, & B. Kahana (Eds.), *Human adaptation to extreme stress* (pp. 245–279). New York: Plenum Press.

Racker, H. (1968). *Transference and countertransference.* New York: International Universities Press.

Scurfield, R. M. (1993). Treatment of post-traumatic syndrome disorder among Vietnam veterans. In J. P. Wilson & B. Raphael (Eds.), *The international handbook of traumatic stress syndromes* (pp. 879–889). New York: Plenum Press.

Simpson, M. (1993). Traumatic stress and the bruising of the soul: The effects of torture and coercive interrogation. In J. P. Wilson & B. Raphael (Eds.), *The international handbook of traumatic stress syndromes* (pp. 667–685). New York: Plenum Press.

Slatker, E. (1987). *Countertransference.* Northvale, NJ: Jason Aronson.

Styron, W. (1979). *Sophie's choice.* New York: Random House.

Wilson, J. P. (1988). Understanding the Vietnam veteran. In F. Ochberg (Ed.), *Post-traumatic therapy and victims of violence* (pp. 227–254). New York: Brunner/Mazel.

Wilson, J. P. (1989). *Trauma, transformation, and healing: An integrative approach to theory, research, and post-traumatic therapy.* New York: Brunner/Mazel.

Wilson, J. P., & Raphael, B. (Eds.). (1993). *The international handbook of traumatic stress syndromes.* New York: Plenum Press.

Winnicott, D. W. (1949). Hate in the countertransference. *International Journal of Psycho-Analysis, 30,* 69–74.

Winnicott, D. W. (1960). Countertransference. In *Maturational processes and the facilitating environment* (pp. 158–165). New York: International Universities Press, 1965.

2

Empathic Strain and Therapist Defense: Type I and II CTRs

JOHN P. WILSON
JACOB D. LINDY
BEVERLEY RAPHAEL

It is the purpose of this chapter to develop a framework for understanding modes of empathic strain and countertransference reactions (CTRs) in the study and treatment of survivors of trauma, so as to spell out the interaction between affect and cognition and to point the way toward empathic growth and CTR resolution. As such, this chapter builds on the conceptual framework developed in Chapter 1. Although our focus is primarily to illuminate the various ways that CTRs occur during the course of post-traumatic therapies (e.g., psychoanalytic approaches, peer support groups, hospital inpatient programs, cognitive-behavioral therapies, stress inoculation, critical incident stress debriefing, graded exposure), much of what we conceptualize in terms of CTRs will generalize to clinical work and research efforts with other populations.

Advancements in the assessment, diagnosis, and treatment of post-traumatic stress disorder (PTSD) have been significant (Wilson & Raphael, 1993). Now we must elucidate the role and dynamics of specific feelings evoked by the treatment situation, *affective responses* (therapist's emotional state) and the *cognitive processes* (both defensive and integrative) that attempt to contain them. Because clinical work with victims of PTSD commonly elicits strong affective reactions (ARs) in the therapist, which may cause a rupture of empathy, a disruption in the treatment process, or treatment failure, it is especially important to understand ARs.

These critical considerations arise because survivors of extraordinarily difficult and often life-threatening events (experiences that leave a narcissistic wound to the fabric of the self) bring to the therapeutic setting an emotional intensity and level of distress that touches, surpasses, and transforms the empathic sensitivity of the listener. Many mental health and other professionals are at risk for strong empathic strains—for instance, psychologists, nurses, social workers, physicians, paramedics, police officers, research interviewers, firefighters, trauma counselors, teachers, and members of the victim's circle of significant others.

The special nature of the interaction between a traumatized person and a therapist sets the stage for a broad range of empathic strain in the treatment situation. As noted in Chapter 1, the spectrum of affects ranges from overidentification with the client's plight to minimization or avoidance of the traumatic impact to the self-structure of the survivors. Further, when empathic strains adversely affect the therapist's professional role, they leave him or her with a distorted or incomplete understanding of the victim's intrapsychic dynamics. It is, therefore, a fundamental premise in post-traumatic therapy (PTT) that empathic strains are natural phenomena in working with survivors with PTSD and allied forms of stress reactions or psychopathology. While such strains are expectable, indigenous, and an integral part of treatments, they pose a potential threat to treatment outcome when they develop into more complex CTRs.

This chapter is organized around five themes and uses eight figures and tables to illustrate these central issues in the treatment of trauma survivors. First, we discuss the psychobiology of empathy and empathic strain and the relationship to developing the therapeutic structures that are critical for containing trauma-specific transference. Second, we discuss a general model of the mechanisms underlying the primary forms of countertransference in PTT. Third, we elaborate modal variations in empathic strain in the treatment of trauma victims as a preface to a more extensive discussion of the continuum of Type I (avoidant, counterphobic, detachment) over Type II (overidentification) CTRs. Fourth, we examine how therapists develop critical therapeutic structures through *empathic stretching*, a counterpart to empathic strain, and the psychological mechanisms that allow the therapist to sustain empathic attunement throughout treatment in a mutual alliance with the client. Fifth, we discuss the nature and role of transference projections in the course of treatment.

THE PSYCHOBIOLOGY OF EMPATHY AND COUNTERTRANSFERENCE

There are several reasons why empathic strains occur in work with traumatized clients suffering from PTSD. Foremost is the fact that, at their core, all empathic strains are forms of the therapist's response to the distress and pain manifested by the trauma survivor. The capacity for empathic response refers to a psychobiologically based capacity (i.e., one which is highly adaptive in nature for the welfare and existence of the species) to recognize and respond to other individuals who suffer emotionally from stressful life events that have adversely affected their psychological and physical sense of well-being. Viewed from this perspective, it is an intrinsic human capacity and even propensity to empathically experience a trauma survivor's distress and his or her personal efforts to restore a sense of coherency, equilibrium, and well-being. In PTT, both the client and therapist experience states of disequilibrium in the dual unfolding process of transference and countertransference in treatment (Maroda, 1990). The survivors' disequilibrium stems from an altered sense of the self (e.g., overwhelmed and numb) caused by the particular trauma they have experienced. The therapists' disequilibrium, however, emanates from their efforts to sustain empathic attunement with the traumatized client.

It is our view that the psychobiological capacity to experience empathy, originating in part from personal experiences with anxiety and psychic injury to the self, may either facilitate recovery or, when strained, impede the process by which the survivor transforms trauma and heals. Many factors, such as the personality and defensive style of the therapist, determine the particular forms of empathic strain that occur in work with traumatized persons. The counterpart to biologically based empathic reactions generated in response to the characteristics of the survivor, the trauma story, and the survivor's life history (Mollica, 1988; Wilson, 1988, 1989) is a set of cognitive and ego-defensive processes in the helper (see Danieli, 1988, for a discussion). We consider these various forms of cognitive, defensive, and belief structures and their efforts to contain trauma-specific ARs to be simultaneous psychobiological processes. The capacity for affect modulation associated with empathic strain does not exist in a vacuum. As professionals, therapists react psychologically to the events that occur in work with traumatized clients (Ochberg, 1993). Their expectable ARs give rise to thought processes in the therapist about what has been said by the client and how that affects the therapist. But it must be made clear that although ARs may strain the empathic potential of the treatment, they are not the same phenomena as CTRs. The empathic reactions, cognitive attributions, and defensive enactments only become CTRs when they cause the therapist or helper to leave the therapeutic role, leading to empathic strain or a rupture of empathy. The critical significance of our need to understand affect modulation, cognition, and CTRs in PTT is that the identification and successful management of empathic strain will permit therapists to appropriately examine and interpret their own reactive styles and use them as insights to reengage a helpful posture toward the client. A safe therapeutic environment with clear and appropriate role boundaries, in which the survivor's affects and the therapist's empathic strain are successfully managed, provides the *critical therapeutic structure* that enables the vulnerable and traumatized person to do the work of recovery. In agreement with Ochberg (1988, 1993), we believe that in PTT the therapist can actively bring to the forefront of his or her awareness the most troublesome issues associated with victimization, as an effort to avoid CTRs. In this way, the therapist uses his or her own normative reactions to the trauma to gain insight about the client's dynamics in the stress recovery process. As such, the insights gained become part of the dual unfolding process in the therapeutic context. When successful, the client will be able to experience new vulnerabilities and previously unspoken fears without excessive protection of the parts of the self injured by the trauma.

In PTT the relationship between the therapist and the survivor is a complex and subtle interpersonal relationship that centers around trauma-specific transference. These transferences place the therapist in various roles, such as failed protector, and they give rise to modes of empathic strain. When CTRs arise in therapy, they have the potential to disrupt recovery due to the therapist's loss of empathic role stance. If this rupture occurs, a new disillusionment with the therapist confirms the client's past disillusionment during and after the trauma, retarding his or her ability to work through the many-faceted transference issues encountered in therapy. On the other hand, the successful management of empathic strain and CTRs facilitates the maintenance of an empathic stance. To suggest that this very human process is easily accomplished would be misleading; at the very least it demands that therapists be open to their own feelings and experiences and that they rely on collegial consultation and supervision to ensure a successful course of treatment. In a sense, this process requires of the therapist an honest self-scrutiny that parallels the client's struggle with the difficulties associated with victimization and traumatic exposure.

A CONCEPTUAL FRAMEWORK OF AFFECT AND CTRs IN PTT

Figure 2.1 outlines a conceptual model of common countertransference processes in PTT. This framework builds on the earlier and seminal contributions to understanding CTRs in PTSD treatment by Haley (1974), Danieli (1984, 1988), Parson (1988), Wilson (1989), and McCann and Pearlman (1990), and the important contributions by psychoanalytically oriented therapists (Brandell, 1992; Gear, Liendo, & Scott, 1983; Giovacchini, 1989; Maroda, 1990; Natterson, 1991; Slatker, 1987; Tansey & Burke, 1989).[1]

In an examination of Figure 2.1, the schematic diagram should be viewed as a way of thinking about the structure, dynamics, and "flow" of the therapist's ARs, cognitions, and CTRs in PTT. The schema is not intended to be a blueprint or mechanistic reduction of some of the most intricate and central features of clinical work with PTSD. Rather, it is an attempt to identify and define the central processes in the therapist's experience of their psychotherapy with victims of trauma. In order to do this, it is necessary to begin by categorizing somewhat artificially the major themes, issues, and reaction styles that interact in very complex ways during therapeutic sessions.

To establish a conceptual framework, we will list the core elements that underlie CTRs and ARs in the therapeutic process. After identifying these elements, we will describe their dynamic interaction effects as they influence the major forms of empathic strain, CTRs, ARs, defensive re-actions, and cognitive schemas—that is, Type I (avoidant, counterphobic, and detachment responses) and Type II (overidentification, enmeshment, and rescuer responses). It is important to recognize that these two forms of therapist reactions are not mutually exclusive. Although one response tendency may be more prevalent for a particular therapist, it is not only possible but likely that a range of empathic strain and CTRs will occur in the course of treatment or even in a single session.

Elements of Affect and Countertransference in PTT

Treatment as an Event

The client suffering from PTSD typically presents with intense affect and discernible distress or, alternatively, psychic numbing, confusion, and depression. Traumatized clients seek out treatment in an attempt to un-derstand their personal distress, and they commonly hold two interrelated beliefs at the beginning of treatment: (1) They secretly fear that they are "going crazy" because of the presence of distressing intrusive recollections of the traumatic event, emotional flooding, or other PTSD symptoms; and (2) they believe that it will be difficult for anyone, including the therapist,

---

[1]Psychoanalytic contributions to understanding CTRs' defensive operations in the therapist have been referred to by various terms which include projective iden-tification, concordant reactions, introjective identification, complementary identifica-tions, objective and subjective countertransference, as well as other concepts (see Brandell, 1992, and Tansey & Burke, 1989, for reviews).

POST TRAUMATIC THERAPY

PTSD & Co-Diagnosis

TRAUMA STORY OF CLIENT:
AFFECTIVE INTENSITY AND DISTRESS

Therapist Empathic Strain
and Personal Reactions

Counter-Transference Reactions

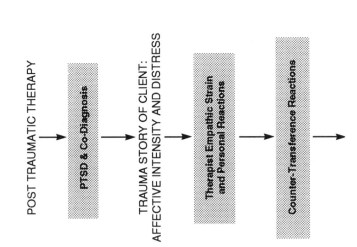

Therapeutic Sanctuary:

Safe Holding Environment

Therapeutic Alliance

Critical Therapeutic Structure

Trauma Victim (Transference)

Therapist Reactions (Counter-Transference)
Dual Unfolding Process

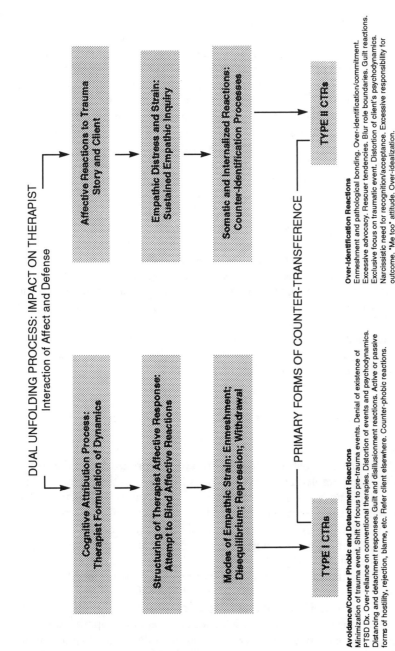

DUAL UNFOLDING PROCESS: IMPACT ON THERAPIST
Interaction of Affect and Defense

Affective Reactions to Trauma Story and Client

Empathic Distress and Strain: Sustained Empathic Inquiry

Somatic and Internalized Reactions: Counter-Identification Processes

TYPE II CTRs

Cognitive Attribution Process: Therapist Formulation of Dynamics

Structuring of Therapist Affective Response: Attempt to Bind Affective Reactions

Modes of Empathic Strain: Enmeshment; Disequilibrium; Repression; Withdrawal

TYPE I CTRs

PRIMARY FORMS OF COUNTER-TRANSFERENCE

Avoidance/Counter Phobic and Detachment Reactions
Minimization of trauma event. Shift of focus to pre-trauma events. Denial of existence of PTSD Dx. Over-reliance on conventional therapies. Distortion of events and psychodynamics. Distancing and detachment responses. Guilt and disillusionment reactions. Active or passive forms of hostility, rejection, blame, etc. Refer client elsewhere. Counter-phobic reactions.

Over-Identification Reactions
Enmeshment and pathological bonding. Over-identification/commitment. Excessive advocacy. Rescuer tendencies. Blur role boundaries. Guilt reactions. Exclusive focus on traumatic event. Distortion of client's psychodynamics. Narcissistic need for recognition/acceptance. Excessive responsibility for outcome. "Me too" attitude. Over-idealization.

FIGURE 2.1. Common countertransference processes in PTT.

to understand what they experienced in the trauma unless that other person was there at the time or has suffered a similar event (Wilson, 1989). Although it is a truism, it is important to properly recognize that PTT constitutes a powerful interpersonal event, one that includes (1) the client's initial perception and transference to the therapist, and (2) the therapist's initial reaction to the client, the nature of the client's trauma, and first accounts of the trauma story. Next, as noted in Chapter 1, for PTT to progress successfully, a safe–holding environment must be created, a milieu that is perceived by the client as a sanctuary where self-disclosure can occur without undue anxiety, fear, or guilt. A safe–holding environment exists when the client feels that the therapist is not only a trusted ally, but someone who, in fact, understands the client's unique experience of PTSD and the various ways it has impacted on his or her adaptive behavior and psychopathology. In Figure 2.1 we refer to this as a *critical therapeutic structure*. As the therapeutic alliance strengthens, especially with regard to the unfolding trauma story, the process of treatment begins in earnest. During the patient's disclosure of more detailed and more genuine affect, complete with memories and images, the therapist is confronted by his or her own reactions to the trauma story and the unique qualities of the client's self-presentation. It is at this point that the psychobiological process of empathy is set in motion; it is at this same point that therapists may experience distress as they search their own memory for material by which to understand and perhaps match the distress presently experienced by their clients.

The Trauma Story, Transference Projections, and Their Impact on the Therapist

Figure 2.1 further illustrates that, as treatment progresses and evolves over time, it inevitably has different types of impact on the therapist. The influence a client has on a therapist may vary but is an intrinsic and integral part of the treatment process. The transference impact of a trauma victim typically evokes complex feelings in the therapist, such as wishes to hold and comfort; wishes to reassure, resume, and make whole; and wishes to share the profound feelings the helper experiences upon hearing the trauma story. These interactions, when pronounced, actually determine the nature and content of countertransference and defensive processes. The trauma-specific transference issues of the client evoke counterreactions in the therapist, who seeks to remain empathic but may experience a broad range of affect and images while attempting to understand the complexities of the client's self-presentation. In Chapter 1, we referred to four specific modes of empathic strain: (1) enmeshment, (2) disequilibrium, (3) repression, and (4) withdrawal. We will elaborate on these reactive styles later in this chapter.

Biological Parameters in CTRs

The nature of psychobiologically based dispositions underlying empathy is such that, at different levels of awareness, therapists respond automatically and instinctively to the degrees of pain, distress, or numbing being manifested by the client. The biological basis of empathy can be demonstrated clinically by laboratory procedures in which a student trainee or a therapist is attached to measuring devices for physiological reactivity (e.g., galvanic skin response, heart rate, muscle tonus, respiration rate) and then asked to respond *in vivo* to a trauma client or watch a videotaped presentation of a patient describing a trauma story. Such a procedure demonstrates the physiological manifestation of empathy and empathic distress: As trainees or therapists listen to the trauma story, their indices of autonomic nervous system (ANS) arousal increase in frequency and amplitude as do other indicators of physiological reactivity. Such biologically based reactions are experienced by therapists in somatic reactions or in specific emotional states, ranging from anxiety and numbing to feelings of sadness and guilt. When such reactions become intense, distressing, or inhibiting, the listeners manifest both empathic and defensive responses in an attempt to contain their own levels of distress or reactions to the client's self-disclosures. It is often the case that the therapists' defensive processes actually occur simultaneously with empathic reactions; they take the form of cognitively framing their reactions and interpersonal events experienced in the therapy session. As noted in Chapter 1, the therapist's personality style moderates the specific types of cognitive attributions that are generated as part of the transference–countertransference matrix.

The Cognitive Structuring of Affective Responses: Therapist Attempts to Bind Empathic Strain in Therapist Disequilibrium

Figure 2.1 illustrates that when there is excessive or unmodulated affective arousal associated with empathic strain (i.e., therapist disequilibrium), a rupture in empathy can occur. This rupture of the empathic stance toward the client may lead to different forms of CTRs, classified in Figure 2.1 as Type I: avoidant, counterphobic, and detachment reactions, and Type II: overidentification reactions. These will be discussed below more fully. Here, however, we wish to indicate that Type I reactions (counterphobic, avoidant, and detachment CTRs) primarily involve forms of denial and withdrawal from the empathic stance toward the client. At the level of defense, such CTRs typically are associated with forms of intellectualization, rationalization, isolation, and denial. In contrast, Type II reactions (overidentification and excessive empathy) involve forms of overinvolvement, overcommitment, guilt reactions, and overidealization of the client. The primary defenses associated with these CTRs are projection, denial, and counteridentification (introjection). In both Types I and II CTRs, the primary defenses serve the function of attempting to bind both the anxiety associated with ARs and the somatic states generated by empathic distress.

A similar position has been taken by Tansey and Burke (1989) in their discussion of signal-affect during the course of treatment.

> Defensive activity is then set in motion unconsciously by the therapist, blocking from consciousness the potential signal value of the affective impact of the identificatory experience. This defensive posture, for example, may surface in the therapist's becoming "too nice" in an attempt to compensate for unconscious guilt, anger, or sadistic impulses toward a patient. On the other hand, a therapist who feels gratified by a patient's idealization may block his pleasure from awareness by an excessively stiff or formal approach. For the therapist, the unfortunate outcome of his defensive activity is a countertransference impact without the absolutely vital awareness that this impact has occurred. Although a projective identification transmitted by the patient has taken hold within, the therapist cannot move forward in the Internal Processing phase without becoming more aware that this critical event has in fact taken place. The empathic process may simply arrest at this point. If the disruption is severe, a regression in the empathic process may also occur in which the therapist reacts to the unconscious identificatory experience by abruptly resisting, in one form or another, further interactional pressure without even becoming aware of the underlying emotions that have been blocked from consciousness. A regression from this level may also disturb and disrupt a therapist's heretofore intact mental set. (p. 82)

MODES OF AFFECT AND DEFENSE IN CTRs

Modal Variations of Empathic Strain in Treatment

Empathic Withdrawal (Type I CTR)

Therapists at risk for withdrawal tendencies are likely to have been spared personal catastrophic trauma; their world view preserves the ideas that life is decent and just; their formal psychological education may be extensive, but not in the trauma area. The client's traumatic stressors often include loss, disillusionment, and threat to life. Hearing about these experiences commonly evokes unpleasant affects, such as horror, dread, fear, hostility, or vengeance. Therapists unconsciously, and in order to avoid pain and preserve their world view, distance themselves from this affect by such mechanisms as denial, disbelief, disavowal, and isolation. The therapist engages the CTR coping mode of *empathic withdrawal* in its several forms: blank screen facade, intellectualization, and misperception of dynamics. Given the strength of his or her educational background, the therapist may deny the response or rationalize it on the basis of theory and technical orthodoxy. The major approach to altering withdrawal is education about trauma and PTSD.

Empathic Repression (Type I CTR)

Unlike withdrawal, therapists at risk for the repression mode are likely to be those who have experienced and continue to suffer from their own related traumas. In fact, there is an overlap here between the work the therapist must yet do and an area of the client's trauma wound. While other aspects of the trauma may become productively engaged in a treatment process, this area remains out of bounds in an *unconscious collusion* between the two victimized survivors. For example, one unresolved traumatic stressor may involve loss, so that grief, the corresponding affect state, is not engaged, acknowledged, or expressed. It is as though the therapist's inability to work through this component or his or her trauma is projectively identified onto the client. In the limited area of the psychic wound, the therapist exhibits empathic repression, featuring withdrawal, denial, and distancing. The therapist feels no need to explain the absent segment of work; he simply does not "see" it or appreciate its significance. Identifying the area of repression is the work of supervision; working through may be the tack of the therapist's own treatment.

Empathic Enmeshment (Type II CTR)

Therapists at risk for the enmeshment mode are largely those with considerable trauma of their own. Typically such therapists' formal education may be incomplete, although they usually engage with trauma survivors quickly and well. The original traumatic stressor in the client might be a dysfunctional family; a thread to life, such as war; or violation of bodily integrity, such as rape or incest. In this case, it is not the story or image that evokes the response so much as a current-day reenactment of danger. As clients repeat their fears in current-day circumstances, they evoke feelings of fright, overprotectiveness, guilt, and excessive responsibility in the therapist. Efforts to rescue the client feel rewarding and lead to a counter-transference coping mode of enmeshment, with special features including loss of boundaries, overinvolvement, and reciprocal dependency. Here the therapist has unconsciously identified with the protective or rescuing role in the trauma predicament as a way of discharging the tensions that continue to come from his or her own wounds. Therapists will vigorously explain these actions as prosocial, despite their leading to overdependence and a halt in the recovery process. In some cases, supervision may be sufficient to adjust the stance, provided the therapist is open to it.

Empathic Disequilibrium (Type II CTR)

Therapists at risk here are primarily those who are naive about this component of the trauma. Often the intrusion of grotesque images, multiple traumas, and impossible choices will set empathic disequilibrium in motion. In some cases, especially in extremely stressful events, the inhumanity present in the trauma images evokes existential shame. Defenses elude the therapist as he or she reels in a state of uncertainty, vulnerability, and unmodulated affect. No explanation integrates this new reality, and the therapist's world view is ruptured; there is only fatigue, despondence, and despair. Unlike other expectable reactions, empathic disequilibrium is less likely to be a stable state but more often will move toward empathic withdrawal or enmeshment. Over time, it may lead to "burn out" and subclinical depression. Effective management includes rest and recuperation, limiting exposure, and support.

Type I: A Continuum of Avoidant, Counterphobic, and Detachment CTRs

Type I CTRs fall along a continuum of avoidant responses in which the therapist leaves the empathic stance toward the client. As Figure 2.2 indicates, the continuum ranges from denial of the level of the client's traumatization, at one end, to actual withdrawal from the therapeutic relationship, at the other end. What activates the various forms of avoidant CTRs is a set of psychobiological processes, which are commonly experienced either consciously or unconsciously as an uncomfortable sense of uncertainty, anxiety, and insecurity in terms of how to best help the person suffering from PTSD and associated symptoms.

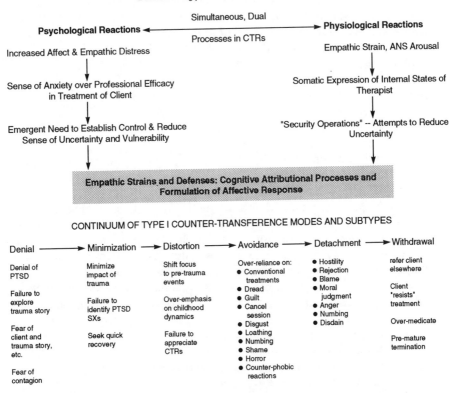

THERAPIST REACTION TO TRAUMATIC EVENT AND CLIENT'S TRAUMA STORY

Psychological Mechanisms of Counter-Transference
Dual unfolding processes in client and therapist

Psychological Reactions ← Simultaneous, Dual Processes in CTRs → **Physiological Reactions**

Increased Affect & Empathic Distress

Empathic Strain, ANS Arousal

Sense of Anxiety over Professional Efficacy in Treatment of Client

Somatic Expression of Internal States of Therapist

Emergent Need to Establish Control & Reduce Sense of Uncertainty and Vulnerability

"Security Operations" -- Attempts to Reduce Uncertainty

Empathic Strains and Defenses: Cognitive Attributional Processes and Formulation of Affective Response

CONTINUUM OF TYPE I COUNTER-TRANSFERENCE MODES AND SUBTYPES

Denial → Minimization → Distortion → Avoidance → Detachment → Withdrawal

Denial	Minimization	Distortion	Avoidance	Detachment	Withdrawal
Denial of PTSD	Minimize impact of trauma	Shift focus to pre-trauma events	Over-reliance on: • Conventional treatments • Dread	• Hostility • Rejection • Blame • Moral judgment	refer client elsewhere
Failure to explore trauma story	Failure to identify PTSD SXs	Over-emphasis on childhood dynamics	• Guilt • Cancel session • Disgust	• Anger • Numbing • Disdain	Client "resists" treatment
Fear of client and trauma story, etc.	Seek quick recovery	Failure to appreciate CTRs	• Loathing • Numbing • Shame • Horror		Over-medicate
Fear of contagion			• Counter-phobic reactions		Pre-mature termination

FIGURE 2.2. Type I CTRs in PTT: Counterphobic, avoidant, and detachment reactions.

As Figure 2.2 shows, the psychobiological responses are simultaneous processes that reflect physiological as well as psychological reactions that are interactive in nature. In response to the client's distress about having been victimized, the therapist may experience empathic distress, which, in turn, leads to a sense of anxiety about professional efficacy in the therapeutic process. The experience of anxiety may then lead to a need to establish control over distressing affect and to attempts at reducing an inner sense of uncertainty and vulnerability. We have labeled these attempts to reduce uncertainty as *security operations* to indicate their role as efforts to enhance the therapist's sense of control and predictability in the therapeutic process. As conceptualized here, these efforts are primarily defensive in nature; they attempt to contain forms of empathic strain and distress indigenous to the therapeutic process.

The continuum of Type I CTRs illustrates some of the ways in which therapists experience counterphobic reactions and detach from their clients. Denial as a CTR often is expressed by a counterphilosophical stance that PTSD does not exist; that it is an experimental diagnosis in the *Diagnostic and Statistical Manual of Mental Disorders*; that it is simply a popular fad. More subtly, denial of PTSD is associated with failure to explore the trauma story or with having fears of the client or fears of contagion. Similarly, another form of denial is to focus primarily on pre-trauma personality functioning and to minimize the potential impact of the traumatic event to the self-structure of the victim. Generally, such defensive tactics reflect the therapist's discomfort with intense affect, a response arising because (1) the therapist finds it difficult to listen non-judgmentally and empathically to the description of traumatic events and their effects on the patient's psychopathology (Wilson, 1988), and (2) the therapist realizes that if clients can be rendered vulnerable emotionally and can be physically injured by a traumatic event, then by implication the therapist himself or herself could vicariously experience such vulnerability to extreme stress. As a security operation, the therapist may shift the focus of treatment away from the injured ego-states of the victim to other issues that are safer for the therapist to address in the session.

Although the line between defensive denial and avoidance may be arbitrary, at least six major modes of Type I avoidance CTRs are apparent:

1. Forms of denial;
2. Minimization reactions;
3. Distortion of the client's psychodynamics;
4. Forms of avoidance;
5. Detachment and overreliance on conventional therapies, or the overuse of the "blank screen" of therapeutic neutrality; and
6. Forms of withdrawal from the treatment situation.

As a Type I CTR, distortion of the client's psychodynamics is often related to forms of denial. The therapist shifts attention away from the traumatic event and places greater emphasis on other relationships or experiences in the individual's life. The result is usually an unbalanced and inaccurate perception of the client because of a lessening of both the empathic stance and the willingness to experience the person phenomenologically in an open, sensitive manner. If distortion of the client's functioning and psychodynamic issues continues for a significant period of time, the therapist may become disillusioned about himself or herself as a therapist. This may result in secret fears about professional competence or, alternatively, a hostility, condemnation, or denigration of the client, among other possible reactions.

As noted by Danieli (1988), Wilson (1989), and Ochberg (1993), the blank screen facade in PTT is potentially a very destructive stance to assume with a client suffering from PTSD. This is so because the survivors need to be validated in their conviction that the traumatic event caused them emotional injury and adversely affected their coping and adaptive behavior. Maintaining a blank screen facade is likely to impede progress in treatment and, as a result, to cause the client to mistrust the therapist, resulting in less self-disclosure about current feelings and behavior. Ochberg (1993), among others, suggests that PTT must be a more active and participative therapeutic process, which eschews the "tabula rasa" therapist style.

There are other Type I CTRs that result in detachment from the client with PTSD. These include, but are not limited to, overmedication with antidepressants and other drugs, and forms of minimization, hostility, and guilt reactions.

Overmedicating clients with PTSD may be an attempt by the therapist to establish a greater sense of control in the treatment process, especially if the helper is uncomfortable with the intense affect associated with the trauma story (Roth, 1988). Even in cases where medication may be indicated for reducing some of the biologically based symptoms of PTSD (Friedman, 1993), the belief that medication may attenuate the florid symptoms that adversely affect adaptive functioning can be a subtle way of detaching from a more active form of therapeutic involvement that demands the maintenance of an empathic attunement to the patient's psychodynamics.

In her research with psychotherapists treating survivors of the Nazi Holocaust, Danieli (1988) found that the development of CTRs of anger, rage, or hostility were not limited to transference reactions but extended to the trauma as a historical event by itself. Beyond countertransference to social events, therapists experience other reactions that result in distancing and detachment, such as hostility, rejection, condemnation, blame, minimization, humiliation of the client, and the passing of moral judgments. In essence, these types of CTRs are expressions by the therapists that they are troubled by what they are hearing and experiencing during treatment. It is as if they are saying to the client, "Don't tell me about your pain and what happened to you. It is too much for me to bear at this time." From our perspective, forms of hostility, minimization, moral judgment, or similar disengaging reactions are also security operations, which attempt to control the level of tension, anxiety, and distress that permeates the treatment process. In time, such reactions may be associated with guilt reactions over professional inadequacy and may result in referring the client elsewhere or, perhaps, to inappropriate disclosure of the CTR feelings in the therapeutic process (Maroda, 1990).

Referral to another therapist or mental health agency after the initial contract with the patient is formulated simply constitutes a withdrawal from PTT.

Type II: A Continuum of Overidentification CTRs

Although Type II CTRs fall along a continuum of attempts to maintain an empathic engagement with the client (see Figure 2.3), they too can lead to a rupture in empathy and a loss of the therapeutic role in a manner that parallels Type I CTRs. The primary difference between them is that, in avoidance, the therapist is overwhelmed by the patient's pain and abandons the empathic stance as a way of finding relief from his or her own

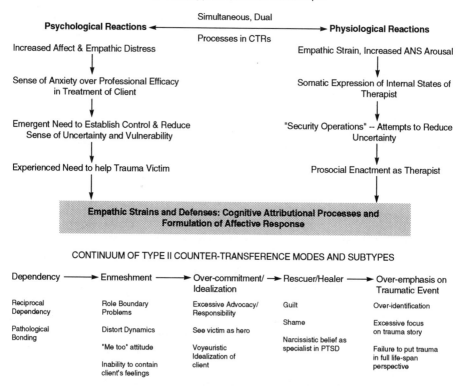

FIGURE 2.3. Type II CTRs in PTT: Overidentification reactions.

pain, whereas in enmeshment the therapist actively wants to help the client with PTSD but in the process loses control over the role boundaries necessary for sustaining empathic inquiry. The loss of therapeutic boundaries then results in five forms of Type II CTRs: (1) dependency, (2) enmeshment, (3) overcommitment and overidealization, (4) rescuer/healer, and (5) overemphasis on the traumatic event.

The therapist's own trauma history may thrust him or her into the midst of one component in the survivor's trauma story, thereby resulting in an enmeshment CTR. Alternatively, a repressed part of the therapist's own trauma story may function to repress that in the survivor. Viewed in a different way, in their attempts to find a comparable wound, therapists face the dilemma of being close but never exact in their empathic understanding of how it is the client relives trauma.

An Intrapsychic Summary of Type I and Type II CTRs

Type I (withdrawal) and Type II (overinvolvement) CTRs can be usefully examined along several additional intrapsychic dimensions, specifically:

- Passive (autoplastic) versus active (alloplastic);
- Ego-syntonic versus ego-dystonic;
- Complementary versus concordant; and
- Structural specificity.

In Type I CTRs, a spectrum of avoidant postures may arise, most but not all of these being passive: Trauma from the patient may fail to register on the therapist (denial, disbelief); trauma may register but be prevented from being an affective presence (isolation, intellectualization); trauma may register in the therapist but drive him or her away because of its power (withdrawal); and trauma may evoke harsh judgments that drive the patient away through blaming and condemning attitudes (rejection). Although most avoidant responses are a passive turning away, some are carried out actively by the therapist's rejection.

Conversely, the Type II CTRs of overinvolvement are primarily active. They include a range of defensive behaviors along an intrapsychic diffusion of behavior: taking on, through loss of boundaries, the ego tasks of the patient; acting out on behalf of the survivor; and counterphobic insistence on getting things done too quickly. Finally, reaction to the trauma story and the various complementary roles in it, such as perpetrator or witness, may activate an even more troubling set of alloplastic tendencies: sadomasochistic impulses, excitement, voyeurism, or murderous vengeance leading to states of overstimulation in the therapist and identification with the aggressor. These states, which feel ego-alien to the altruistic therapeutic role, are among the most difficult for the therapists to recognize and tolerate as part of their human repertoire. Finally, therapists tend to rationalize these differing countertransference coping modes in a variety of ways.

Psychological Dimensions of Type I and Type II CTRs

The delineation of the continuum of Type I and Type II CTRs common to psychotherapy with trauma survivors enables us to further discern their psychological dimensions. Tables 2.1 and 2.2 presents a summary analysis of common reaction patterns in Type I and Type II CTRs, classified by five primary factors:

1. *Affect*—the types of affect and impulses experienced during treatment sessions and afterwards;
2. *Defense*—defensive processes in the therapist associated with empathic strain and efforts to contain affect experienced during sessions;
3. *Coping mode*—behaviors by the therapist that are an effort to cope with the transference dynamics of the client and the affective reactions experienced to them;
4. *Impaired role boundary*—the effects that empathic strain exerts on the therapist's capacity to maintain effective roles and boundaries; and
5. *Theoretical rationale*—the therapist's theoretical or personal beliefs about the client and the therapeutic process that rationalize the above behaviors.

The five factors that comprise the psychological dimensions of Type I and Type II CTRs are, of course, interrelated processes. As discussed earlier, affect and defense are dual simultaneous processes that lead to different forms of coping with trauma-specific transference reactions. The coping modes employed by a therapist have the potential to affect the structure or frame of therapy and its role boundaries. On the one hand, rigidification of boundaries, for example, may result in a loss of empathic attunement and a failure to fully explore the trauma story as it unfolds during treatment. On the other hand, excessively malleable or weak boundaries may result in a rupture of empathy due to an inability to adequately contain the client's affect and a disposition to overidentify with the client through enmeshment.

The five factors that underlie Type I and Type II reactions in PTT

TABLE 2.1. The Psychological Dimensions of Type I CTRs: Common Configurations (Avoidant, Counterphobic, and Detachment)

	Insecurity Anxiety Uncertainty	Fear of client Fear of contagion	Overload Disequilibrium Exhaustion	Hostility Anger Sadism	Guilt Dread	Disdain Numbing Agitation	Shame Horror	Disgust Loathing Exasperation	Annoyance Irritability Resentment
Affect									
Defense	Denial of PTSD Minimize trauma Excessive secrecy	Counterphobic reactions Avoidant reactions Denial	Distort dynamics Withdrawal Inattention	Identification with aggressor Suppression	Excessive detachment Distancing	Intellectualized affective reactions			
Coping mode	Denial of responsibility Excessive detachment	Moral judgments Condemnation	Maintain blank facade Institutionalize responsibility	Reject client Feigned indifference	Passive rejection				
Impaired role boundary	Failure to explore trauma story	Failure to identify PTSD symptoms	Failure to appreciate CTRs	Cancel session Miss appointments	Rigidification of conventional roles	Denial of need for supervision			
Theoretical rationale	Seek quick recovery Pre-morbid focus	Shift focus pre-trauma Overemphasize childhood	Overreliance on conventional treatment	Refer client elsewhere Apply improper diagnosis	View client as resistant Justify by rule-bound behavior	Stereotyping Diffuse responsibility			

49

TABLE 2.2. The Psychological Dimensions of Type II CTRs: Common Configurations (Overidentification)

Affect	Psychic overload Disequilibrium Vulnerability	Insecurity Anxiety Uncertainty	Grief Sadness Disillusionment	Shame Guilt Discouragement	Dread Horror Frustration	Numbing Fear Confusion	Somatic reactions, helplessness, etc.	Hyperaroused states Exhaustion	Anger Felt "pressure" Voyeuristic reactions
Defense	Distort dynamics Overidentification	Exclusive focus on trauma	Narrow focus Projection	Vicarious vigilance	Introjection Somatization	Grandiosity Entitlement	Denial Suppression		
Coping mode	Enmeshment Pathological bonding	Excessive advocacy Overresponsible	Overidentification Overidealization	"Me too" reactions Alienation	Inappropriate self-disclosure Reciprocal dependency	Over-commitment Reenactment			
Impaired role boundary	Inability to contain clients' affect	Role boundaries excessively malleable Acting out	Excessive empathy Empathic rupture	Overschedule clients	Allow intrusion in personal life	Overly distressed Under-modulated affect			
Theoretical rationale	Failure to place trauma in whole life perspective	Narcissistic belief as trauma specialist in PTSD	Adherence only to trauma-specific therapeutic approach	View client as "hero" or special	Adherence to institutional procedures for treatment				

illustrate the enormous complexity of countertransference as a dynamic concept. The broad range of possible ARs to traumatized clients, with the various defensive styles and coping modalities that can be activated, points to the large number of possible interaction effects between a client and therapist in terms of attempts to maintain role boundaries.

To illustrate a few of the possibilities in Type I and Type II reactions, let us consider the example of a therapist working in a country where torture is used as a political tool of oppression by a government (see Agger & Jensen, Chapter 10, this volume). The client in this case was accused of collaborating against the government and subjected to torture, which included electric shock, cigarette burns, beatings, rape, sensory deprivation, and mock execution, and was forced to watch others being tortured in horrific ways. Upon release from internment, the torture victim sought treatment to help him with the post-traumatic aftermath of the torture and internment experience.

The treating therapist, a resident of the same country as the client, confronted a moral dilemma at the beginning of treatment. By offering professional help as a mental health expert the therapist ran the risk of being identified as an antigovernment sympathizer by offering assistance to someone who was tortured for being "subversive." Thus, a therapist prone to Type I countertransference tendencies may react to the torture survivor with fear of contagion, personal guilt as to whether or not to offer treatment, or bystander guilt as a noninvolved party. Additionally, the therapist may experience horror and dread at the description of the torture experience, and he or she may manifest phobic defenses, which results in a failure to fully explore the trauma story. In response, the therapist may overrely on medications as the primary method of treatment or refer the client elsewhere.

In contrast, a therapist prone to Type II countertransference tendencies may react to the torture survivor by being overwhelmed and shocked by the details of the torture experience to the point of feeling angry, horrified, and numb. The therapist's ARs to the torture accounts may then lead to a need to rescue the client based on overidentification with the ordeal that the survivor endured at the hands of his oppressors. As a result, the therapist may overidealize the client as a courageous survivor and develop a need to advocate on behalf of torture victims. In the course of treatment, the empathic strain experienced may then weaken role boundaries and result in a failure to fully understand how the torture experience affected the pre-trauma personality structure of the client or the special way the client has construed the torture experience in his life. Certain trauma experiences are more likely to evoke particular countertransference configurations, as the repetition strikes selected aspects of the treatment frame. So, for example, incest survivors evoke blurred boundaries, political prisoners evoke extra therapeutic rescue efforts, and Holocaust survivors convince therapists that separations are inevitable.

It is important to underscore the fact that either a Type I or Type II CTR may cause a rupture in the empathic stance toward the client and the capacity to adequately contain trauma-specific and associated forms of transference. When empathic strain results in a loss of therapeutic role and boundaries, there is a risk that the stress recovery process will be retarded, delayed, halted, or in some other way injured (see Chapter 1, this volume, for illustration). As Tables 2.1 and 2.2 illustrate, the five primary factors that comprise CTRs also have many variations as common reaction patterns. Given the indigenous nature of Type I and Type iI reaction in work with PTSD, it is important to recognize and identify the possible configurations of the different ways these five primary factors (affect, defense, coping mode, role boundary, and theoretical rationale) can combine within a modal countertransference style.

Maintenance of an Empathic Stance

PTSD therapists who work through their own CTRs can sustain empathic inquiry, engage in effective PTT throughout the phases of the stress recovery process, and, through the dual unfolding process (Maroda, 1990), help clients eventually integrate traumatic events into the self-structure in ego-syntonic ways. The disturbing events are reappraised, given meaning, and are now seen as part of the client's life story and progression of epigenetic development.

As Figure 2.1 illustrates, efficacy in the therapeutic role implies maintenance of an empathic stance toward the client and does not result in a rupture in empathy, despite the expectable "trials and tribulations." There are, of course, many factors that affect whether or not a therapist is able to maintain the necessary empathic stance in PTT. These include adequate education and training in PTSD, the number of years of experience in treating traumatized clients, proper supervision, collegial peer support, and particular personality traits, such as resilience, flexibility, and sensitivity. Clearly, efficacy in the process of PTT is the most important feature in creating a safe–holding environment in which a client can establish a therapeutic alliance. It is our belief that when the client with PTSD feels safe and begins to trust the therapist at deeper levels, healing can begin and the victim/survivor can experience idiosyncratic vulnerability (without excessive defensiveness), which permits integration of the traumatic experience. Although Figures 2.2 and 2.3 summarize two primary forms of CTRs, it is important to recognize that they are not mutually exclusive. Indeed, it is quite possible for a therapist to manifest both Type I and Type

II CTRs in the course of treatment, and for one type of reaction (e.g., guilt, anger) to precipitate a compensatory reaction of the other type, such as overidentification or detachment. As noted in Chapter 1, the personality of the therapist determines whether the helper is more disposed toward the Type I or Type II reactions. Nevertheless, both types of CTRs can adversely affect the process of treatment.

Type II CTRs, paradoxically, can facilitate transference reactions during the early stages of treatment, especially if the client has had previous treatment that was unsuccessful (Horowitz, 1986). The therapist's excessive empathy and overidentification may make the client feel that the therapist is highly attuned to existing PTSD symptoms and behaviors, and the client may therefore feel a false sense of security about the recovery process. Horowitz (1986) has noted that overidealization of the therapist in the early phases of treatment may facilitate a therapeutic alliance. However, a false sense of security can be experienced by the therapist and can potentially lead to treatment failure because other forms of Type II reactions can blur the boundary role distinctions, which are critical for maintaining a focus on the issues that motivated treatment in the first place. When this blurring occurs through pathological bonding and enmeshment, overidentification, overcommitment, overidealization, or feeling excessively responsible for the patient's recovery, the therapist leaves the empathic stance, thereby intensifying such transference reactions as fear of abandonment or fear of betrayal (McCann & Pearlman, 1990).

DEVELOPMENT OF A CRITICAL THERAPEUTIC STRUCTURE TO CONTAIN TRAUMA-SPECIFIC AND ASSOCIATED FORMS OF TRANSFERENCE

Table 2.3 presents an illustration of the relationship of empathic strain experienced in the treatment of trauma victims to the development of Type I and Type II forms of countertransference.

In our view, the identification and open acknowledgment of normative (objective) and personal (subjective) countertransference processes is an integral part of ability of the therapist to effectively manage such reactions in the service of creating a *critical therapeutic structure*. This structure contains the client's traumatic experiences by changing the holding configuration of the therapist's internal structure, and it constitutes a special relationship with a trusted ally who provides the pathway to the healing and transformation of trauma (Wilson, 1989). Moreover, central to the creation of a critical therapeutic structure, one which can effectively contain trauma-specific and associated transferences, is the idea of *empathic stretch*. Specifically, this concept implies that survivors' trauma-

TABLE 2.3. Development of Critical Therapeutic Structure to Contain Trauma-Specific Transference

Function	Dynamic process: Empathic strain in treatment process
Therapist affect during treatment	Modes of empathic strain: Disequilibrium, withdrawal, repression, and enmeshment. Modes reflect interactional communication.
Reaction/defense	Type I (avoidance) and Type II (overidentification) CTRs: Affect, defense, coping mode, role boundary, theoretical rationale. Indigenous reactive processes.
Containment	Identification, acknowledgment, and management of affect and countertransference in treatment versus role boundary problems. Attempt to maintain empathy.
Critical therapeutic structure and sanctuary of trusted alliance	Evolution of critical therapeutic structure: Sanctuary to contain trauma-related memory, imagery, and affect versus empathic break. Dual unfolding process in reception, processing, and communication of interaction sequence.

specific transferences produce an interactional communication that is associated with empathic strain. To regain sustained empathic inquiry therapists are forced to stretch their capacity for empathy, in order to maintain sensitive attunement to the needs of the client. A critical therapeutic structure thus evolves when the therapist succeeds in sustaining empathic inquiry to the trauma-specific transference dynamics of the client.

Empathic stretch in a therapist is part of a growth process occurring through the shared task of assisting the trauma survivor to reformulate the meaning of their particular traumatic experience. As such, the capacity for empathic stretch is closely allied to empathic strain because the trauma-specific transference processes constantly tax the therapist's capacity for empathic attunement. A similar conclusion has been reached by Tansey and Burke (1989) who state:

> The therapist's capacity to entertain various trial identifications is correlated with his tolerance for what may be difficult self-experiences. This capacity is critical in the achievement of an empathic outcome. A corollary of this important relationship is that the therapist's degree of conscious awareness of his internal state at any point in the processing sequence depends largely on his capacity to tolerate the image of self that is aroused by the interactional communication from the patient.
>
> Optimally, the therapist is a willing recipient of the introjective identifications that are induced by the patient's interactional pressure. However, therapists differ in their willingness to tolerate potentially

uncomfortable self-states, depending on the particular dynamic involved and the intensity with which it is transmitted. (pp. 67–68)

As noted in Chapter 1, countertransference processes have the potential to cause an empathic break or rupture in the therapeutic structure at any point in the phases of stress recovery and integration of the traumatic experience into the self-structure and life history of the client. Thus, to continuously maintain an effective therapeutic structure, the sources of empathic strain in the therapists should be acknowledged, identified, and managed, so as to prevent the possibility of damaging the sanctity and material of the structure, thereby impeding the client's opportunity for recovery. Similarly, developing the capacity for sustained empathic inquiry through insight into empathic strain lays the foundation for empathic stretch which, deepens the therapist's ability to understand the complexity of the trauma survivor's inner distress, pain, and psychic scarring associated with unpleasant memories and difficulties in affect regulation. The mutuality of the therapeutic process in the treatment of trauma survivors is such that both therapist and client experience ego-states of vulnerability and uncertainty. For the trauma survivor the state of vulnerability is typically a part of PTSD or is a residue from previous trauma that is reexperienced from time to time in daily life. For the practitioner, the state of vulnerability is part of the empathic strain intrinsic to the responsibility of being a psychotherapist. Thus, the successful creation of a critical therapeutic structure to contain the powerful affects of the trauma survivor is the precondition to an alliance of mutual trust in a process devoted to the transformation of extremely stressful life experiences into a new configuration within the self-structure of the survivor. During this therapeutic process, empathic stretch causes a transformation in the therapist, which can range from vicarious traumatization (McCann & Pearlman, 1990) to a more generative orientation (Erikson, 1968) toward the meaning of life and the existential nature of personal relationships.

TRANSFERENCE PROJECTIONS AND THEIR IMPACT ON COUNTERTRANSFERENCE PROCESSES

The delineation of the underlying dimensions to Type I and Type II CTRs (affect, defense, coping mode, role boundary, theoretical rationale) now allows us to further understand *transference projections* in the therapeutic process. Figure 2.4 illustrates the relationship between transference projections and the development of specific role enactments by the therapist as a form of countertransference (e.g., rescuer, judge, failed protector). It is important to understand this relationship to countertransference be-

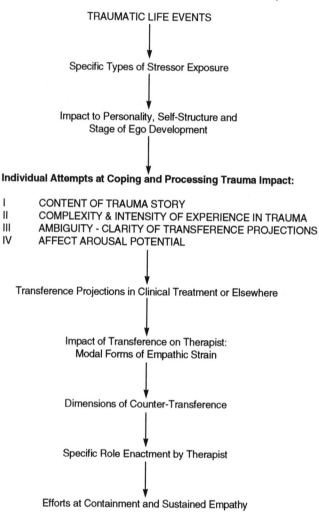

TRAUMATIC LIFE EVENTS

Specific Types of Stressor Exposure

Impact to Personality, Self-Structure and
Stage of Ego Development

Individual Attempts at Coping and Processing Trauma Impact:

I   CONTENT OF TRAUMA STORY
II   COMPLEXITY & INTENSITY OF EXPERIENCE IN TRAUMA
III   AMBIGUITY - CLARITY OF TRANSFERENCE PROJECTIONS
IV   AFFECT AROUSAL POTENTIAL

Transference Projections in Clinical Treatment or Elsewhere

Impact of Transference on Therapist:
Modal Forms of Empathic Strain

Dimensions of Counter-Transference

Specific Role Enactment by Therapist

Efforts at Containment and Sustained Empathy

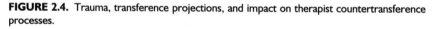

FIGURE 2.4. Trauma, transference projections, and impact on therapist countertransference processes.

cause it has direct implications for the clinician's ability to sustain empathic inquiry.

The contents of Figure 2.4 indicate a dynamic process between the trauma client and the therapist. Traumatic life events impact on the personality, self-structure, and stage-of-life ego development (Wilson, 1980). In response to a particular traumatic event, victims manifest their particular forms of coping and processing of the stressful life event, which have at least four central features: (1) the content of the trauma story, (2) the complexity and intensity of their experience in the trauma, (3) the degree to which there is ambiguity or clarity in transference projections during treatment, and (4) the *affect arousal potential* of the trauma-specific transference. In our view, these four components of traumatization as *ego-stages* in the client determine the specific forms of transference projections at various stages in the stress recovery process. The resulting transference projections, which include trauma-specific transferences thus have the potential to lead to the four modal forms of empathic strain and different manifestations of Type I and Type II CTRs. As such, the therapist then may assume specific role enactments within the Type I or Type II CTRs. The awareness of such role enactments within a Type I or Type II reaction then enables the clinician to attempt to contain both the client's transference projections and his or her own CTRs in an attempt to sustain empathic inquiry. Figure 2.5 summarizes this process and adds two additional factors that provide a more holistic view.

Figure 2.5 adds to the information contained in Figure 2.4 by indicating that a fuller understanding of the determinants of countertransference begins by classifying the ten major categories of traumatic events (i.e., typology of traumatic events), especially those most likely to be associated with the onset of PTSD and comorbid conditions. In Figure 2.5 we have indicated that the types of traumatic events and the specific stressors experienced interact, in a dynamic sense, to determine the elements that will form the nucleus of transference projections. As noted above, the specific types of transference projections have the potential to elicit Type I and Type II CTRs. Finally, the figure ends with a listing of common themes in countertransference role enactments that, if successfully managed, can lead to therapeutic effectiveness and the development of a critical therapeutic structure, which enables the client to work toward resolution and integration of the traumatic experience within their self-structure and life course.

CONCLUSION

It is our view that recognition and management of Type I and Type II CTRs is essential for the successful treatment of PTSD. It is possible to view CTRs as intrinsic to the process of therapy and associated with a psychobiologically based capacity for empathy. Furthermore, although CTRs are not avoidable, they can be successfully managed in order to maintain an effective therapeutic stance of empathy. To the extent that well-defined role boundaries are established, a critical therapeutic structure is established as a safe–holding environment in which the traumatized person can heal. The integration and transformation of trauma into a new

TRAUMA EXPERIENCE

A. Typology of Traumatic Events $\overrightarrow{(A \times B)}$

I. Childhood abuse/family violence
II. Wartrauma/civil violence
III. Natural disaster
IV. Technological/toxic disaster
V. Political oppression, torture, internment
VI. Duty related (military, EMS, police, fire)
VII. Mass genocide/Holocaust
VIII. Physical health/terminal illness
IX. Work/industrial trauma
X. Anomalous trauma

B. Traumatic Stressors: Direct or Indirect/Experience and Impact

I. Harm or injury to self, personality and belief system
II. Harm or injury to others
III. Harm or injury to personal relationships, attachments and social networks
IV. Harm or injury to Earth, biosphere, and physical structure
V. Harm or injury to physical integrity, bodily function or physical health

INDIVIDUAL ADAPTATION AND PROCESSING OF TRAUMA

Psychological Structure and Dimension of Post-Traumatic Adaptation Influencing Transference/Counter-Transference Dynamics →

I. Content Imagery of Trauma Story
II. Complexity/Intensity of experience in Trauma (stressor level exposure)
III. Ambiguity - Clarity of Transference Projections
IV. Trauma Specific Transference Themes
V. Affect Arousal Potential

POST-TRAUMATIC THERAPY: COUNTER-TRANSFERENCE PROCESS

Modal Forms of Empathic Strain →

A. AVOIDANCE
Type I - Withdrawal
Type I - Repression

B. OVER-IDENTIFICATION
Type II - Enmeshment
Type II - Disequilibrium

C. EMPATHIC CONTAINMENT
Empathic stretch and growth leading to critical therapeutic structure

Psychological Dimensions of Counter-Transference Reactions →

I. Affect
II. Defense
III. Coping
IV. Impaired Boundary
V. Theoretical Rationale

Common Counter-Transference Role Enactments of Therapist

Failed Protector
Collaborator
Rescuer
Comforter
Judge
Conspirator
Perpetrator
Fellow Survivor
Victim
Authority Figure
Others

FIGURE 2.5. The relation of traumatic events to individual forms of post-traumatic adaptation influencing transference and CTRs in treatment.

configuration within the self is the central task of treatment. To the extent that the critical therapeutic structure allows the therapist to maintain a genuine empathic stance unduly complicated by either Type I or Type II CTRs, the patient will be able to tolerate such inner states as vulnerability, narcissistic injury, degradation, defilement, humiliation, affective flooding, distressing intrusive imagery of the trauma, and so forth, without the overuse of defenses. When this occurs, the phases of recovery from trauma proceed naturally in the direction of integration and completion (Horowitz, 1986). On the other hand, CTRs have the potential to disrupt the stress recovery process and intensify transference dynamics. It is for this reason that we have referred to PTT as an interpersonal event, which contains many subtleties in the trauma-specific transference–countertransference dynamics that may affect the nature of the balance in the relationship. Managing CTRs is vitally important in maintaining a nurturing therapeutic structure: one that is experienced by the client as safe, firm, supportive, clear, trustworthy, and helpful. A similar conclusion was reached by Giovacchini (1989), in regard to analytic forms of therapy:

> The degree to which the analyst allows himself to internalize the patient, and it may be minimal, represents a countertransference element that is an intrinsic part of the therapeutic interaction. Inasmuch as an effective interpretation requires the patient to fuse with the therapist, all interpretations occur within a transference–countertransference context. This formulation is in accord with the recent emphasis that has been placed on empathy. But there is nothing mysterious and esoteric about empathy; it is simply another way of describing subtle and sometimes complex transference–countertransference interactions.
>
> I have given countertransference reactions a central position in the therapeutic interaction and have viewed them as an integral part of any technical maneuver. They cause technical problems and they become a means of resolving them. Whether good or bad, countertransference reactions are ubiquitous. (pp. 334–335)

As the knowledge of PTSD continues to grow at an exponential rate (Wilson & Raphael, 1993), the understanding of CTRs in the treatment process will assume an increasingly important role. One of the central implications is that the PTSD training of mental health professionals must include information regarding CTRs and their management in the clinical setting.

Beyond Countertransference: Empathic Growth

It is our belief that CTRs are not only intrinsic processes in PTT, but an expression of a very human tendency to experience empathy and feel the distress of the trauma survivor. The interpersonal process in treatment is that of two individuals working together to understand how a traumatic event altered the vitality and sense of well-being of the survivor. In the process, the therapist empathically shares the distress and pain that pervades the treatment. The effective containment of empathic distress and the successful management of CTRs are essential to the development of a therapeutic structure in which a survivor transforms and resolves the painful legacy of an experience that altered the individual's sense of coherency and well-being. As part of this process, the therapist may experience forms of empathic stretch as part of their effort to understand the inner world of the trauma victim by removing an empathic block to progress. One therapist in supervision observed that her client interpreted a dimension of honor to being raped as a child and commented, "I don't know if I stretch that far." Through the development of deeper insight and with adequate supervision, empathic growth can occur, which strengthens the therapist's capacity to continuously recognize empathic strain and CTRs, thereby transforming such processes into creative modalities of psychotherapy.

REFERENCES

Brandell, J. R. (1992). *Countertransference in psychotherapy with children and adolescents.* Northvale, NJ: Jason Aronson.
Danieli, Y. (1984). Psychotherapists' participation in the conspiracy of silence about the Holocaust. *Psychoanalytic Psychology, 1*(1), 23–42.
Danieli, Y. (1988). Confronting the unimaginable: Psychotherapists' reactions to victims of the Nazi Holocaust. In J. P. Wilson, Z. Harel, & B. Kahana (Eds.), *Human adaptation to extreme stress* (pp. 219–237). New York: Plenum Press.
Erikson, E. H. (1968). *Identity, youth, and crisis.* New York: W. W. Norton.
Friedman, M. (1993). Psychobiology and pharmacological approaches to treatment. In J. P. Wilson & B. Raphael (Eds.), *The international handbook of traumatic stress syndromes* (pp. 785–795). New York: Plenum Press.
Gear, M. C., Liendo, E. C., & Scott, L. L. (1983). *Patients' and agents' transference and counter-transference in therapy.* New York: Jason Aronson.
Giovacchini, P. L. (1989). *Countertransference: Triumphs and catastrophes.* New York: Jason Aronson.
Haley, S. (1974). When the patient reports atrocities. *Archives of General Psychiatry, 39,* 191–196.
Horowitz, M. (1986). *Stress response syndrome.* New York: Jason Aronson.
Maroda, K. (1990). *The power of countertransference.* New York: Wiley.
McCann, I. L., & Pearlman, L. (1990). *Psychological trauma and the adult survivor.* New York: Brunner/Mazel.
Mollica, B. (1988). The trauma story: The psychiatric care of refugee survivors of

violence and torture. In F. Ochberg (Ed.), *Post-traumatic therapy and victims of violence* (pp. 295–314). New York: Brunner/Mazel.

Natterson, J. (1991). *Beyond countertransference.* New York: Jason Aronson.

Ochberg, F. (Ed.). (1988). *Post-traumatic therapy and victims of violence.* New York: Brunner/Mazel.

Ochberg, F. (1993). Post traumatic therapy. In J. P. Wilson & B. Raphael (Eds.), *The international handbook of traumatic stress syndromes* (pp. 773–785). New York: Plenum Press.

Parson, E. (1988). Theoretical and practical considerations in psychotherapy of Vietnam war veterans. In J. P. Wilson, Z. Harel, & B. Kahana (Eds.), *Human adaptation to extreme stress* (pp. 245–261). New York: Plenum Press.

Roth, W. (1988). The role of medication in post traumatic therapy. In F. Ochberg (Ed.), *Post-traumatic therapy and victims of violence* (pp. 39–57). New York: Brunner/Mazel.

Slatker, E. (1987). *Countertransference.* New York: Jason Aronson.

Tansey, M. J., & Burke, W. F. (1989). *Understanding countertransference.* Hillsdale, NJ: Analytic Press.

Wilson, J. P. (1988). Understanding the Vietnam veteran. In F. Ochberg (Ed.), *Post-traumatic therapy and victims of violence* (pp. 227–254). New York: Brunner/Mazel.

Wilson, J. P. (1989). *Trauma, transformation, and healing: An integrative approach to theory, research, and post-traumatic therapy.* New York: Brunner/Mazel.

Wilson, J. P., & Raphael, B. (Eds.). (1993). *The international handbook of traumatic stress syndromes.* New York: Plenum Press.

3

Empathic Strain and Countertransference Roles: Case Illustrations

JACOB D. LINDY
JOHN P. WILSON

CLINICAL THEORY AND PSYCHOANALYTIC PERSPECTIVES

In this chapter we examine and illustrate a range of countertransference roles and reactions and their management at different points in the treatment process as outlined in Chapter 1. We shall use these illustrations to demonstrate the multiple layers through which countertransferences appear and the complex trauma-specific roles evoked in the treatment. Finally, we shall illustrate the possible use of countertransference in the working through of trauma. Throughout this discussion, and central to it, is the principle that unremembered components of the trauma story are vividly reenacted in the treatment situation. In psychoanalytic theory, the irrational, persistent psychopathology is seen as an unconscious repetition of psychological tensions (conflicts, deficits, traumas) unresolved from earlier times or life-events. The repetition compulsion infuses current-day perceptions, relationships, and self-esteem. As a consequence, the repetitions dictate fixed configurations of affects, defenses, and object relations that do not adapt well to changing current circumstances. These repetitions then become organizers of the ongoing psychic life of affected individuals.

Trauma is one such unresolved earlier tension. And nowhere is the repetition compulsion more clearly demonstrated than in post-traumatic stress disorder (PTSD), where trauma and attempted efforts to cope with it are the essence of the repetition. Gradually, as a treatment alliance is formed, repetitions of the trauma or reenactments take place in vivid form between therapist and survivor. To paraphrase the theologian Martin Buber, these are the "I–thou" components of traumatic therapy. Psychoanalytic psychotherapy seeks to address these repetitions as they play out within the therapist–patient interaction and the transference–countertransference matrix of the treatment itself.

Other clinical constructs must be addressed in the therapeutic situation in order for the transference and countertransference to be available for clinical work. These include establishing a therapeutic split in the ego (Sterba, 1934) and a working alliance (Greenson, 1967); managing and interpreting efforts to shift the therapeutic frame (Langs, 1982); maintaining a neutral, empathic, nonjudgmental therapeutic stance (Strachey, 1934); and respecting the valuable role of interpreting/understanding rather than resorting to action in the therapeutic interplay (Gill, 1983).

Within the clinical construct of transference–countertransference, a variety of differing meta-psychological psychoanalytic theories may be brought to bear, given the specifics of the case and formulations of the therapist. Unremembered components of the trauma reexperienced in the treatment situation may have been (1) *disavowed* by the survivor and retrieved by introspection, intuition, and empathy on the part of the therapist (Kohut, 1959) (see Case Example Two, below); (2) *dissociated* or split off by the survivor but recovered by the therapist's awareness of projective identification and introjective identification (Kernberg, 1965) (see Case Example Four, below); or (3) *denied* or suppressed subsequent to the trauma, then retrieved by the therapist's recognition of displaced superego identifications (Freud, 1914) (see Case Example Six, below). We include all of these phenomena in our comprehensive definition of trauma-specific countertransference.

The terms *transference* and *countertransference* are clinical working assumptions. While these concepts have a theoretical basis within psychoanalytic theory, they are more widely relevant in that, as working clinical assumptions, they in fact help to organize material into useful, manageable form, which can inform us with regard to the management and care of our patients. As noted in Chapter 1, transference is broadly defined as a ubiquitous, unconscious phenomenon in which patients tend to repeat significant psychological experiences of the past with current-day figures. Transference in its more specific form refers to the narrowing of this general phenomenon into the area of greatest conflict and the expression of it within the psychotherapeutic situation or onto the person of the therapist. Similarly, countertransference refers to psychodynamic phenomena in therapists rather than patients. In its general sense, a countertransference is any emotional response on the part of the therapist consciously or unconsciously derived and arising out of the dual unfolding aspects of treatment between client and therapist. Viewing countertransference

> requires the therapist to direct what Freud (1912) called his evenly suspended attention not only to the patient but also to the full range of his own thoughts and feelings, even if such thoughts and feelings at first blush seem irrelevant, inappropriate or unacceptable. . . . The therapist is encouraged to treat all thoughts and feelings as potentially important sources of information about the interaction with the patient . . . the therapist . . . strives to appreciate the ways in which he is being acted upon by the patient. (Tansey, & Burke, 1989, p. 41)

Countertransference in a more specific sense derives from pathognomonic transference and its complementary emotional response. Here the therapist seems unwittingly drawn, by the circumstance of the transference–countertransference fit, into specific roles such as victim, perpetrator, or judge, with associated affects. Countertransference tendencies and thoughts become distinguished as countertransference responses, symptoms, and behavior when they divert the therapist from an empathic, role-specific task and keep the therapist from listening, empathizing, and interpreting.

Within the trauma role paradigm outlined here, the therapist's inner positions may be (1) *concordant* or in consonance with a given survivor's role, such as outraged but helpless victim; (2) *complementary* to the survivor position, such as condemning judge as "complement" to guilty survivor; or (3) *dysjunctive* with the survivor position because the therapist's inner position derives from unique personal trauma circumstances, such as counterphobic comforting and rescuing response that fails to appreciate the survivor's position of avenging rage at the perpetrator. Figure 3.1 depicts a schema for common trauma roles in which therapists unwittingly find themselves despite efforts to remain relatively empathic, neutral, and nonjudgmental when treating trauma victims/survivors. The therapist may be cast in potentially positive roles within the trauma membrane, such as protector, rescuer, comforter, or fellow victim, or in negative roles outside the trauma membrane, such as perpetrator or fellow victim turned enemy (e.g., Nazi prison guard/*Kapo*). The therapist may be feared as a judge, or aspects of the therapist's attitudes or working conditions may be seen as noxious extensions of the same social, environmental, and/or governmental policies that permitted or encouraged the trauma. Paradoxically, in the unconscious effort to turn passive into active, a therapist may find himself or herself attacked by a patient such that

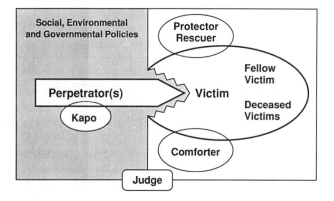

FIGURE 3.1. Trauma-specific countertransference roles.

the patient has assumed the perpetrator role and the therapist is now victim. Determining which role is active within a given countertransference tendency plays an important part in permitting the treatment to resume its atmosphere of empathic enquiry rather than aborting in a repetition of the trauma.

FORMS OF COUNTERTRANSFERENCE DURING TREATMENT AND RECOVERY

Building on the conceptual model developed in Chapter 1 (see Figure 1.2), we now wish to illustrate the countertranferences that are likely to rupture empathy in the different phases of a trauma therapy: (1) therapist's bias, which inhibits trauma engagement; (2) therapist's defenses, which collude against engaging traumatic material; (3) therapist's vicarious traumatization, which incapacitates the therapist once the trauma imagery is engaged; (4) therapist's experiencing split-off parts of the client's trauma experience as it is being reenacted; and (5) therapist's experiencing of different trauma roles as aspects of the client's working through of multiple facets of the trauma experience (Racker, 1968).

Examining countertransference response in the psychotherapy of survivors of catastrophe has a few more steps than in the psychotherapy of neurotic and character disorders (see "rupture in empathy," Figure 1.2, this volume) First, massive events, such as the Holocaust or the Vietnam War, are historical occurrences. They in some way define not only the patient/survivor but also define the identity of the therapist as participant in or witness to these historical forces. The same is true of regional tragedies, such as the dam collapse at Buffalo Creek, West Virginia, in the

United States, or the King's Cross fire in England, and of epidemics of individual catastrophic events, such as rape and incest. In the course of the work, each therapist is absorbing and working through his or her own affective response to events of the times, attributing personal meaning to community trauma as a necessary part of his or her evolving identity. Yet this is a separate, intrapsychic task from that of the survivor/patient. Because the therapist's preoccupation with this internal work (or its avoidance by defense and stereotype) may interfere with empathic listening to the patient's processing of his or her own unique, intrapsychic world in relationship to those trauma events, we include these reactions as potential countertransference responses. As the first case reveals, however, sometimes the trauma is not engaged because the survivor judges that the therapist is unable to go beyond his or her own limited or defensive misconceptions.

Case Example One: Latrine Duty at Auschwitz

Mr. K., feeling encouraged by his beginning analysis, lapsed into a vivid memory of learning that he and his brother had been assigned to clean the latrines at Auschwitz. Dr. N. unable to hear the positive tone of this memory. Her reaction was limited to the images and smells of feces, which stirred in her reactions of disgust. Dr. N. commented, "Analysis will be a difficult 'assignment' in which truly untouchable things from childhood will need to come to light." But Mr. K. was referring to the life-saving nature of the latrine assignment there. He and his brother would remain clear of the ovens. SS guards, now wishing to avoid the offensive smell on him and his brother, would choose to avoid rather than randomly beat them. The assignment had been good news within the trauma context.

Dr. N.'s failure to hear his memories accurately, in this and similar encounters, led Mr. K. to reason that his analyst could not bear to understand his memories and metaphors from Auschwitz. "Although she is trying to help me," he concluded, "she would rather we talked of childhood memories than Holocaust memories. I can sense how uneasy that trauma is for her; I will protect her by keeping the trauma inside."

Once therapist and survivor have agreed to include trauma experience as central to their joint venture, the task of bearing witness to unthinkable happenings begins. The survivor tries haltingly and in rushed fragments, to tell the remembered trauma story. Yet the striking, evocative images that emerge set off powerful reactions in the therapist. The simple listening and processing of the *stories* of traumatic happenings and their images often stirs powerful countertransference responses.

Case Example Two: Dismembered Torso

As Frank, a combat veteran from Vietnam, was telling his story of coming upon the bodies of American soldiers in the Vietnam War who had been overrun and slaughtered, he described, in a distant voice, the surreal image of a dismembered torso propped against a tree. This image stirred powerful feelings in Dr. B. He experienced nausea followed by rapid breathing. Later that night, he noted agitation and "pressure to talk." Once home, he looked to alcohol for relief, yet was continually aware of the intrusive image of the torso. Finally, that night he experienced a nightmare of his own traumatic experience as a child: his own apparently cutoff torso that he saw upon waking from anesthesia after the open heart surgery that had frightened him so terribly. Thus, Dr. B. became aware that his own *annihilation anxiety* had been set off by the patient's story.

Yet, this understanding of his response was incomplete, and it was followed by a period of feeling disturbed, preoccupied, and distant from the patient. Dr. B. was only vaguely aware of his mechanical effort to prod both himself and the patient to continue on track. "You have to go back to the hill," he said to the patient. These words were meant for himself as well. For the patient, however, these were the wrong words. Even though Dr. B. was in a position to empathize with Frank's annihilation anxiety and disillusionment, he had to pay the price for the mechanical intervention he had made while trying to keep the treatment on track. For Dr. B. unwittingly repeated the words of the inexperienced lieutenant who, defending against *his* anxiety, commanded the patient, then an experienced infantry sergeant, to take a hill that was untakable. The result, in war, had been disaster. Trying to follow his therapist's instructions, Frank dissociated (as he emotionally went "back to the hill") and his inability to pull out of his clinical regression required hospitalization. The sequence here was from trauma image (dismembered torso) to countertransference defense (withdrawal/dissociation) to intervention (mechanical leadership), which ironically reproduced the original trauma, including disillusionment with the leader.

As difficult as it sometimes is to truly hear the remembered trauma story and to manifest empathy with the patient's experience of its central features, it is often only the beginning of the work for many trauma survivors. Much still remains unremembered, split off, dissociated, disavowed, or denied. Sometimes recall may be facilitated by the therapist's experience and understanding of the transference–countertransference reenactment within the treatment situation. In the next illustration, a supervisor assists the therapist whose defenses were identical with and thereby colluded with those of the survivor, in order to keep the trauma from being explored.

Case Example Three: Clenched Hands

Dr. V. found Mr. R. to be a difficult and uninvolved patient. Dr. V. reported becoming sleepy in sessions and acknowledged to the supervisor that the treatment did not seem to be getting anywhere. The supervisor correctly heard in the history that this rescue worker's trauma story involved the horrendous act of sawing apart the clenched hands of a man and woman who died from toxic fumes at a supper club fire while celebrating their 50th wedding anniversary. Both Mr. R. and Dr. V. had colluded to keep trauma material out of the therapy. In this case, the defenses have split off the trauma affect. The therapist, in the countertransference, identified with the patient's defense (isolation) and joined in the collusion (Type I, repression). The horrific memory was dissociated both by the survivor and the doctor in a concordant identification. It was as though Dr. V., too, pretended that the trauma story, although told, did not exist. The power of the countertransference alludes to the power of the disassociation that occurred at the time and the isolation that preserved its sequestered position.

Case Example Four: Forgetting the Children

In the following vignette a trauma story is relayed only partially in words. The most telling element is conveyed through action. The therapist, a recipient of projective identification, feels the split-off affect that the survivor denies.

Mrs. J., a well-organized and efficient mother of four, experienced the sudden accidental death of her youngest child 1 year prior to the beginning of treatment. In therapy, Mrs. J. was characteristically efficient, having taken care of administrative matters relating to the treatment and being prompt for each of her sessions. It was therefore unusual when, following the end of the fourth session, Mrs. J.'s son knocked on the therapist's door, asking where his mother was. The therapist became alarmed that the mother had walked out of the clinic while leaving her children in the waiting room. In the 20 minutes or so that it took to trace Mrs. J. down, the therapist found herself infuriated. Overtly, she was angry that her schedule had been interrupted and that she had misjudged this woman whom she had thought to be so reliable. But the therapist's supervisor was also able to point out that Mrs. J.'s forgetting of her children within the treatment context could also be seen as a trauma reenactment. At the time of her son's death, she had diverted her attention to other matters. The unbearable part of her loss was that at the time of the accident she had neglected her son. The therapist's countertransference response of extreme anger at the patient was understood within the trauma-specific transference–countertransference matrix, namely, that the therapist's anger could be seen as a complementary countertransference. She was functioning as the split-off superego of the patient, who could herself not tolerate the full intensity of blaming herself for her child's death. Although Mrs. J. had given an apparently thorough description of the traumatic events, she had unconsciously avoided any mention of her inattention or guilt.

At times, countertransference may provide more than clues to disavowed traumas that are being reenacted in the treatment: it may provide the *only* vehicle by which the patient can translate a horrendous story from action to narrated form.

Case Example Five: It's Your Turn

Spike was being seen in connection with his Vietnam War-related PTSD and his current violent fantasies of destruction toward Asians. A pattern had evolved at the beginning of the sessions, in which Spike tensely leaned forward in his chair and, making eye contact, would insist to Dr. R. that "it's your turn." The therapist had for a number of sessions been trying to understand the patient's reluctance to begin the session. He would try to empathize with the discomfort that beginning might arouse, but continued to insist that it was the patient's role to begin each hour. On this occasion, the therapist also became aware of the enormous tension that was present in the room during the silence that followed "it's your turn." Focusing on the almost explosive silence in the room, he found himself thinking: "Something terrible happened when it was somebody's turn." Using his own countertransference associations, Dr. R. turned this observation back as a question/statement: "When you were in Vietnam, something terrible happened when it was someone else's turn." Spike responded, "Yes, his face disappeared." Going on, he clarified: "He was hit in the back of the head by a sniper. All the features of his face disappeared in the bloody explosion." In the trauma, Spike and his buddy had been jostling each other in "horseplay"; it was first one, then the other's "turn." In fact, seated in the back of the $2\frac{1}{2}$-ton truck, neither was performing the assigned role of keeping an eye out for snipers, and as result, Spike's buddy was killed.

Some weeks later, the grief work around this friend's traumatic death seemed less central, yet tension remained high between doctor and patient. Dr. R. gradually entertained another set of associations.

Here the line of thinking was slightly different. As he identified with the man whose face was destroyed in the trauma he was aware that a struggle was still occurring between Spike and himself as to how the sessions should start. Spike's enactment could be interpreted as: "If you continue to conduct this treatment in a way that I find dangerous, I will blow your face off." This countertransference fantasy seemed to capture Dr. R.'s affective state during the sessions, during which he felt intimidated, as though he were being held hostage, threatened with death. Placing this countertransference within the trauma context, Dr. R. (himself a former Army officer) hypothesized the affectively plausible situation that Spike had "fragged" (hurt, maimed, or killed) American officers in Vietnam whose views and procedure enlisted men had deemed dangerous. In the present, he felt deprived of the ultimate, intense discharge of affect provided in Vietnam by killing those whom he opposed, as well as frightened and guilty lest his wishes be reenacted in civilian life. With this new formulation in mind, Spike's persistent, dangerous conflict with authorities in his contemporary world made more sense. Dr. R. later said to Spike, "I know it would be difficult or even impossible to say to me that you were asked to frag American officers in Vietnam, but I believe that that occurred." Spike appeared surprised and relieved. The treatment had turned an important corner.

Thus, countertransference responses during the course of treatment have a range of effects: they may delay or impede the telling of the trauma story; they may reproduce defenses from the time of the trauma; they may reveal complementary components of the trauma story that are too painful to remember. Finally, in certain circumstances, countertransference processes may be the only available road to otherwise unacknowledgeable truths.

DIAGNOSING COUNTERTRANSFERENCE IN PTSD

Diagnosing the developing countertransference tendency *in vivo* is often not an easy matter. Indeed, because countertransference is largely an unconscious phenomenon, it is easily rationalized as professionally justified or prosocial behavior. The supervisor, the peer study group, or even the patient may recognize its presence before the therapist does.

In this section, we shall examine some of the elements in the treatment relationship that the therapist should monitor, and that, in turn, become grounds on which to conclude that countertransference is actively at work. This is especially important in that the clinician undergoing such experiences is likely to be attributing the phenomena to other explanations.

Countertransference reactions (CTRs) may be recognized on the basis of (1) dysphoric and excessive affects that effect the core of the therapist; (2) defenses against those affects that distance the therapist (Type I CTR) or spur overinvolvement (Type II CTR); (3) empathic strain characterized by withdrawal, regression, disequilibrium, or overidentification tendencies; or (4) breakthrough of defenses with (a) symptom formation or ego-alien thoughts or feelings arising in the therapist, (b) impairment of at least one component in the therapist's usual, empathic, neutral function, and (c) loss of some aspect of professional boundary or therapeutic frame.

Figure 3.2 aligns the several layers active in a trauma-specific CTR. The chart is intended to begin at the center with a unique affective experience on the part of the vicariously traumatized therapist (McCann & Pearlman, 1990), which we think of as shame and despair (Danieli, 1981). Clusters of powerful affects such as dread, horror, or fear accompany the core reaction. These in turn are defended against by efforts to

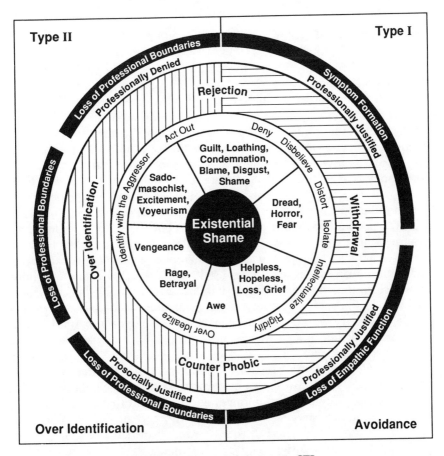

FIGURE 3.2. Layering of elements in CTR.

control the feelings, such as denial, or through unconscious efforts to discharge the feelings, such as acting out. The resultant state of empathic strain is usually withdrawal (Type I CTR) or overidentification (Type II CTR). Efforts to rationalize the empathic strain may conform to limitations of professional theory or technique, or the imperative for prosocial action. When in fact these tensions have led to a CTR, these rationalizations can no longer successfully hide therapist's loss of professional boundaries, loss of empathic function, and/or personal succumbing to trauma-related symptoms.

The following case illustrates the diagnosis of CTR on the basis of excessive dysphoric affect, impaired empathy, a skewed frame, and transient identification with the perpetrator.

Case Example Six: "I'll Make You Pay For This"

Mrs. T., a victim of prolonged and violent childhood incest by her stepfather, was in treatment with Dr. H. Mrs. T. asked Dr. H. to extend his hours to see her in the evening as no other time seemed possible. Aware that late hours might reduce the sense of safety, but not wishing to repeat the harsh treatment of childhood, Dr. H. reluctantly complied despite compromising his own private time. After several months, Mrs. T. confided that the fee she had agreed to was beyond her means. Fearing he would be seen as a sadistic stepfather if he did not comply, Dr. H. reduced the fee at some sacrifice to himself. Soon it became clear that Mrs. T. could not pay at all. She explained that she had hidden an earlier debt that she would need to pay off first. Meanwhile, her dreams and associations became filled with terrifying and overwhelming sexual images and feelings, which could be understood as allusions both to her past trauma and to impending danger in the transference situation. She gradually became aware of intense feelings toward the therapist, a powerful mixture of admiration, fear, and arousal. Dr. H. felt paralyzed. As he monitored his own associations he noted that irritability was intruding on conscious wishes to be liked. He was drawn to the vulnerable, needy side of Mrs. T., yet he was angry with her for not paying her bill. Reflecting on his own state of mind, he became aware of an erotically gratifying fantasy of wanting to spank her.

In earlier supervisory sessions it had been easier for the supervisor than for Dr. H. to observe how uninterpreted pressures were resulting in boundary shifts (time of appointment and fees), and that these shifts indicated countertransference behaviors on the part of Dr. H. With the spanking fantasy, Dr. H. agreed with his supervisor that a complex, complementary countertransference was occurring. Despite powerful efforts to stave off such thoughts and wishes, he was feeling some of the very impulses that her abusing stepfather had felt in connection with the trauma.

The grounds for identifying the above clinical vignette as countertransference include (1) excessive dysphoric affect, (2) the pressure on the therapist in managing these affects and the therapist's overresponsiveness, (3) an impaired therapeutic frame, (4) impaired therapeutic functioning (empathy and neutrality being impinged upon by sadomasochistic fantasies), and (5) recognition that the complex shifts and feelings plausibily describe a dimension of the perpetrator role within the trauma context. We shall examine each component in the diagnosis of countertransference trauma work in more detail, illustrating them with some of the case vignettes already presented in this chapter.

THE RANGE OF DYSPHORIC AFFECT IN THERAPISTS

Even if their patients have suffered quite different traumas, the therapists who work with them find that they share a similar range of dysphoric affect. Table 3.1 categorizes empirically derived excessive affect which was described in two studies, one by Danieli (1981), working with Holocaust survivors, and the second by this author (JDL) and his colleagues, working with Vietnam veterans (Lindy, Green, Grace, MacLeod, & Spitz, 1988). In Table 3.1 affects are grouped as autoplastic (experienced as subjective distress) and alloplastic (experienced as discharged behaviors). They are also subdivided into ego-syntonic (acceptable to the therapists' anticipated feelings in their roles) and ego-dystonic (incompatible with feelings about themselves as therapists in the therapeutic role).

In the case illustration above, Dr. H., at least in retrospect, was able to diagnose a specific constellation of excessive affects including those that were dystonic for him as therapist. He felt too guilty regarding fee and time pressure to set limits, and he anticipated the patient's morbid

TABLE 3.1. Excessive Affects

	Ego-syntonic		Ego-dystonic
Autoplastic	Fear	Hopelessness	Disgust
	Horror	Helplessness	Contempt
	Dread	Grieving	Loathing
	Betrayal	Shame	
	Rage	Guilt	
Alloplastic	Prosocial action		Excitement
			Voyeurism
			Sadomasochism

sexual fantasies and dreams with dread, as well as excitement and sado-masochistic thoughts. Spike's and Frank's therapists felt a different range of affects, including horror, dread, betrayal, and helplessness, as they reacted to events disclosed within their treatments, the "dismembered torso" and the "blown-off face." These were dysphoric but were ego-syntonic in terms of acceptable feelings in the therapeutic role.

Managing Affect by Withdrawal as Therapist (Type I CTR Responses)

Often the unconscious response of the therapist to the strong affects illustrated in Table 3.1 is to withdraw. For example, analysts like Dr. N. (Case Example One) and those described in the preface of this book withdrew from the power of trauma stories by intellectualizing. They prematurely interpreted affects linked to trauma with the less disturbing conflicts of childhood or, more destructively, they preferred to believe stories to be fantasies rather than reality. These verbal actions, taken in the midst of the transference–countertransference response, drove their clients away from engaging their trauma in the treatment.

In the case of the rescue worker above (Case Example Three), Dr. V. was aware only of feeling bored. This was the particular form that disengagement and numbing took in this instance. The numbing also represented a temporary amnesia or disavowal of the actual traumatic circumstance, the events of which were well known to him. In our Vietnam study (Lindy et al., 1988), it was most apparent in the interrupted cases that defenses against strong affects led to constricted therapeutic responsiveness.

Managing Affect by Overresponsiveness as Therapist (Type II CTR Responses)

Overresponsiveness may arise as a defense in the countertransference, as in Dr. H.'s overcompliance (Case Example Six) with the potentially seductive shifts in the frame, or as in another therapist's counterphobic wish to see his client more frequently, even though he was actually frightened by his client.

Symptoms

When the empathic strain is strong, countertransference symptoms may emerge in the therapist working with trauma patients. The manifestation of these symptoms varies with the personality features and past trauma history of the therapist, but it also reflects the patient's failed effort to manage both his or her own intrusive symptoms and the denial components of the PTSD dilemma, and the symptoms may parallel the actual symptomatology of the client's PTSD. For example, Dr. B. (Case Example Two), reacted to trauma of his patient (with the intrusive image of the dismembered torso) by experiencing many of the cardinal symptoms of PTSD himself. He could not concentrate as he listened to his patient and in fact psychologically distanced himself from the therapeutic setting. He felt a stormy physical sensation of nausea followed by rapid breathing, agitation, pressure to talk, a need to seek relief in alcohol, and finally a traumatic nightmare. This therapist's reaction is not unique. Frequently, at crucial moments in the treatments, other therapists describe developing one or more PTSD symptoms, such as nightmares, intrusive images, reenactments, memory lapse, irritability, and other psychological reactions.

A therapist after the first several sessions with a PTSD patient dreamt that an old locker trunk was about to be opened. Its contents were vaguely dangerous, explosive, and unending. The therapist felt he somehow had to keep the trunk closed and yet allow some of the pressure inside it to be released. The task appeared impossible, and he awoke as from an anxiety dream. This therapist interpreted the dream as his concern that the pent-up pressure and anxiety in his patient would explode in a destructive fashion. He thought that it was his job to contain the power of this explosion. The dream portrays the therapist's struggle to contain his own anxiety as he exposed himself to his patient's trauma.

Another therapist, while taking a summer vacation from his ongoing work with a traumatized Vietnam veteran, learned that his pet dog had been run over by a train. He found himself insisting that he go with the forest ranger to identify his pet. There, he confronted not only the impact of the grotesque image but also a great sense of loss. He sensed that the loss involved not only memories and experience connected with the pet but an identification with the loss of innocence and profound regret that his patient had experienced when his truck ran over a little girl in a war zone.

One doctor discovered himself walking more than 5 miles through difficult weather in order to meet his patient. Only in retrospect did he discover that his behavior was an unconscious reenactment of one of his patient's experiences during the Vietnam War.

Transient forgetfulness is common in work with trauma survivors. In supervision, therapists often cannot remember the details of the trauma material the patient reported even in the previous hour. It is common to be unable to retrieve vital information that had been reported in the previous supervisory session. Therapists often identify strongly with the sense of estrangement and alienation that the survivors feel, and at times act this out, for example, by fighting against the Department of Veterans Affairs, a governmental agency responsible for veterans' health care.

Therapists become irritable working with survivors commonly finding it difficult to contain the affect of the individual hours. This state of irritability sometimes spills over, and presents the therapists from concentrating on the material of patients who follow or proceed trauma patients. The therapist sometimes brings the irritability home, and it may lead to increases in alcohol consumption. Although they do not report startle reactions, therapists report an increased sensitivity to certain trigger stimuli; those working with Vietnam veterans found themselves with a heightened responsiveness to the sound of a helicopter, humid weather, Asian people, and/or walking single file in the woods with their children, and some had the need to sit in public places with their back to the wall in order to survey possible escape exits.

Such physical phenomena as nausea, lightheadedness, and headache often indicate more denial in the countertransference, such as Dr. D.'s migraine (Case Example Eight below).

IMPAIRED FRAME AND IMPAIRED PROFESSIONAL BOUNDARIES

We turn next to aspects of the therapeutic situation or frame that are likely to be strained when countertransference to the survivors' unresolved feelings connects with the trauma. These aspects include (1) management of separations, such as the ending of a session, and the management of missed sessions and vacations; (2) setting and maintaining limits, such as the fee and negotiations about it; (3) maintaining confidentiality; (4) the relative activity and inactivity of the therapist; (5) maintaining clear and consistent boundaries; (6) consistency as to time and place of appointment; and (7) constancy of professional bearing. Each becomes a potential focal point around which a transference–countertransference event can form.

Case Example Seven: "I Have to Be Able to Reach You"

Dr. E.'s patient was a child Holocaust victim. Because of a series of adult decisions beyond her control, she had been traumatically separated from family members. In each case, the separation turned out to be permanent and the family member killed. In the treatment, separations, especially those occasioned by the therapist's travel, became unbearable. Between appointments, the patient would call with apparently invented crises that seemed to resolve only when she heard the therapist's voice. Although initially Dr. E. was understanding, she grew weary of these ever-increasing interruptions, but she inhibited limit setting out of a fear of the patient's regression. However, Dr. E.'s anger grew more intense. When she finally set a limit, it was as if she were lashing out at the patient. Unwittingly, the therapist's frustration over boundaries activated her client's separation anxiety in their transference–countertransference matrix and reminded the client of the brutalizing Nazi. Separations in the treatment frame were the fulcrum of the reaction.

Other cases in this chapter point to different elements of the therapeutic frame. In Spike's (Case Example Five) treatment, countertransference focused on who would control the therapist's relative activity or inactivity in the sessions. In the incest illustration (Case Example Six), the transference–countertransference focused on the safety of the session and painfulness of the fee. Inconsistency of spatial configurations, for example, are particularly important in evoking transient transference–countertransference responses in work with Vietnam veterans. A rearranged chair in an office, a new landscaping in the building, a new item on a desk can become potential sources of fear of espionage, stirring strong reactions in both patient and therapist.

Impaired Therapeutic Functions

By definition, a countertransference tendency becomes a countertransference event when the thoughts and behavior of the therapist fail to attend to the therapeutic frame or when some aspect of therapeutic function is temporarily disturbed. For example, Dr. N.'s withdrawal from engaging her patient's Auschwitz memories interfered with her empathizing. Dr. E.'s harsh words revealed a loss of her nonjudgmental stance. Dr. R., finding himself paralyzed in the transference tension, failed to set limits regarding fee and time of session, as did Dr. E. regarding frequency of telephone calls.

Finally, although it is not the focus of this book, it is crucial to remember that countertransference tendencies and reactions may also reflect figures from the early childhood of both the patient and therapist. Of special interest to the trauma therapist are two types of childhood transferences that evoke complementary countertransference. The first is when the therapist represents early parent figures, comforters, and containers of strong tensions in the childhood home. The second is the therapist as childhood figure in a trauma-related context, such as problem-solver, protector, persecutor, victim, or innocent friend.

TRAUMA-SPECIFIC COUNTERTRANSFERENCE ROLES AND WORKING THROUGH TRAUMA

By now it should be clear that the transference–countertransference matrix with trauma patients is always active; discovering and identifying the countertransference tendency or even a symptom should come as no shock to the therapist. Having identified its presence, the therapist's toughest job begins. What meaning does the dysphoric affect, specific defense, or breakthrough of symptom or action have with respect to the trauma to the patient? Why is it that this particular part of the frame, such as the time boundary or spatial configuration, has acted as the fulcrum of the reaction? What dynamic sequences is the therapist playing out and how does that complement the trauma context by elucidating plausible human reactions within the trauma event (perhaps countertransference feelings allude to the response of an enemy, a perpetrator, a dying friend, or a failed protector)? The final section is a more detailed examination of how the therapist works once the countertransference has been identified, and how the countertransference replays these various roles in the trauma event.

Countertransference of Trauma-Specific Roles

During the working through of the trauma, the trauma configuration is reenacted in multiple forms within the treatment. This is sometimes seen through the countertransference, so that the therapist may at one time be forced into the victim role, as though he or she is being held prisoner, for example, or being destroyed or raped endlessly. Yet within the same treatment, the therapist, by enforcing previously agreed-upon limits, may feel to the survivor like the perpetrator. Again, within the same treatment, the therapist may be thrust into the failed protector role or the role of judge and prosecution. The following case illustrates how, in the countertransference, the therapist's unconscious involvement in different trauma roles became clarified and available for increased empathy.

Case Example Eight: The Migraine Headache

For some weeks, Jeb, a Vietnam War combat veteran who had had extensive activity in long-range reconnaissance, had been reliving separate missions in each of succeeding sessions. Dr. D. had found himself energized by the danger and excitement of these missions, as each had unfolded. But Dr. D. was shaken when Jeb took him on "his most horrendous mission." This was a My Lai-type massacre in which Jeb was in charge and the first to pull the trigger. The session ended in enormous tension, as Jeb avoided Dr. D.'s eyes. Dr. D. was at first only mildly dysphoric and irritable. Images of the massacre intruded. He was relieved when Jeb failed to show up for his next appointment. Several days later, Jeb called under the influence of alcohol, asking for medication. Dr. D.'s dysphoric mood broke into a crashing migraine headache, in which he feared he would lose consciousness and might die. With the breakthrough of this symptom, Dr. D. knew he was in the midst of a delayed counter-transference response to Jeb's reliving the massacre experience. In an almost mechanical manner, he fielded the request for mediation by phone with his policy, that he would need to see Jeb first before he could make a judgment regarding medication. Jeb seemed relieved simply to have heard Dr. D.'s voice and agreed to meet at their regular time. Although there was further cautious exploration of the "My Lai" experience in the next several weeks, the content of the session actually decreased in intensity and focused more on familiar, current-day, external issues. However, Dr. D.'s internal world was reeling with the trauma.

Dr. D.'s first task was to make sense of the migraine, especially the feature of nearly passing out and his thoughts "nearly dying." He knew from past experience that for him the migraine often connoted rage. Later that week, in a burst of unexpected fury, he assailed his work with Vietnam veterans, wishing to be rid of it, because it demanded that he empathize with murder. Focusing on the missed session and his own relief, Dr. D. became aware of the following "forbidden" thought: "I am glad Jeb is not here today. I'm enraged at his murderous role in the massacre; I hope he never returns to treatment; I wish he were dead." Perhaps the symptom had broken through when this forbidden thought pressed too close to awareness. Once Dr. D. realized that he felt "righteous" in his vengeful state, he wondered who might have such a reaction within the trauma context. Then he recalled Jeb's self-reference to being an SS man in an American uniform; and Dr. D. thought of his own Jewishness, which Jeb had correctly guessed. Dr. D.'s identity, then, as kin of those murdered by the SS in the Holocaust, would make him a likely representative of the Vietnamese families whose kin were slaughtered in Jeb's massacre. Dr. D represented the rageful witness and the surviving family members of the victims.

Although this level of understanding brought some clarification regarding Jeb's guilt and desire for execution, the dysphoric mood continued, and Dr. D. felt this explanation for his outrage was still too distant. Next, he focused on his disillusionment with Jeb and his own earlier excitement when he looked forward to "joining" Jeb on these missions as they were revived in the treatment. Painfully, Dr. D. realized he was involved in yet another way. He was a comrade-in-arms with Jeb during the treatment. He had looked forward to their missions together, anticipating Jeb's leadership as danger appeared. Jeb had referred to the two of them as Israeli soldiers. Dr. D. had been lapsing into the younger brother's role with Jeb so that his disillusionment with Jeb, therefore, was immense; it was as if his own brother had fired the shot and set off the massacre. But why did Dr. D. feel such chagrin and shame? Dr. D. continued his painful logic: he asked himself how he would have responded when there was motion in the village and his trusted leader chose to fire. It grew clear to Dr. D. as he faced his own impulses to follow Jeb in the massacre; he would have pulled the trigger as second in command, and he could have blamed Jeb for his own murderous action. In the second countertransference role Dr. D. was a fellow perpetrator.

Some weeks later, Dr. D. decided his work on this countertransference response was not yet done. Earlier in the treatment, he had been the accuser, the Nuremburg trial prosecutor; next he was the kin of the massacred; and then the junior buddy in the unit. But he had not yet fully walked through the moment of the massacre in Jeb's boots. Here Dr. D. had the greatest difficulty. As he imagined the massacre, might he as leader also have pulled the trigger? As Dr. D. placed himself in this situation, he became aware of a powerful self-loathing, which he identified as Jeb's core dilemma. Dr. D. concluded he could have done what Jeb had done and the internal consequences would have been devastating.

In the above clinical illustration, the therapist finds himself in multiple countertransference roles and uses his understanding of them to reestablish empathic connection with the survivor.

CONCLUSION

In summarizing some of the steps necessary for therapists to work with such countertransference problems, we may conclude that (if the countertransference is acted out) therapists must first discontinue out-of-role behaviors. Next, we should examine the tension states within the transference–countertransference matrix that precipitated the out-of-role behaviors, defenses, or affects. Here we must give free rein to examining our associations and affect states aroused by the patient's verbal and nonverbal material, moving into our own past and back again to the patient's trauma, many times. We should examine our own reactions as complementary or concordant with the trauma events themselves. In this way we can spell out new hypotheses about the motives, drives, behaviors, and defenses used by the survivor and those intimately engaged with the trauma around him. Without necessarily stating these new ideas, we can listen to further material from the patient in light of the above hypotheses. We can then respond to this new material with the insights gained and await the patient's further reactions with (1) enlarged areas of empathy, (2) more complete reconstruction of the trauma and its nuances, and (3) use of our internally gained knowledge of the tension state that occurred in us as a vehicle for these new understandings.

The operational structure of the working alliance, the therapeutic frame, transference and countertransference, the complementary associative pathways between patient and doctor, and the unconscious resistances to recognizing these phenomena are useful concepts in the psychotherapy of trauma survivors. They help us organize *expectable* emotional pitfalls in the work for the therapist.

Ideally, we as dynamic therapists entering a world of empathic strain will examine our own affects, associations, and memories to clarify evocative affect states that are set off in the treatment, which are likely to be related to the trauma itself. This self-examination helps us to recognize split-off components of the trauma and reactions to it, and it lays the groundwork for deeper, more comprehensive understanding.

REFERENCES

Danieli, Y. (1981). Therapists' difficulties in treating survivors of the Nazi Holocaust and their children, *Dissertation Abstracts International, 42,* 4927-B.

Freud, S. (1912). Recommendations to physicians practicing psychoanalysis. *Standard Edition, 12,* 111–120.

Freud, S. (1914). Remembering, repeating, and working through. *Standard Edition, 12,* 146–156. London: Hogarth Press, 1953.

Gill, M. M. (1983). The interpersonal paradigm and the degree of the therapist's involvement. *Contemporary Psychoanalysis, 19,* 200–237.

Greenson, R. (1967). The working alliance. In *The technique and practice of psychoanalysis* (Vol. 1, pp. 190–215). New York: International Universities Press.

Kernberg, O. (1965). Notes on countertransference. *Journal of the American Psychoanalytic Association, 13,* 38–56.

Kohut, H. (1959). Introspection, empathy, and psychoanalysis: An examination of the relationship between mode of observation and theory. *Journal of the American Psychoanalytic Association, 7,* 459–483.

Langs, R. (1968) *Transference and countertransference.* New York: International Universities Press.

Langs, R. (1982). *Psychotherapy: A basic text.* New York: Jason Aronson.

Lindy, J. D., Green, B. L., Grace, M., MacLeod, J. A., & Spitz, L. (1988), *Vietnam: A casebook.* New York: Brunner/Mazel.

McCann, I. L., & Pearlman, L. A. (1990). *Psychological trauma and the adult survivor.* New York: Brunner/Mazel.

Racker, H. (1968). *Transference and countertransference.* New York: International Universities Press.

Sterba, R. (1934). The fate of the ego in analytic therapy. *International Journal of Psycho-Analysis, 15,* 117–126.

Strachey, J. (1934). The nature of the therapeutic actic.1 of psychoanalysis. *International Journal of Psycho-Analysis, 50,* 275–292.

Tansey, M., & Burke, W. (1989). *Understanding countertransference.* Hillsdale, NJ: Analytic Press.

PART II

Countertransference in the Treatment of Victims of Sexual, Physical, and Emotional Abuse

Part II focuses attention on the difficulties therapists encounter when working with children, adolescents, and adults who were subjected to sexual, physical, or emotional abuse in their formative years. Although the age at the point of entry into treatment may vary in proximity to the traumatic experience, the insidious and intrusive nature of the abuse, which violates trust and integrity, inevitably leaves injuries to the core of the self. Clinicians working with patients suffering from the deleterious consequences of abusive relationships are especially prone to counter-transference reactions (CTRs), because these clients have a fundamental mistrust of others, inevitably have significant problems with boundaries, and have developed defensive structures erected to protect deep-seated feelings of vulnerability, fear, insecurity, rage, depression, and other man-ifestations of low self-esteem and narcissistic injury. As is to be expected, the damaged self transfers object relations in unconscious ways and this creates an unfolding process in treatment that is likely to stir either a Type I or Type II countertransference.

In Chapter 4, I. Lisa McCann and Joseph Colletti describe the in-tricacies of the transference–countertransference process as "the dance of empathy," a metaphor that characterizes the alternating tendencies of movement toward and away from therapeutic encounters. The authors employ a hermeneutic model to characterize the dynamics of trauma-specific transference and the forms of countertransference in working with adult patients who suffered abuse in childhood. Through case ex-amples, McCann and Colletti illustrate the use of the hermeneutic approach, which is laid out in four basic steps: (1) listening, (2) being aware of CTRs, (3) monitoring CTRs, and (4) completing one phase of the humanistic spiral. Included in this chapter is a transcript of a very intense therapy session in which McCann annotates her CTRs during a session with a woman who was brutally sexually victimized in childhood by a sadistic father.

In Chapter 5, Richard P. Kluft presents an extensive review of the phenomena of countertransference in clinical work with dissociative disorders, especially multiple personality disorder (MPD). Based on over 20 years of research, consultation, and psychotherapy, Kluft and his study group have identified eight predominant and recurring countertransference concerns: (1) frustration/exasperation with the world of MPD; (2) frustration/exasperation with the patient's preoccupation with pain evasion; (3) frustration/exasperation with the patient's preoccupation with controlling the therapist; (4) the price of empathy; (5) the rebuffing of the healer; (6) the loss of a sense of efficacy and the pressure to misguided repair; (7) the frequent absence of collegial appreciation for, or validation of, one's efforts; and (8) feeling entrapped in reenactment of the patient's past with the discounting/invalidating personality's contemporary personal reality. Each of these themes is discussed in the chapter, which concludes with observations about what happens to therapists who work primarily with MPD or post-traumatic stress disorder patients. This interesting discussion takes the idea of countertransference into an uncharted area of investigation, that is, the long-term consequences to the therapist's sense of self, professional identity, and world view.

In Chapter 6, Erwin Randolph Parson discusses one of the least studied and most pressing problems in the United States today: inner city violence and its impact to the sense of self and well-being of children and adolescents. Parson introduces a new term to the literature "urban violence traumatic stress response syndrome (U-VTS)," a concept that broadens the definition of PTSD. More specifically, the U-VTS phenomenon is characterized by at least seven interrelated features: (1) the damaged self syndrome, (2) trauma-specific transference, (3) adaptation to danger, (4) cognitive and emotional stress response, (5) impact on moral behavior, (6) post-traumatic play, (7) PTSD, and (8) post-traumatic health outcomes. After a discussion of each of the components of U-VTS, Parson describes innovative techniques of treatment and the specific problems of CTRs. Based on clinical research, he details specific forms of countertransference in work with children who have suffered urban violence, which include minimizing responses, counterphobic reactions, passionate parenting reactions, raciocultural countertransference, and organizational forms of numbing and unresponsiveness. Parson concludes the chapter with a discussion of the long-term consequences of the failure to properly treat children who suffer from U-VTS, the spectrum of transgenerational cycles of violence, and the absence of morality.

In Chapter 7, Kathleen Nader discusses countertransference in the treatment of acutely traumatized children. The insights contained in this chapter stem from Nader's ongoing research with Robert Pynoos at the UCLA Neuropsychiatric Institute and Hospital. The UCLA Prevention Intervention Program in Trauma, Violence, and Sudden Bereavement has provided both national and international consultation to child victims of natural disasters, violence, accidents, warfare, and many other forms of traumatization. As such, this chapter is rich in knowledge about the impact of traumatic events on the inner world of the child. Therapists working with traumatized children need to know when to intervene to provide treatment, as well as how to recognize CTRs that are forms of resistance in the provider. Various countertransference themes are discussed that are common to clinical work with children (e.g., fantasies of reversal of outcome), and Nader points out potential traps and pitfalls for the therapist that can sabotage treatment.

In Chapter 8, Carol R. Hartman and Helene Jackson discuss rape and countertransference. To illustrate the range, severity, and complexity of CTRs in clinical work with victims of rape and sexual assault, many case examples are provided, along with transcriptions of a therapy session. This material provides a "window" into the active process of treatment and creates a foundation for discussion of subtypes of Type I and Type II countertransference in work with this victim population. Among the many important findings in this chapter, the authors indicate that providers are at risk for vicarious traumatizations. Clearly, the risk potential to the well-being in clinicians working with PTSD currently lacks a data base, in a part because the field of trauma studies is so new. Nevertheless, Hartman and Jackson make a strong case that training programs must include preparation for understanding and managing countertransference.

4

The Dance of Empathy: A Hermeneutic Formulation of Countertransference, Empathy, and Understanding in the Treatment of Individuals Who Have Experienced Early Childhood Trauma

I. LISA McCANN
JOSEPH COLLETTI

Over the past 10 years, there has been a growing awareness of the profound psychological impact of early childhood trauma, including emotional, physical, and sexual abuse, on personality development and adaptation (e.g., Courtois, 1988; Herman, 1981). Most recently, researchers have discovered a relationship between early childhood trauma and the later development of severe personality disorders, such as borderline personality disorder (Herman, Perry, & van der Kolk, 1989; Westen, Ludolph, Misle, Ruffins, & Block, 1990) and multiple personality disorder (Braun, 1984). To date, the etiology of borderline personality disorder remains controversial. However, converging evidence suggests that such "disorders of the self" (Kohut, 1971) and related disturbances in identity, affective regulation, and interpersonal relationships may have their origins in highly traumatic childhood experiences.

The therapeutic process with adults who have experienced serious childhood traumas is often a challenging, complex, demanding, and protracted process. Early childhood trauma usually occurs within a relational context. It is often associated with serious boundary violations, intrusions, betrayals, and assaults on the sense of self. Thus, the "dance of empathy"

requires the utmost skill and delicacy in managing the complex transference–countertransference issues that inevitably emerge (see Wilson &
Lindy, Chapter 1, this volume). Patients who have experienced early
childhood trauma will often reexperience and reenact their role in previous abusive relationships within the context of the therapy relationship
(Ganzarain & Buchele, 1986; van der Kolk, Boyd, Krystal, & Greenberg,
1984). These roles shift from being a victim to being identified with the
aggressor, and, for the patient who has experienced intrafamilial abuse or
incest, to being the "favorite" or "special" child (Ganzarain & Buchele,
1986). According to Finell (1986), projective identification describes an
enactment or actualization wherein the therapist is unconsciously drawn
into playing a role in the patient's reenactment of prior and or current
abusive relationships. McCann and Pearlman (1990a) describe various
trauma-specific transference reactions that may emerge within the therapy
relationship. These may include fears that the therapist will recapitulate
experiences of threat, terror, and boundary violations, a transference
reaction that relates to a disruption in one's sense of safety and security.
Likewise, the patient may fear that the therapist will repeat experiences in
which the patient is betrayed, abandoned, and unsupported, reflecting
transference themes related to previous violations in trust and dependency. The patient's ability to develop a safe and trusting relationship with the
therapist will depend on the therapist's ability to genuinely listen, be with,
and understand the patient's conflicted internal experience and malevolent objective world. This, in turn, challenges the therapist's capacity to
"contain" intolerable affects (Parson, 1988) within a "safe–holding environment" (Winnicott, 1965) while modulating his or her own reactions
of revulsion and shock to the often intense, affectively charged trauma-
related material.

Over the years, increased attention has been given to the importance
of countertransference reactions (CTRs) when working with traumatized
individuals (e.g., Danieli, 1981; Haley, 1974; Herman, 1981). These
reactions are important due to their impact on the nature and quality of
the empathic stance of the therapist toward his or her patient. The pitfalls
of either significant fluctuations in empathy or empathic failures have
been well documented in the psychoanalytic literature (e.g., Kohut, 1977;
Langs, 1974).

The dance of empathy between the therapist and the patient who has
experienced early childhood trauma is conceived of here as choreographed and guided by the quality and accuracy of empathic responses, as
determined by the countertransference of the therapist. As we will demonstrate in this chapter, this dance is a crucial factor for the successful
treatment of individuals who have experienced early childhood trauma
and abuse.

The first section of this chapter will explore and explain the importance of managing CTRs with patients who report early childhood trauma. Next, we will present a hermeneutic formulation of the relationship between countertransference, empathy, and understanding in treating individuals who have experienced early childhood trauma and abuse. This formulation is embedded within a psychoanalytic perspective. Finally, clinical examples will be presented to clarify and explicate the hermeneutic formulation of the dance of empathy.

CLASSICAL AND CONTEMPORARY FORMULATIONS OF COUNTERTRANSFERENCE

There are two types of CTRs: classical formulations, which refer to subjective reactions on the part of the therapist; and contemporary formulations, which refer to objective reactions on the part of the therapist (see Wilson & Lindy, Chapter 1, this volume). Classical formulations of countertransference refer to reactions on the part of the therapist that are specific, personal, and subjective, and that resonate with his or her prior understanding and experience. Contemporary formulations of countertransference refer to reactions on the part of the therapist that are universal. These reactions are universal in that anyone exposed to this material is likely to have characteristic responses. Likewise, these reactions are objective, in that they are related to specific trauma-embedded images and recollections conveyed by the traumatized patient.

In the classical conception of countertransference, the patient's transference reaction activates unresolved unconscious and conscious conflicts within the therapist, arising from his or her personal history (Freud, 1910). Freud also believed that the CTRs of the therapist could be useful to the extent that "everyone possesses in his own unconscious an instrument with which he can interpret [and understand] the utterances of the unconscious in other people" (cited in Marcus, 1980, p. 286). Marcus (1980) goes on to explain that the early view of the analytic process "was characterized as the resonance which takes place between the patient's unconscious and that of the analyst" (p. 287). CTRs of which the therapist is unaware oftentimes are a hindrance to establishing empathy within the therapeutic relationship. However, those personal reactions and feelings of which the therapist is aware are important tools that he or she must use to understand a patient's inner experience (Kohut, 1971).

Case Example One
   Patient A. was a 36-year-old divorced mother who was referred for major depression and chronic fatigue. After a series of medical evalua-

tions, no physical cause for her condition was diagnosed. She reported being emotionally and physically violated by her hypercritical, volatile, and emotionally explosive mother. In an early session, the patient recalled a vivid memory of her mother repeatedly "stalking" her with a knife, then tying her up and locking her in a closet for hours at a time. The therapist became anxious and preoccupied in one of these sessions but was unaware that the patient's material had activated her own, as yet, unresolved rage toward her own controlling and capricious mother.

In a supervisory session, the supervisor noted that the therapist had defensively "moved away" from the patient's emotional experience and then refocused the patient on the material related to her mother's family background. This inquiry on the part of the therapist was understood as representing an intellectualized defense against her own unresolved history of victimization. Until the therapist was able to work through her CTRs aroused by the patient's material, the patient was unable to spontaneously produce further recollections of her own abuse.

Contemporary formulations of countertransference refer to universal reactions to the patient's presentation of traumatic imagery and recollections, a process described as secondary victimization (Figley, 1983) and vicarious traumatization (McCann & Pearlman, 1990b). Within this perspective, McCann and Pearlman (1990b) have described pervasive countertransference themes that often emerge in working with individuals who have been traumatized. These may include disruptions within the therapist's internalized object world. For example, the therapist's inner experience of his or her own sense of safety and power may be threatened by exposure to the patient's traumatic imagery. Likewise, the therapist's internal experience of other people as trustworthy and benevolent may be disrupted by the patient's vivid accounts of cruelty, violence, and betrayal perpetuated by other human beings. Exposure to the traumatic imagery and recollections of traumatized individuals thus has a profound effect on the emotional life of the therapist. Powerful affective responses may include horror, repulsion, shock, guilt, grief, and rage (Danieli, 1981; Ganzarain & Buchele, 1986; Lindy, 1988). Defensively, the therapist may react with disbelief, numbing, detachment, avoidance, and intellectualization of the patient's traumatic disclosure (see Wilson & Lindy, Chapter 1, this volume).

Vicarious traumatization, as distinct from classical conceptions of countertransference, is conceived of here as a "universal" reaction. Here the therapist's reaction is elicited by the material itself. In contrast, the classical view of countertransference presumes that the reaction of the therapist results from a resonance with his or her unconscious wishes and fantasies. Although vicarious traumatization does include a resonance with the therapist's own prior understanding and experience, we believe that these reactions are universal and are therefore common reactions to horrific and shocking accounts of traumatic material.

Case Example Two

Patient B. was a 37-year-old mother of two who had recently discovered that her 4-year-old child had been sexually molested and ritually abused in a local day care center. She was suffering profoundly from rage, shock, revulsion, and guilt at what had been done to her child. She came into therapy as her depression worsened months after the disclosure and she was overcome by "irrational" guilt that she had failed to keep her child safe from harm. The patient's view of herself as a "good mother" was massively violated and she questioned whether she was capable of keeping her children safe. She even had thoughts of killing herself because she believed her children might be better off if she were dead. Her obsessive preoccupation with issues related to safety had become so extreme that it was interfering with her ability to function in her daily life.

The therapist, who herself was a mother, identified strongly with her patient's maternal feelings and reacted to the patient's trauma by becoming anxious and preoccupied about her own children's safety. She developed intrusive thoughts that her children would be harmed and suffered from terrifying nightmares that they had been kidnapped and killed by a stranger. In supervision, the therapist was ultimately able to use her own vicarious traumatization to empathize with her patient's deep guilt and despair at having "failed" her child.

CONJUNCTIVE AND DYSJUNCTIVE COUNTERTRANSFERENCE PROCESSES

According to Atwood and Stolorow (1984), there are two processes by which the therapist comes to understand and empathize with the patient by utilizing the CTRs. The first of these is considered *conjunctive*. Here, feelings and experiences shared by the patient readily resonate with and are assimilated into the internal experience of the therapist. These experiences, by definition, are easily accepted, empathized with, and understood by the therapist. The interpretation and understanding that result from conjunctive countertransference processes enhance empathy and facilitate the therapeutic process.

Case Example Three

Patient C. was a 23-year-old male graduate student who was referred for depression and anxiety. He complained of being unable to concentrate and focus on his studies due to a preoccupation with vivid and violent fantasies and intrusive thoughts of destruction to himself and others. Shortly after entering therapy, early memories of his father beating him while in a drunken rage began to emerge. He was able to recall numerous instances of his father sadistically teasing and verbally tormenting him and his siblings until each was in a state of absolutely overwhelming fear and terror. His father would then in a systematic and brutal fashion sadistically beat each child with an extension cord until one was forced to confess to the father's psychotic, fantasized accusations.

The therapist of this patient himself had an alcoholic father and had experienced frequent beatings by him. Initially his CTR was to experience revulsion and anger at having to reexperience his own abuse through his patient's report of horrendous torture. Being aware of and modulating his own intense feelings allowed the therapist to "be with" and empathize with the patient's emotional experience of helplessness and vulnerability. The therapist was then able, by analyzing his CTR, to correctly interpret the violent fantasies of the patient as a defense against these painful memories and associated affects. In this case the therapist's ability to resonate with the experience enhanced his ability to readily understand and empathize with the patient.

The second process by which the therapist comes to understand the patient by utilizing a CTR is considered *dysjunctive* (Atwood & Stolorow, 1984). Here again, there is a resonance of feelings and experiences shared by the therapist and patient. The therapist "takes in" the patient's material, but then alters the configuration of the patient's experience in accordance with his or her own prior experience and understanding. The therapist may then react to or interpret the information from the patient in a way that leads to a misunderstanding of the patient's experience, a Type I CTR (see Chapter 2, this volume). Using the metaphor of the dance, the therapist misses a beat, and thereby incurs a possible failure of empathy and understanding of the patient. The resulting loss of empathy and understanding can result in the patient experiencing feelings of rage, rejection, abandonment, and estrangement. These failures in processing CTRs often lead to a recapitulation of a traumatic assault to the sense of self, in which the patient feels that he or she is not seen, heard, understood, and acknowledged by significant others. It is now understood that these mismanaged dysjunctive countertransference processes may lead to a retraumatization of the patient. If these processes are not carefully considered, understood, and monitored within the emotional life of the therapist, the resulting reactions may precipitate a rupture of the empathic stance of the therapist. More importantly, if left unaccounted for, these reactions may undermine and threaten the therapeutic relationship as a whole.

With an awareness of when and how a dysjunctive CTR occurs, the therapist can correct his or her reaction. By recognizing how his or her own subjective experience and prior understanding taints and distorts his or her understanding of the patient's experience, the therapist can experience a more accurate and empathic understanding of the patient's subjective experience. Thus, by utilizing the reaction of the patient to an incorrect or threatening formulation based on a dysjunctive CTR, the therapist's corrected dysjunctive awarenesses can effectively aid in clarifying for the therapist the internalized object world of the patient.

Case Example Four

Patient D. was a 34-year-old married mother of three who was self-referred for treatment due to depression and "chronically low self-esteem." She reported that her father died in an auto accident when she was 7 years old. Patient D. described her mother as an "able-bodied caretaker" but emotionally cold and distant when interacting with her and her siblings. On numerous occasions the patient described waking up in her bed at night to find her mother fondling her. These experiences, while terrifying and confusing for the patient, were also the only times she felt any warmth from her mother.

In an early session the patient reported a dream in which she was being chased and then devoured by a large female bear. The therapist interpreted the dream as meaning that the patient wished to merge with and be nurtured by a fiercely protective, maternal object. Her empathic response, aimed at decreasing the anxiety and arousal caused by the material, only seemed to increase the patient's agitation and discomfort. Clearly, the interpretation and reassurance precipitated a highly traumatic experience for Patient D. Only when the therapist came to understand that her own desire to be closer to her own mother was incorrectly assimilated into her understanding of the patient's experience, was she able to step back, listen, and understand the meaning of this incident.

When the therapist corrected her dysjunctive CTR, she then understood the patient's internal experience as one in which she feared encroachment and annihilation by a devouring mother. Only when she shifted her understanding to the meanings conveyed by the patient, was the therapist able to construct an effective intervention based on the patient's inner experience and object world.

In summary, a breakdown in empathy (empathic strain) precipitated by unconscious or unresolved CTRs poses a serious threat to the therapeutic process when treating patients who have experienced early childhood trauma. Possible consequences include premature termination of treatment, retraumatization, and/or a repetition of earlier experiences of confusion, misunderstanding, and neglect within significant interpersonal relationships.

What has not been fully explicated is a conceptual formulation of the exquisitely complex process by which a therapist develops and maintains a consistent empathic stance with patients who report detailed accounts of vivid and horrific traumatic experiences.

HERMENEUTICS AND THE DANCE OF EMPATHY

What will be explained here is a theoretical model that describes the circular process of monitoring CTRs to individuals in psychotherapy. The process is metaphorically conceived of as a spontaneously choreographed dance in which the therapist and patient move forward together in a fluid but deliberate pattern of interaction. It is this delicate process that creates the rhythm and tempo required for a patient to effectively work through and integrate threatening experiences. This model subsumes the primary functions of empathy, understanding, and countertransference.

Instead of a rational or empirical method for explaining this process, a hermeneutic conceptualization of understanding will be used to describe how to maintain an effective empathic stance with individuals who have experienced early childhood trauma. This hermeneutic conceptualization allows a more precise description of the complex processes of understanding and interpretation that are involved in psychotherapy.

Two important side notes need to be mentioned here. First, this hermeneutic formulation is broadly conceived within psychoanalytic and developmental frameworks. These frameworks allow for the most articulate description of the process. Second, the terminology used here is not entirely consistent with the formal terminology of philosophical hermeneutics. The goal here is not to create a major contribution to philosophical hermeneutics but to utilize the hermeneutic paradigm to describe in detail an important facet of the therapeutic process.

A Philosophical Hermeneutic Conceptualization of Understanding

Philosophical hermeneutics is the study of interpretation and understanding (Polkinghorne, 1983). In a hermeneutic inquiry, understanding, interpretation, and knowing are conceptualized as occurring in a circular or, more accurately, in a spiral organization (Polkinghorne, 1983). The inquirer approaches the object to be understood not with a preconceived notion or theory of what exists but with an openness that allows a natural unfolding of the phenomenon in order that it become revealed and understood. Yet to know and understand an object or phenomenon, it must resonate with what the inquirer or interpreter already knows and understands from his or her prior experience (Palmer, 1969; Polkinghorne, 1983). In order for this to occur, however, the inquirer must approach the phenomenon or object empathically (Mueller-Vollmer, 1989). According to the philosopher Wilhelm Dilthey, it is from an empathic position that the unknown phenomenon can resonate, resound, and move with what is already known and understood by the inquirer (Mueller-Vollmer, 1989).

Figure 4.1 shows the internal movement of the inquirer or "knower" to the object to be understood or "known." The arrows in the diagram demonstrate the reciprocal interaction of the part to whole configurations (spiral) between the inquirer and the object to be understood. It is through this process that an understanding of the phenomenon can emerge. According to the hermeneutic paradigm, it is only through repeated experience with and exposure to a phenomenon from an empathic position that a true understanding of that phenomenon can emerge within the inquirer. In other words, the reciprocal interaction is an ongoing, repetitive process that includes a constant revision of and/or reconsideration of the phenomenon due to new information obtained about it during each exposure.

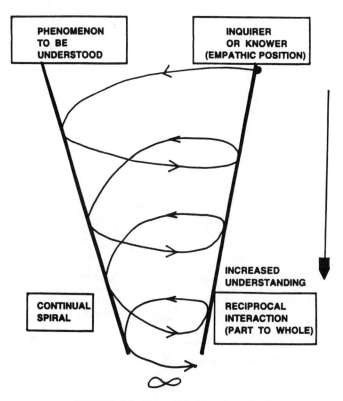

FIGURE 4.1. Philosophical hermeneutics.

A Hermeneutic Conceptualization of Therapeutic Countertransference and Empathy

This philosophical conceptualization of hermeneutics will now be described within the context of psychotherapy. This same empathic position is essential in understanding the inner experience of another person. Effective empathy allows the therapist the openness to experience and eventually understand previously unknown and unfamiliar material offered by the patient. The therapist achieves this effective empathy by allowing the experience of the patient to resonate, resound, and move with what is already known and understood by the therapist. In this formulation of understanding, then, contrary to philosophical hermeneutics, it is essential that the emotional and subjective experience of the therapist be considered. Now countertransference becomes an essential element for the therapist to consider when attempting to understand the patient.

Figure 4.2 shows the movement of the therapist as he or she first encounters the patient to be understood. The therapist approaches the patient not with a preconceived judgment of the patient's experience but

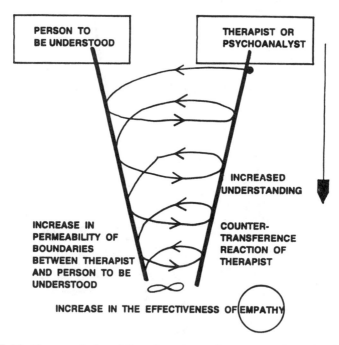

FIGURE 4.2. Hermeneutic formulation of countertransference, empathy, and understanding.

rather with an openness that will allow for an unfolding and revealing of that patient's inner experience. Through a consistent monitoring and evaluation of CTRs, the therapist can modulate his or her responses so that the most effective and appropriate empathy is maintained. As there is an increase in appropriate empathy, the patient will more freely explore and reveal material about himself or herself. Now a greater understanding of the patient's experience can emerge.

In the early stages of psychotherapy, a solid, impermeable boundary often exists between the therapist and the patient. That solid, impermeable boundary effectively blocks the therapist from entering into and understanding the inner experience of the patient. In effective psychotherapy, however, as the therapist's understanding of the patient and accuracy of the empathy increase, the once solid and impermeable boundary between the therapist and patient becomes permeable. Now the therapist can more effectively "be with" the person (Heidegger, 1962) and can continuously engage with him or her when it is appropriate. In this fashion, threatening experiences can be explored, revealed, understood, and then worked through. Although the boundary is conceptualized here as becoming more permeable, it is never to be broken or threatened by the therapist. Boundary loss will most assuredly lead to a retraumatization and a threat to safety and containment for the patient.

The Completion of the Hermeneutic Spiral: The Dance of Empathy

Within the hermeneutic spiral, the dance of empathy is choreographed through a mediation between (1) the quality of empathy, (2) the depth of the therapist's understanding of the patient, and (3) the therapist's awareness of his or her CTRs aroused by the patient's material. It is through this dance that the fluctuations in the empathic position remain beneficial for the patient.

The therapeutic process of understanding is considered to be the movement from the therapist's initial judgment of the meaning of the patient's internal experience to a qualitative change in that meaning due to a reciprocal interaction between the detailed parts of the patient's internal experience, and the whole of his or her life story. The proper empathic stance enables the therapist to secure a more profound understanding of the patient's experience. It is through effective empathy and the monitoring of CTRs that an understanding of another person's inner experience is possible. The hermeneutic process of understanding involves the therapist deriving a preliminary understanding of the patient and then revising and considering new possibilities through a reciprocal engagement with the patient. The goal of this dance, as exemplified in the hermeneutic spiral, is twofold: for the therapist there is a greater understanding of the patient's internal experience and an increase in the permeability of the boundary between him or her and the patient; for the patient there is a greater understanding of himself or herself and a safe, contained environment in which to work through threatening material.

This more complete understanding and empathic stance allows the detailed parts of the patient's experience to be understood in terms of the whole person. Now those previously differentiated and separated parts can be more precisely defined, understood, and eventually integrated by the patient. For the patient there is an increased sense of feeling safe, cared for, and understood. The reemergence of threatening memories and affects will be experienced as less threatening and toxic and therefore, more readily accessible.

Understanding as the Mediation of Part-to-Whole Configurations

A lucid application of the hermeneutic principle is offered by Barker (1963), who described aspects of a person's behavior as tesserae, the tiny squares of marble or glass used in constructing a mosaic. Utilizing tesserae to construct a mosaic is analogous to the process by which the therapist comes to understand the experience of traumatized patients or any other patient for that matter. A therapist is exposed to tiny fragments or isolated parts of a person's experience. If the therapist attempts to understand the whole person from this fragmented piece of experience, little, if any, overall understanding will be possible.

Likewise, the whole person is understood only in relation to those parts of his or her experience. This repeated formulation and mediation of part-to-whole experience, and then whole-to-part experience, is essential for an overall understanding of the person. Thus, the therapeutic process with patients who have experienced childhood trauma is analogous to the process in which the tiny tesserae are utilized to construct and create the mosaic.

Implicit within the spiral of the hermeneutic process is the idea that an understanding of the patient's experience is never complete. In the dance of empathy, the therapist needs to both "be with" the patient and, at the same time, maintain separateness from the patient's experience. Crossing the boundary and resonating too closely with the patient's affective experience can result in a breakdown and threat to the empathic position. The therapist may then defensively move away from the patient's experience. The therapist, being led by his or her CTRs, either approaches or avoids his or her own emotional reactions to the material presented by the patient. Consequently, the therapist may use his or her CTRs to move closer to, or away from the patient's emotional experience.

The Dance of Empathy and "Two-Stepping"

The dance of empathy involves a circular, reciprocal process of "being with" or moving closer to the patient's experience, and moving away from the material in order to maintain an appropriate boundary, empathic stance, and level of understanding. The choreography of the dance is determined by the therapist's awareness of and management of the countertransference. When an effective empathic stance is maintained over the course of therapy or within an individual session, the patient is able to freely "be with" the therapist and work through threatening experiences. In the dance of effective empathy the approach–avoidance of the therapist does not parallel the defensive processes of the patient. Instead the movements of the therapist complement the movements of the patient.

Utilizing the metaphor of a dance, this process resembles a ballet with Mikhail Baryshnikov and Twyla Tharp, each a seasoned, expert dancer. Although they had never danced together, it took only a few steps for each to anticipate, react to, and move with the other in a graceful, flowing motion. Here the partners moved together and away from each other in an intricate, spontaneously choreographed rhythm when no motion was prearranged, preplanned, or even rehearsed.

Applied to therapy, when the patient approaches threatening material, the therapist remains with him or her throughout the emergence of this material. Likewise, when the patient needs to step away from the material in order to regroup and work through the experience, the therapist reacts in such a way as to complement this movement and yet remain with the patient. This organized movement is determined, in part, by the therapist's ability to empathically "be with" both the patient and the material, while at the same time remaining separate from the experience. Within the context of this safe–holding environment, recovery can take place. This is the dance of empathy and understanding as choreographed by the countertransference.

CLINICAL APPLICATIONS OF THE HERMENEUTIC FORMULATION OF THE DANCE OF EMPATHY: A "FOUR-STEP" PROCESS

In this section, a "four-step" process for maintaining an effective empathic stance will be explicated. Table 4.1 outlines this process.

TABLE 4.1. Four "Steps" for Maintaining a Maximal Stance for Empathy and Understanding

Step 1: Listening
    a. Words (behavior)
    b. Feelings (affect)
    c. Transference projections and object relations

Step 2: Awareness of CTRs
    a. Past history, including traumatic experiences (classical formulations)
    b. Vicarious traumatization (contemporary)
    c. Conjunctive and dysjunctive CTRs
    d. Monitoring for CTRs
      1. Thoughts/ideation
      2. Feelings and visceral reactions
      3. Fantasies/dreams

Step 3: Monitoring of how CTRs are affecting effective empathic stance toward the patient
    a. Increased level of understanding of presented material
      1. Greater spontaneity
      2. Greater trust
      3. Increased insight on part of the patient
      4. Movement into areas that were previously threatening
      5. Less resistance to approaching traumatic material
    b. Increased permeability of boundary between therapist and patient
      1. Quality of therapeutic relationship
        a. Safety
        b. Containment
        c. Analytic "holding"

Step 4: Completion of one cycle of the hermeneutic spiral: the "dance"

Step 1: Listening

Listening is an important facet of psychotherapy that receives relatively little attention in the contemporary psychotherapy literature. Here we will explicate the complex, delicate process of listening. We conceptualize the therapists' process of listening as it occurs on three levels of psychological experience: the words, feelings, and object relations the patient reveals during the therapy hour (B. Dujovne, personal communication, November 7, 1992).

The first level of listening concerns the words the patient uses to communicate his or her experience. The second level is indicated by those feelings expressed in the session, both verbally and nonverbally. The third and deepest level of listening is the level of transference projections and object relation revealed by the patient in his or her interactions with the therapist. It is clear that in order for the therapist to fully listen to the patient, words, feelings, and object relation must be considered. Listening on these levels requires that the therapist approach the patient not with a preconceived notion of the patient's experience but instead with an openness to the material as experienced by the patient. In accordance with a psychoanalytic, object relations perspective, CTRs are an essential tool for understanding the patient, rather than an obstacle for the therapist to overcome.

The First Level

In the first level of listening, the therapist listens to the words and nonverbal behavior of the patient in order to understand that patient's experience. The language used by the patient often reveals complex motivations, unconscious conflicts, and meanings. Words are more powerful in therapy than is sometimes recognized. Words define inner experiences and selfobject representations. More important than the definition of words is the meaning of the words to the person. If a therapist presumes to understand the psychological significance of the words conveyed by the patient, he or she runs the risk of misinterpreting and misunderstanding the patient's experience. Horner (1985a) writes:

> The use of words that are assumed to have consensual meaning when it is more likely to have specific meaning for the patient should be clarified. Words like "rejection" in particular lend themselves to this kind of obfuscation. What constitutes a rejection for this person? What is the fear? the fantasy? the reaction? (p. 78)

Psychoanalytic listening involves fully exploring the meanings of the words and the patient's associations to those words in order to more accurately understand what the person is communicating to the therapist about his or her inner experience (S. Appelbaum, personal communication, November 17, 1992).

One prevalent example of listening gone awry is when therapist presume to understand the meaning the terms patients use when they first come to therapy. These include such ambiguously defined terms as "survivor" and "multiple personality disorder" (MPD). Frequently individuals who come to therapy refer to themselves as a "survivor" or a person with "MPD." Yet even in the professional community little if any shared meaning or understanding exists for these terms. The therapist may presume that the term "survivor" means the patient identifies with living through an experience of trauma and that he or she has "survived" the experience to tell about it. Yet, this term may have different meanings for different people. Listening more carefully to how patients understand the term "survivor" may reveal numerous other meanings such as being unique, special, and part of a group. Vulnerable people who in the past have felt disconnected and alienated may now feel a sense of belonging and connectedness because they can identify with others who also see themselves as "survivors." Now the term means more than merely living through a traumatic incident or abusive past. It may signify that the patient is searching for something, such as belonging, specialness, and a sense of identity.

The following example illustrates the meaning of the term "MPD" for a young woman in ongoing psychotherapy. The therapist, not presuming to "understand" what the term meant to the patient, inquired as to what the term meant to her. The patient offered the following reflections in a letter to the therapist:

> "I talked to someone after the group and she sounds like a clear case of it [MPD]. It has been bothering me . . . because I really do not think that I have MPD and yet I am meeting people who really do and I feel out of place . . . I'm almost jealous of the ones who do have it . . . I'm afraid if I don't have it, then I will just be another ordinary patient with problems and I won't be anyone. . . . And if I don't have it, maybe you won't want to see me anymore because I won't be as important to you as your other patients who do have MPD . . . I think I am trying hard to produce it . . . but I do not have it. . . . It's crazy even to want to have it, I know . . . but you wanted to know my fantasy . . . my fantasy has been to be special in any way I can . . . and having MPD would make me special. It would make me be somebody . . . but I'm nobody and I'm not connected inside or out . . . maybe I'm making that up too. No I'm not . . . I just want to feel good about me and I don't."

Clearly what a term means to the patient is more important than the therapist's preconception and understanding of the terms and what implications it may hold for the patient. In therapy, words are powerful symbols by which patients reveal their inner experience and reality.

The Second Level

At the next level of listening, the therapist considers those feelings the patient reveals through his or her use of language and nonverbal behavior. Words reveal how the person has structured his or her affective experience and to what extent feelings are consciously recognized or defensively avoided. The therapist's ongoing inquiry into the patients' feelings leads to a deeper exploration of meanings and associations. In the dance of empathy, the therapist uses his or her CTRs to understand the emotional experience of the patient. The emotional experience of patients with histories of childhood sexual abuse is conflicted, and it includes defended-against wishes, fantasies, and impulses. These patients may reveal feelings of shame, disgust, fear, and helplessness, as well as sexual arousal and longings for closeness. Understanding the complex constellation of feelings and their nuances requires that the therapist listen to the "music" and resonate with the deeper level of the patient's affective experience. The language used by the patient must be carefully considered as a symbolic reflection of his or her inner reality.

Case Example Five

   A 40-year-old patient who had amnesia for most of her childhood reported a series of repetitive nightmares she had first experienced at age 9. These dreams involves being chased by a monstrous figure whose features would become swollen and distorted. This patient rarely expressed emotion in therapy and was very intellectualized. The therapist noted the use of the following words in a therapy session as the patient associated to the meaning of the dream: desperate, boxed in, trapped, smothered, choking, consumed, threatened, fleeing. The therapist reflected the words and commented that they were very strong and powerful terms. The patient looked startled but then spontaneously reflected upon the emotions underlying her inner experience.

The Third Level

At the deepest level of listening, the therapist considers the patient's object relations and internalizations as revealed through the transference projections. We believe that the ongoing relatedness of patient to therapist is the most important indication of the internal structure of the patient. This level of listening involves the greatest degree of inference on the part of the therapist. The accuracy of the therapist's listening at this level is dependent on his or her awareness of countertransference feelings as they are activated in the therapeutic relationship. Patients with histories of early childhood sexual abuse will unconsciously reenact their earlier abusive relationships within the therapy relationship. These patients often experience other people as malevolent, untrustworthy, and overpowering (e.g., Westen, 1989). The therapist may be aware of wishes and fantasies toward the patient that are in some way complementary to the projections and projective identifications of the patient. In the dance of empathy, the therapist must pay attention to and monitor his or her feelings elicited in interactions with the patient. The therapist thus comes to "know" and understand the patient's object relations and transference projections through an awareness of his or her countertransference responses.

Case Example Six

Early in her treatment, a 34-year-old female patient with a history of verbal abuse and neglect by her father came to therapy session and immediately provoked the therapist by informing him that she did not want to talk about herself. The patient sat quietly for the next 20 minutes staring at a wall and playing with a piece of string in her hands. The therapist initially felt irritated and agitated, and then felt a strong pull to reprimand and demand that the patient tell him how she was feeling or why she was being provocative. Reflecting on his countertransference feelings the therapist noticed that this may have been exactly what the patient wanted him to feel. Now the therapist better understood what her experience had been like with her father. The therapist offered the following interpretation to the patient: "I wonder if your silence isn't a way to make me prod and poke at you to talk in a similar way that your father used to do to you?" The patient, feeling understood and "listened to" proceeded to freely express the feelings about her father whom she experienced as cruel, intrusive, and demanding.

Below, we describe the awareness of CTRs as the next "step" in understanding the patient's inner experience.

Step 2: Awareness of CTRs

In his work with Holocaust survivors Krystal (1984) said that therapy with traumatized patients is difficult at best. He states: "When dealing with individuals who have lived in a psychotic world and whose reality was beyond the scope of ordinary life and expectable environment . . . the therapist must be prepared to deal with extraordinary events, extraordinary ideas, and extraordinary feelings and responses on his or her own part" (p. 22).

As depicted in Figure 4.2 there is initially an impermeable boundary or significant psychological distance between the therapist and the patient. The therapist seeks to know and understand the patient initially by listening to the patient's words, feelings, and transference projections in an attempt to achieve an effective empathic stance. After listening to what the patient offers, the therapist then monitors his or her CTRs. In this way, the therapist comes to "know" and understand the patient's experience. It is the therapist's reaction to his or her feelings of countertransference that then determines the quality of the empathy. If the therapist resonates too closely with the patient's experience, he or she may react with a defensive withdrawal from the patient or an incorrect interpretation. The patient will consequently feel misunderstood, attacked, rejected, abandoned, violated, or otherwise retraumatized. The therapist's task is to use his or her CTRs to "listen" at a deeper level to the meanings underlying the patient's communications about his or her inner experience. The therapist thus monitors his or her own ongoing reactions, adjusts his or her empathic stance, and therefore moves closer to an understanding of the patient's inner experience.

In terms of the hermeneutic spiral, the boundary between the therapist and the patient must be permeable enough for empathy to develop so that the therapist can come to "know" and understand the patient. However, empathic strain (see Wilson & Lindy, Chapter 1, this volume) develops when the boundary between patient and therapist becomes too permeable. The following is a description of the types of CTRs that must be monitored by the therapist in order to maintain a maximally effective empathic stance.

Thoughts/Ideation

The therapist may be aware of spontaneous, intrusive thoughts or images about a patient or the material during or after the therapy session. As the boundary between the therapist and the patient becomes more permeable and the therapist moves closer to an understanding of the patient's experience, the therapist's spontaneous thoughts may occur as a prelude to further disclosures by the patient. As the empathic connection between the patient and the therapist deepens, the spontaneous ideation of the therapist may represent a parallel process with the patient.

Case Example Seven

A therapist in supervision reported being deeply engrossed in listening to a female patient speak about her deep feelings of shame and disgust about her body during sexual intercourse with her husband. The therapist then reported being aware of a spontaneous, intrusive image of a young child being anally penetrated by a man's finger. This ideation was initially shocking and repulsive to the therapist but the therapist understood it to mean that the patient was trying to communicate something important about her experience. The therapist, being aware of and monitoring her CTRs, commented to the patient that the patient appeared to be struggling with something that felt shameful and dirty. Moments later, the patient revealed for the first time a memory of being anally penetrated by her father at the age of 4 while he was giving her a bath, an experience that was both stimulating and frightening.

If the boundary between the therapist and the patient becomes too permeable, and the CTRs are not monitored, vicarious traumatization may result. As described earlier, the therapist may experience intrusive thoughts, trauma-related visual imagery, and reexperiencing phenomena.

Feelings and Visceral Reactions

Powerful affective experiences on the part of the therapist who works with traumatized patients have been well documented in the literature (e.g., Danieli, 1981; Lindy, 1988). These feelings include guilt, rage, dread, horror, grief, sadness, shame, and the inability to contain intense emotions. Likewise, powerful visceral reactions such as nausea, diarrhea, headaches, and other somatic reactions may be experienced by therapists who work with these patients. The emotional responses and visceral reactions on the part of the therapist, if monitored and understood, can be used to facilitate the correct empathic position and a deeper understanding of the patient's emotional experience. Patients with a history of early childhood trauma often grew up in an environment in which their emotional experience could not be shared, listened to, or understood within the context of a safe, empathic relationship. These patients often report growing up with caretakers who were oblivious to their deep feelings of sadness, shame, fear, loneliness, and anger. In families in which incest occurred, deep emotional experiences had to be denied and, at times, split off from conscious awareness. Patients who grew up in these unresponsive, emotionally neglectful environments may report the development a "false self" (Winnicott, 1965). Here the deeper self-experience was masked by an external appearance of happiness and well-being. In terms of the hermeneutic spiral, then, the therapist comes to "know" and understand the patient's experience first by listening, and then being aware of his or her emotional reactions to the patient. The patient, unconsciously, may need to know that the therapist will be able to "hold" and tolerate these painful emotions before he or she is able to consciously acknowledge these experiences.

Case Example Eight

A therapist reported being aware of intense feelings of rage coupled with abdominal distress in sessions with a patient who reported being sadistically abused by her father. The therapist was not aware of the activation of her own unresolved anger. In supervision, she began to understand that the patient, who presented as extremely passive, helpless, and childlike, was terrified of her own angry feelings. The therapist understood that the patient needed her to hold and tolerate these intolerable affects before she could acknowledge these feelings herself. The therapist did not prematurely interpret the patient's anger. Instead, the therapist used her CTRs to correctly empathize with the patient's terror of being killed should she express her rage. The patient gradually came to name her own emotional reactions and the therapist reported a decrease in her own rageful feelings during the sessions.

Fantasies, Dreams, and Other Symbolic CTRs

Therapists must be aware of fantasies, wishes, and dreams that emerge when they work with traumatized patients. Narcissistic wishes to be seen as "special," the only one who genuinely understands the patient, or the all-good, nurturing object are common Type II CTRs when working with these patients (see Chapter 2, this volume). In the case of therapists who themselves have an unresolved history of childhood abuse or neglect, an unconscious fantasy of undoing and/or transforming one's own traumatic history may be activated.

Sexual fantasies, voyeuristic impulses, and merger wishes may also be activated in work with these patients. The reality of eroticized or romanticized CTRs has long been recognized in psychoanalytic writings, with some authors suggesting that these reactions can be productively used by the therapist in long-term psychoanalytic therapy with deeply disturbed patients (Searles, 1959). In childhood development, early wishes and fantasies of being closed to, loved, and admired by a male (father) are in large part essential for females as they work through the developmental issues of relating to, loving, and being loved by a man (Horner, 1985b). In the case of father–daughter incest, infantile sexuality and oedipal wishes and fantasies are exacerbated, resulting in a tremendously ambivalent sense of power and shame in having won the father and destroyed the mother (Colletti & McCann, 1992). Some of these patients, then, may unconsciously seek to recapitulate or repeat these experiences in a relationship with a therapist who is unconsciously perceived as God-like and all-powerful. Likewise, homoerotic fantasies may emerge within the context of same-sex therapy relationships. Powerful wishes of the patient to merge with, be nurtured by, and protected by mother or father may activate strong, parental, loving feelings from the therapist. These complex transference and countertransference feelings pose potential hazards for both the therapist and the patient. The countertransference dilemma here is that the therapist may defensively move away from the patient and avoid exploring the patient's wishes and fantasies. These countertransference feelings are often conflictual for the therapist and therefore not readily acknowledged by him or her unless CTRs are carefully monitored in supervision (Courtois, 1988). At the same time, however, the therapist's awareness of and monitoring of these CTRs can be utilized to enhance effective empathy for the patient's experience and conflicted object world.

Countertransference Activation

If the therapist's CTRs are not modulated and worked through in personal therapy or supervision, a phenomenon we call *countertransference activation* may result. Countertransference activation is described here as the therapist breaking the frame of therapy in the service of his or her own countertransference feelings of protectiveness and security. This is an important CTR that we have observed in our own work with traumatized patients as well as in our supervision and consultation with colleagues. Countertransference activation is most likely to be an issue in work with individuals who appear to be directly threatened by a perpetrator in their current lives. For example, patients with a reported history of cult abuse who describe ongoing harassment and threats by cult members may activate powerful affective reactions on the part of the therapist. These CTRs may include strong maternal/paternal feelings of overprotectiveness, rescue fantasies, and intense fears about the patient's safety. One danger of unmonitored countertransference activation is that it compels the therapist to break the frame of therapy by becoming too active and over-involved in the patient's dilemma as opposed to being reflective and empathic with the patient's experience of being in danger.

Case Example Nine

A patient reported being harassed by telephone on a daily basis by cult members. This patient told her therapist that a "cult-created alter personality" was in danger of returning to the cult. These telephone calls, which presumably came in the middle of the night, were believed by the patient to be activating "programming" to return to the cult. The patient was overwhelmed by fear and terror because of her belief that she would be killed if she returned to the cult. The therapist consulted one of the authors of this paper after she had become "stuck" in her work with the patient. The therapist reported feeling fearful, distressed, helpless, and overwhelmed. She felt responsible for the patient's safety. She reported several experiences that represented a breakdown in boundaries between she and the patient. For example, the therapist agreed to be "on-call" 24 hours a day for crisis calls. Many of these calls occurred in the middle of the night and involved prolonged conversations in which the therapist tried to convince the various alter personalities not to respond to the cult members. On one occasion, the therapist agreed to meet the patient at her office late at night because the patient reported that she was in immediate danger of leaving her house and meeting with a cult member. The therapist was exhausted, depleted, and "burned out" in her work with this patient and was on the verge of terminating the therapeutic work.

The above case, although extreme, is not an uncommon example of Type II countertransference activation gone awry in therapists who work with patients who perceive themselves to be in danger. The powerful pulls on the therapist to be actively nurturing, helpful, supportive, and so forth impose an important therapeutic dilemma that needs to be openly addressed in the professional community. Too often, therapists may become overextended before they seek supervision and consultation because initially these responses appear to be supportive and helpful to the patient. Once overextended, therapists may feel ashamed at their overinvolvement with the case and thus avoid consultation for fear of their colleagues' disapproval. These types of countertransference dilemmas emphasize the need for ongoing supervision and support in working with these complex, difficult cases.

Clinical Case Analysis of Countertransference and Vicarious Traumatization

The following segment of a transcript is from a session with a female patient who reported severe early childhood trauma. The transcript will be explicated in terms of the hermeneutic conceptualization of countertransference, empathy, and understanding as described above. This transcript demonstrates how the case material produced intense CTRs and vicarious traumatization on the part of the therapist, which needed to be continually monitored in order to maintain effective empathy. Those shifts in empathy due to CTRs and vicarious traumatization will be highlighted.

The patient was a 27-year-old single woman who worked as a clerk in a department store. She had been in weekly psychotherapy with the first author of this chapter (ILM) for approximately 6 weeks. The patient had not been in treatment prior to the present time. For the first few sessions it was difficult to believe that the patient was even emotionally present. The patient came into the initial session in an extremely traumatized, regressed, frightened state. The patient was brought to the session by a friend who spoke for her. This woman shared pertinent aspects of the patient's history. Early on it was learned that the patient had regressed significantly over the past year as memories of severe, ritualistic childhood abuse began to emerge, and there was evidence of fragmented internal parts. The patient had been sadistically and ritually abused by her father from age 4 through 16, when the patient moved out of the house to live with an older, male friend of the family. It was not yet known whether this man had also used and exploited her sexually but it was known that the patient had been in a series of horrifying, abusive relationships with men over the course of her adult life. The patient had no previous therapy experience but had been in pastoral counseling at her church. Her friends now appeared to be in over their heads and had finally "insisted" that the patient be referred for psychotherapy. At the sixth session the patient presented herself in a childlike, regressed fashion She spoke in a childish, "sing-song" voice and sat curled up in a fetal position throughout the session. The annotated remarks include the therapist's comments on her CTRs throughout this session.

[I was aware of strong countertransference reactions as soon as I saw the patient sitting in the waiting room that day. Believing that the patient's father sexually, physically, and emotionally tortured and tormented her in a ritualistic way, I was aware of feeling enraged at what her father did to this child. I was aware that I blamed him for her current childlike, regressed, traumatized condition. I was also aware of maternal, protective feelings toward her, intermingled with rage. I felt like a mother lioness who is protecting her young.]

PATIENT: My daddy is coming home and he wants to see me. I told mommy I didn't want to see him. He said he was going to come up when I visit. I haven't seen him for 16 years.

THERAPIST (*gently*): I don't think it's a good idea for you to see him now.

P: One time he called and talked to me. He scared me. He threatened to come and get me.

T: He scared you very much. I don't think it's safe to see him now.

[I was aware of needing to step in quickly to provide support and containment. I was also aware of needing to lend her my ego. I was frightened for her and intensely aware of her extreme vulnerability. She seemed so childlike and unable to defend herself.]

P (*childlike voice*): Do you think he might be all better now?
T: No, I don't believe that.

[I was aware that I directly engaged with her here. I wanted to provide direct, realistic support. Somehow it seemed important to directly address the denial and to let her know that I was right there with her.]

P: I can hide my people [alters] inside if he comes.

[The patient clearly did not accept my offer of reality. She was still in denial and somehow I felt that this was dangerous for her now. I continued to feel concern for her safety.]

T: But they may be scared. He hurt you, he raped you. It's too soon to see him.

[Looking back on the transcript, I was surprised at how early I named the abuse in such straightforward language. However, I felt the need to pull her back for fear of her being hurt and possibly threatening our work early on. I was concerned that in her regressed, childlike state the patient could not see the implications of her choices or make appropriately self-protective judgments on her own behalf.]

P (*sing-song, chanting voice*): It's too soon, it's too soon. But he can't hurt you anymore.

T: He can't hurt you in the outside world but he can hurt you in the inside world.

P: I missed you. (*Starts talking gibberish.*) (*sing-song chanting*) You can't be scared, you can't cry, you have to be strong.

T: You can feel the feelings in here. You're safe now.

[I continued to be aware of a pervasive feeling of anger and horror at what this father must have done to this young woman to damage her to this extent. I was enraged and wanted to protect her, to keep her safe; these feelings for me are maternal and nurturing. I did not want her to see her father. I was more active at this point in the session, and I wanted to be clear in my responsibility to her. I felt encouraged that she appeared to be able to begin taking me in, establishing contact. Her statement that she missed me over the previous 2 weeks appeared to indicate the beginning of transference.]

P: (*Begins to vividly relive memory of ritual abuse.*) Blood on the wall. Baby hurts . . . it's dead. Poor baby. Someone killed the baby . . . I have pretty flowers in my bedroom.

[Here, the patient suddenly regurgitated bits of unconnected fragments of trauma. It felt a bit like she was vomiting the material from deep within her. It was gruesome, horrible material and I was aware of feeling sick in my stomach, a similar place as where the material seemed to come from in her. I realized my reaction and felt that I could stay with her through it.]

T: And the flowers comfort you now when you are in pain. It's safe here now. . . . I'm sorry for what happened to your baby.

[This appeared to be an empathic statement. I was trying to "be with her."]

P (*switching into adult voice*): Are you mad at me?

[This seemed to be a transference reaction. I believed that she may have told others in the past and their reaction was to become angry with her. I felt she was needing to test whether I was safe, or would I recapitulate what others had done to her?]

T: Why would you think I am mad at you?

[In rereading the transcript, I believe my reaction to her transference is due more to my own countertransference feelings than an attempt to maintain empathy. I was taken aback by the adult voice and "pulled away" from her momentarily. Asking her a question here did not acknowledge the immediate process but protected me from my own threatening feelings in response to her adult voice.]

P: For talking about my daddy.

T: You're afraid I'll be angry if you talk about him. . . . Your father hurt you. I feel angry at what he did to you when you were little but I'm not angry at you.

[Reacting to my own defensive pulling back from her, I was aware of wanting to say, "He did this to you, not me." I was aware of not wanting to be the object of her negative projections. This is a difficult countertransference reaction for me as it is painful to be experienced as the perpetrator.]

P: He'll kill me, hurt me.

T: If you tell?

[Ah ha, I felt now like I understood. Of course, she was terrified about having made this disclosure to me. She wanted to know whether I would be able to "hold" and "contain" it for her or whether she would be destroyed. I felt like I can stay with her here.]

P: Yes.

T: You're afraid that you told me the secret.

P: Yes. They will kill me. Mister hurt my baby, the knife, oh the knife. See the pretty candles. God will hate me for what I did. . . . (*a sudden shift*) Daddy didn't hurt me. He loved me, he was very good to me.

[The patient could not quite stay with the material. She needed to pull back and retreat to a defensive, primitive denial.]

T: It's painful to face what happened but your father hurt you. It's safe to talk about it now.

[Engaging here, I made an empathic statement acknowledging her pain. I was aware of wanting to give her support for continuing her disclosure. I wanted to validate her experience and somehow reduce the need for the defensive denial.]

P: (*Becomes very scared, starts speaking gibberish.*) The pipes, the pipes, oh my god. (*curled up, crying, reliving*)

[I was alarmed here. Did I come "too close"? I feared that she might move into a psychotic state. Internally, I wanted to say "Come back!" On the other hand, perhaps this was a reaction to my validation and a continuation of abreaction of prior traumatic experience and affects.]

T (*feeling like I had to pull her back, in a strong voice I say*): Try to stay connected to me, in here. You're safe now. When you see the pictures in your mind, try to put words to it.

P: In the basement, Daddy, pipes, tight. I hurt. Chains. Water. (*affect shift*) You be good, you can't cry. Don't say no. Don't tell Mommy.

T: Where was your mother?

[I was aware here of distancing somewhat by asking her a question about the context of the experience. Perhaps I could only take so much at this point.]

P: Home.

T: Does your mother know what happened to you when you were little?

P: Some things.

T: Does she know what your father did to you?

P: Yes, but she doesn't understand me, she doesn't want to believe me. Where was my mommy? She tried to kill herself. If I'm mad at my daddy, will God forgive me? Mommy tells me he's my dad, I should forgive him. Should I forgive him? Is God mad at me because I can't forgive him?

[I was aware again of being very angry and needing to feel the anger and protectiveness that her own mother did not feel for her. I was also outraged at whoever made her feel that God would not forgive her and that she was responsible.]

T: You're very angry at your father. What he did was wrong. You were just a little girl. He hurt you very badly. You still feel all the hurt inside.

P: (*major reliving*) He forced me to take a sleeping pill. Oooooh. My tummy hurts. (*childlike voice*) I didn't mean to go to the bathroom. He put me in the car, in the trunk of the car, and he locked me up. I was a bad girl. Bad girl, bad girl, I have to hurt you now.

[I was aware of feeling sick with the horror of it. She needed me to bear the horror for her. It felt like we were stepping into the abyss. I felt ready now, although one is never really ready. But I felt like I could stay with her. At the same time I felt the horror, I was aware of feelings of tenderness for her. She seemed so young, so vulnerable.]

P: He hurt my tummy, he put his penis in my mouth to teach me to listen. He went to the bathroom in my mouth. He put me on the circle rug and took a knife and made it hot and he stuck it into my tummy.

[My heart felt like it would break with the sadness of it. I thought to myself, "Oh God, it's going to be really bad. This is just the beginning. We've just stepped into the abyss."]

T (*soothing sounds*): It hurts, I know. I'm so sorry he hurt you like that. . . .
P: (*Begins to sob and sob.*)
T: I know, it hurts, you need to let it out, you're safe now.

This case example illustrates the need for continual awareness of and monitoring of countertransference feelings on the part of the therapist. As we have illustrated above, unresolved and unmonitored CTRs can result in either of two experiences for the therapist. Defensively, the therapist may move away from the patient's experience as a result of the empathic strain created by the CTR. Thus, the boundaries between the therapist and the patient may be too impermeable. In this case, the therapist may experience detachment, distance, emotional numbing, intellectualization, and a failure to deeply empathize with and understand the patient's experience. Likewise, as described above, too great an increase in the permeability of boundaries between the therapist and the patient may result in countertransference activation, overinvolvement with the patient's experience, and a breakdown in the frame of therapy. An inability to monitor CTRs, leading to empathic strain, will be experienced unconsciously by the patient and may lead the patient to act out, or to feel abandoned, misunderstood, or violated. In other words, the patient is retraumatized. As depicted in Figure 4.2, the dance of empathy occurs when these reactions are monitored in a way that increases the effective empathic stance toward the patient in which the therapist "moves with," but not too close to, the patient's experience.

Step 3: Monitoring of How CTRs Are Affecting Effective Empathic Stance toward the Patient

There will be an increased level of understanding of the material presented by the patient as the therapist corrects his or her empathic position.

The patient, feeling listened to, understood, and respected within a safely boundaried relationship, will begin to "take in" and ultimately internalize the correct empathy as offered by the therapist. This will often result in greater spontaneity and trust on the part of the patient in which further elaborations and details will be freely offered within the session. The patient will be able to move into areas of his or her experience that were previously too threatening to approach, and greater insight on the part of the patient will emerge.

As the empathic position is corrected through monitoring counter-transference feelings, the therapist's understanding of the patient's experience deepens. The permeability in the boundary between the therapist and the patient increases as the therapist comes to understand the complexity of the patient's object world. The quality of the therapeutic relationship is enhanced when the patient feels greater safety, containment, and analytic "holding." In the early phases of therapy, the traumatized patient is often vulnerable, frightened, overwhelmed, and needy. When a patient is acutely traumatized, as in the early phases of therapy or when traumatic material is beginning to emerge, patients may need tools for grounding and safety. Here, education and direct interventions, such as the use of "safe-place" imagery, may be helpful as the patient learns to internalize the empathy of the therapist and develop internal resources for affect tolerance and self-soothing (McCann & Pearlman, 1990a). When the dance of empathy is under way, the patient is able to safely approach threatening material with less anxiety. The patient feels less fear about "telling" or acknowledging what happened. Transference projections begin to be named and understood as recapitulations of earlier, abusive relationships. Now the patient's intolerable or unacceptable affects, wishes, impulses, and traumatic memories are able to be "contained" and thus looked at, "owned," and ultimately worked through. Uncontrolled flashbacks, intrusive ideation, nightmares, flooding, and self-destructive impulses decrease and the patient is better able to regulate the emergence of traumatic material both in and out of the session.

In essence, the patient is able to experience a sense of being "held" and understood. It is important to note that we distinguish analytic "holding" from literal holding. We encourage therapists to never engage in physical touch with patients because of the powerful, conflictual wishes and fantasies that may be activated. Within a broadly psychoanalytic perspective, we believe that patients feel "held" when they feel listened to, respected, and understood within a safely boundaried relationship. Analytic holding is distinct from more direct "nurturing" approaches, such as providing teddy bears, children's toys, and physical holding. One of the dangers of providing direct types of holding is that it encourages regression. We previously described that powerful wishes and fantasies to regress may be activated in the patient as he or she unconsciously seeks to enact these fantasies within the therapeutic relationship. The therapist may experience a resonance with the patient's experience, resulting in a pull to nurture, protect, support, or otherwise "reparent" the patient. These countertransference fantasies must be continually monitored so that regression is minimized for the patient.

Step 4: Completion of One Cycle of the Hermeneutic Spiral: The "Dance"

The therapist and the patient are now able to coordinate their moves and dance together. The dance of empathy involves a circular, reciprocal process of "being with," or moving closer, to the patient's experience and moving away from the material in order to maintain an appropriate empathic stance and level of understanding. The choreography of the dance is determined by the therapist's awareness and management of the countertransference.

The following transcript is a session in which a patient reflects on her reactions to a previous session in which she acknowledged and abreacted a previously disavowed memory of sexual abuse by a stranger in childhood. The exploration of this memory also activated the patient's fears that she may have been sexually abused by her father as well. Transferentially, this patient had also previously found it extremely difficult to acknowledge any angry or negative feelings toward the therapist, despite the fact that her words and feelings suggested profound ambivalence toward the therapist and difficulty establishing trust. The transcript will be annotated to include comments on the four-step process.

The Dance: Case of a Female with a History of Childhood Sexual Abuse

CLIENT: I'm mad . . . I don't want to talk today (*loud laughter*). (*long pause*)

THERAPIST: You're feeling very angry today.

[Step 1: Listening to the words and feelings]

C: I am. (*sadly*) I wish I could just take all my medicine tonight and get it over with but I can't, I have to work tomorrow.

T: It seems as if it doesn't feel safe to be angry in here.

[Step 1: Listening for the object relations]

C: I don't want to talk about that. (*louder voice, looking down at journal*) (*affect shift, softly*) I wish I could just quit thinking about it.

T: Uh huh.

C: I wish I could just take all my pills, every one . . . (*affect shift, louder*) but I can't do that, (*pause*) it just makes me so mad.

T: Mm.

C: (*long pause*) You know what, (*breaks down crying*) if this really happened, then all this stupid shit with my father must have happened too.

[Step 3: Moving into areas that were previously threatening]

T: It hurts a lot to believe that may have happened.

C: (*long sigh*) I just want to scream, I don't believe it.

T (*soothing*): Tell me about it. . . .

C: (*long sigh*) (*voice cracking with tears*) It goes so far back, that memory, 5 years ago, I had a damn flashback of being in the corner of that room, that winter, that man who put his hands between my legs . . . it's been so many years, it's all a memory, it's just a memory and I don't remember anymore but I think he breathed really funny, and it was really scary, and if that's real, all this other stuff may be (*long sigh*). That really hurts.

T: I know it does. . . .

C: (*long sigh, taking deep breaths*) I don't know what to do about this . . . (*sigh*)

T: You're feeling very hurt but you're also feeling very angry, a lot of confusing feelings today. . . .

[Step 1: Listening to the words and feelings]

C: (*affect shift*) Yeah, but mostly I'm mad at my mom and dad . . . bastard, I wish I could kick him you know where, yeah, I'd like to kick him there a million times until it would hurt bad enough, which supposedly it does. (*long releasing sigh*)

T: And very angry at me as well. . . .

[Step 1: Listening for the transference projections]

C (*blast of angry affect*): Yeah, because you're the one who brought it up . . . (*shift into a softer voice*) but you know, after we talked about the memory in our last session, I felt better, I felt older, and it wasn't bad, it was a good feeling, I wrote that to you, I felt like maybe I didn't have to feel so little next to people, like maybe I could be way up there too, grown up like.

T: Perhaps you've felt that in our relationship, that I'm way up here and you've felt little next to me. . . .

C (*softly*): Yeah, sometimes. . . . I mean you are, you're very wise and very sophisticated . . . and everything like that . . . it's not that you put me down, you never do, but sometimes that's just the way I feel (*sigh*) but you know, but you know, when we did the memory, it was like it was not so bad, cause I could just walk out of that room, like I was a woman, it's like, I don't know how to say it, but, it's like I was going to say I'm more complete, but I don't know how to explain that, except it's like, I'm more in control . . . before it was like I was a child terrified of these bits and pieces . . . (*strong voice*) but now it's like, I have looked at you, you son of a bitch, and I've seen what you did to the child that I was and I'm an adult and you'll never touch me again . . . and I feel older, I feel more my own age, probably, and I like it.

T: It feels good, feeling more like an adult, more your own age. . . .

C: It feels *very* good, yeah (*sigh*). It's almost like I don't have to be cute and vivacious every damn minute . . . and I know that sometimes, but it's like, it's like inside me, I don't have to be that way at all . . . I can be serious, if I'm tired I can be tired and that's a good feeling, yeah . . . so I guess something good has come out of it already . . . (*pause*) (*in a whisper*) I didn't want to come tonight (*sigh*).

T: Tell me more about that. . . .

[Step 2: Awareness of own CTRs: having previously monitored wish to be idealized by patient, therapist shows a willingness to genuinely listen to patient's conflicted experience within the therapy relationship]

C: Oh, I didn't want to come, I was mad at you, I didn't want to come, I was too tired, I resented having to come . . . but now it's good to talk with you . . . but I just, I wanted to hurt you (*pause*).

[Step 3: Increased insight on part of the patient about transference reaction and its relationship to the abuse]

T: Sure you did, it's understandable that at times you may experience me as your tormentor, bringing up these painful memories. . . .

C: How can you say that, I mean, that's so awful of me (*breaks down crying*), how can I feel that, you're so nice to me.

T: It doesn't mean that you don't also feel furious at me sometimes and that it's safe to talk about it in here. I imagine you may have wanted me to feel some of the hurt . . . to know how bad it feels. . . .

C: (*long sigh*) Yeah, awful. . . .

T: And can I really understand how deeply hurt you have been. . . .

C: Yeah, you can, you do . . . I mean I've wondered if you were abused . . . you've told me why you won't answer that before so you don't have to answer it . . . but you do understand, when you say, I know, and I know that you know and whether it's because of your work with other women or because you know because it happened to you, it doesn't matter, it's like, it feels nice, no nice is a shitty word, I feel comforted. . . .

[Step 4: The dance; patient reports comfort of feeling understood; therapist able to "be with" patient and understand patient's wish to make therapist understand by making the therapist hurt, to feel how deeply tormented patient feels]

This transcript illustrates the circular, reciprocal process of "being with" the patient's experience through listening and awareness and management of the therapist's countertransference. When an effective empathic stance was achieved, the patient was able to more freely acknowledge her ambivalent feelings and begin to work through threatening experiences.

CONCLUSION

As the dance of empathy unfolds and deepens, the patient is gradually able to experience the therapist as "being there" in a safe, constant way. Over time, the traumatized patient will be able to internalize the therapist, first as part object and later as whole object, and thus consolidate internal resources for tolerating and integrating strong, unacceptable affects and impulses. Thus, object constancy and the internalization of safe "whole" objects can begin to occur. This leads to a decrease in symptoms, and it signals the initiation of a therapeutic alliance. Now the patient can tolerate being alone without feeling distressed and anxious. As the patient begins to internalize the therapist as a whole object, the patient becomes less reliant on transitional objects for comfort and care and instead will begin to show an increased capacity for affect tolerance and self-soothing (McCann & Pearlman, 1990a).

In summary, this chapter explored and explained the importance of understanding and managing CTRs with persons who have experienced early childhood trauma. A psychoanalytic and hermeneutic conceptualization of the relationship between empathy, understanding, and countertransference was presented. This conceptual formulation explicates the intricate and complex process by which the therapist maintains a consistent empathic stance with patients who report horrific, vivid memories of childhood abuse. Through self-monitoring and an increased awareness of his or her internal experience within the therapy session, the therapist is able to more carefully modulate and utilize CTRs to "be with," understand, and empathize with the patient's experience. This process is metaphorically conceived of here as a choreographed dance in which the therapist and patient move forward together in a fluid but deliberate pattern of interaction. This "dance of empathy" is guided by the quality and consistency of the empathic responses as determined by the therapist's CTRs. It is from within this empathic position that the traumatized patient's tortured internal experience and object world can be known, understood, respected, and ultimately transformed.

REFERENCES

Atwood, G. E., & Stolorow, R. D. (1984). *Structures of subjectivity: Explorations in psychoanalytic phenomenology.* Hillsdale, NJ: Analytic Press.

Barker, R. G. (Ed.). (1963). *The stream of behavior: Explorations of its structure content.* New York: Appleton Century-Crofts.

Braun, B. G. (1984). Towards a theory of multiple personality and other dissociative phenomena. *Psychiatric Clinics of North America, 7*(1), 171–193.

Colletti, J., & McCann, I. L. (1992). *Oedipal issues in treating women who have experienced childhood incest.* Unpublished manuscript.

Courtois, C. A. (1988). *Healing the incest wound: Adult survivors in therapy.* New York: W. W. Norton.

Danieli, Y. (1981). Therapists' difficulties in treating survivors of the Nazi Holocaust and their children. *Dissertations Abstracts International, 42,* 4947-B.

Figley, C. R. (1983). Catastrophes: An overview of family reactions. In C. R. Figley & H. I. McCubbin (Eds.), *Stress and the family: Coping with catastrophe* (Vol. 2, pp. 3–20). New York: Brunner/Mazel.

Finell, J. S. (1986). The merits and problems with the concept of projective identification. *Psychoanalytic Review, 73*(Part II), 103–120.

Freud, S. (1910). Future prospects for psycho-analytic therapy. *Standard Edition, 1,* 141.

Ganzarain, R., & Buchele, B. (1986). Countertransference when incest is the problem. *International Journal of Group Psychotherapy, 36*(4), 549–567.

Haley, S. A. (1974). When the patient reports atrocities. *Archives of General Psychiatry, 30,* 191–196.

Heidegger, M. (1962). *Being and time.* New York: Harper & Row.

Herman, J. L. (1981). *Father–daughter incest.* Cambridge, MA: Harvard University Press.

Herman, J. L., Perry, C., & van der Kolk, B. A. (1989). Childhood trauma in borderline personality disorder. *American Journal of Psychiatry, 146*(4), 490–495.

Horner, A. J. (1985a). Principles for the therapist. In A. J. Horner (Ed.), *Treating the oedipal patient in brief psychotherapy* (pp. 75–86). New York: Jason Aronson.

Horner, A. J. (1985b). The oedipus complex. In A. J. Horner (Ed.), *Treating the oedipal patient in brief psychotherapy* (pp. 25–54). New York: Jason Aronson.

Kohut, H. (1971). *The analysis of self.* New York: International Universities Press.

Kohut, H. (1977). *The restoration of self.* New York: International Universities Press.

Krystal, H. (1984). Psychoanalytic views on human emotional damages. In B. van der Kolk (Ed.), *Post-traumatic stress disorder: Psychological and biological sequelae* (pp. 1–28). Washington, DC: American Psychiatric Press.

Langs, R. J. (1974). *Techniques of psychoanalytic psychotherapy: Vol. 2. The patient's responses to intervention, the patient–therapist relationship, the phases of psychotherapy.* Northvale, NJ: Jason Aronson.

Lindy, J. D. (1988). *Vietnam: A casebook.* New York: Brunner/Mazel.

Marcus, I. M. (1980). Countertransference and the psychoanalytic process in children and adolescents. *Psychoanalytic Study of the Child, 35,* 285–298.

McCann, I. L., & Pearlman, L. A. (1990a). *Psychological trauma and the adult survivor: Theory, therapy, and transformation.* New York: Brunner/Mazel.

McCann, I. L., & Pearlman, L. A. (1990b). Vicarious traumatization: A framework for understanding the psychological effects of working with victims. *Journal of Traumatic Stress, 3*(1), 131–149.

Mueller-Vollmer, K. (Ed.). (1989). *The hermeneutics reader.* New York: Continuum.

Palmer, R. E. (1969). *Hermeneutics: Interpretation and theory in Schleiermacher, Dithey, Heidegger, and Giadamer.* Evanston, IL: Northwestern University Press.

Parson, E. R. (1988). Post-traumatic self disorders (PTsfD): Theoretical and practical considerations in psychotherapy of Vietnam War veterans. In J. P. Wilson, Z. Harel, & B. Kahana (Eds.), *Human adaptation to extreme stress: From the Holocaust to Vietnam* (pp. 245–284). New York: Plenum Press.

Polkinghorne, D. (1983). *Methodology for the human sciences: Systems of inquiry.* Albany, NY: State University of New York Press.

Searles, H. (1959). Oedipal love in the countertransference. *International Journal of Psycho-Analysis, 40,* 180–190.

van der Kolk, B., Boyd, H., Krystal, J., & Greenberg, M. (1984). Post-traumatic stress disorder as a biologically based disorder: Implications of the animal shock model of inescapable shock. In B. van der Kolk (Ed.), *Post-traumatic stress disorder: Psychological and biological sequelae* (pp. 124–134). Washington, DC: American Psychiatric Press.

Westen, D. (1989). *Social cognition and object relations.* Unpublished manuscript.

Westen, D., Ludolph, P., Misle, B., Ruffins, S., & Block, J. (1990). Physical and sexual abuse in adolescent girls with borderline personality disorder. *American Journal of Orthopsychiatry, 60*(1), 55–66.

Winnicott, D. W. (1965). *The maturational process and the facilitating environment.* New York: International Universities Press.

5

Countertransference in the Treatment of Multiple Personality Disorder

RICHARD P. KLUFT

Dissociative defenses are closely associated with the experience of over-whelming trauma (Putnam, 1985; Spiegel, 1991). They allow the victim to segregate certain experiences, perceptions, reactions, and memories from others, and to do so in a relatively rule-bound manner (Spiegel, 1986a). They permit the traumatized individual both to detach himself or herself from the full impact of the trauma as it is occurring and to com-partmentalize the warded-off mental contents thereafter. Such attempts to sequester aspects or the entirety of a trauma and its impact may prove extremely useful in defending against the acute overwhelming event and may palliate its immediate effects. They may allow an individual to main-tain a sense of control (however defensive and illusory) during the trauma itself. However, this transient benefit may be more than overbalanced by the psychological sequelae (Spiegel, 1991). If what has been dissociated remains withheld from autobiographical memory, and if it is not pro-cessed and worked through, the short-term gain may be followed by undesirable long-term consequences, which may be described as second-ary loss (Kluft, 1990a). The person who cannot draw upon the full spec-trum of his or her past experiences in life to inform and guide subsequent behavior must make decisions on the basis of a flawed and incomplete data base (Fine, 1988, 1990; Kluft, 1990a). He or she may become vulnerable to revictimization and to entrapment in a vicious cycle of maladaptive responses and behaviors (Kluft, 1990b).

No condition better exemplifies these qualities of dissociation than multiple personality disorder (MPD) and those forms of dissociative disorder not otherwise specified (DDNOS) that most resemble it in form and function. MPD is increasingly appreciated to be a complex chronic post-traumatic dissociative disorder. Many of its features overlap with those of post-traumatic stress disorder (PTSD) per se. It is highly correlated with antecedent child abuse in Western civilization, but may more frequently follow other overwhelming childhood experiences in other cultures (Kluft, 1984b; F. W. Putnam, personal communication, May 1983). Surveys of contemporary North American MPD patients indicate that between 95.1 and 98% of the cases that were studied had indicated that they had suffered abuse during their childhoods (Coons, Bowman, & Milstein, 1989; Putnam, Guroff, Silberman, Barban, & Post, 1986; Ross, Norton, & Wozney, 1984; Schultz, Braun, & Kluft, 1989). A number of investigators have argued that MPD is a specialized form of the post-traumatic response that occurs in highly dissociation-prone children in response to overwhelming childhood experiences (Kluft, Steinberg, & Spitzer, 1988; Loewenstein, 1991; Spiegel, 1991). MPD and allied forms of DDNOS often are difficult to distinguish, because a given patient may fluctuate between manifesting the more overt phenomenology of MPD with the less distinct signs and symptoms of DDNOS (Kluft, 1985, 1991b), and because both respond to the same therapeutic approaches (Braun, 1986). Therefore, the full spectrum of such psychopathologies will hereafter be referred to as MPD.

MPD is an extreme and creative response to intolerable circumstances by a beleaguered child who can neither escape nor fend off the impact of external stressors. Instead he or she takes flight inwardly, creating alternate self-states, many of which endorse different perceptions of the significant persons and upsetting events in that child's life. Once such an adaptation becomes established, it can achieve and sustain a distressing secondary autonomy. A number of recent books and review articles offer excellent overviews of MPD (Kluft, 1991a; Kluft & Fine, 1993; Putnam, 1989; Ross, 1989).

By forming alternate identities, which often have differential access to particular memories, the traumatized individual develops specialized mental structures/entities, traditionally called personalities, that will respond differentially to particular types of situations and will retain specific types of memories from general awareness. The development of personalities and the definition of the concept of personalities have been the subjects of recent discussions (Kluft, 1991a, 1991b). The patient who develops such an adaptation thereby forestalls coming to terms with unpleasant circumstances, realizations, and affects, and he or she attempts to proceed more or less with "business as usual." This remains adaptive when one cannot take leave of a chronically abusive or overwhelming environment (i.e., the circumstances of an abused, dependent child in a dysfunctional family), but is profoundly maladaptive when it persists thereafter, and the traumatized person has forfeited the continuity and integrity of his or her own self and memory.

Elsewhere (Kluft, 1993), I have noted that the combination of different identifies with access to different memory banks and operating upon them with different rules of logic and cognitive distortions generates a virtual "multiple reality disorder" that supports the personalities' virtually delusional beliefs in their own realities and proves to be a major complication of the treatment process.

It is crucial for the student of post-traumatic stress to bear in mind that MPD and its treatment are distinguished from most other post-traumatic states by virtue of the number and variety of the traumata that were endured, by the extent of time over which they were inflicted, and by the nature of the relationship of the victim to the perpetrator or perpetrators (who are usually family members to whom complex ties, some of which are affectionate, persist). Schultz and her colleagues (Schultz et al., 1989, and unpublished research findings) demonstrated that the average MPD patient reports abuse within his or her family of origin over a 10-year period. An example of what I have termed "the mathematics of misery" (Kluft, 1994) may offer a useful insight. If a victim of father–daughter incest is violated twice a week, 50 weeks a year, for 10 years, then approximately 1,000 incestuous violations have occurred. Because a single such violation can lead to significant adult psychopathology (Kluft, 1990c), it should not surprise the student of post-traumatic stress that the average MPD patient suffers considerable misery, and his or her treatment poses many challenges to the clinician.

The purpose of this chapter will be to review relevant literature in the field, and then, by drawing my experience and my consultation with numerous others (Kluft, 1988a, 1988b, 1989a), to offer a discussion and classification of some of the difficulties that therapists encounter in their efforts to help this clinical population. Some thoughts on how to respond to these issues will be offered.

LITERATURE REVIEW AND GENERAL CONSIDERATIONS

Background

MPD itself remains a controversial diagnosis. Many prominent mental health professionals dismiss it from serious consideration, or regard it as an iatrogenic artifact. Among those who accept the legitimacy of the condition, some continue to insist that it is rare and hold that the recent explosion in the identification of contemporary cases represents over-diagnosis and/or misdiagnosis by credulous and/or enthusiastic clinicians. A review of the arguments surrounding iatrogenesis is beyond the scope of this chapter. Suffice it to say that there is, as of this writing, no evidence that full MPD can be induced iatrogenically, but there are data to demonstrate that many of its phenomena can be induced transiently under experimental or clinical circumstances (Kluft, 1991a). To reason that the transient enactment of an MPD role demonstrates the creation of the full condition would be analogous to arguing that because a subject under hypnosis can be induced to cluck like a chicken, he or she would thereby become eligible to be cooked for dinner. The interested reader is referred to the papers of the David Caul Memorial Symposium, which appeared in *Dissociation* in 1989 along with other relevant articles (Braun, 1989; Coons, 1989; Fine, 1989; Greaves, 1989; Kluft, 1989c; Ross, Norton, & Fraser, 1989; Torem, 1989).

This scientific controversy becomes relevant to the study of counter-transferential concerns because the clinician confronted with an MPD patient may be influenced, swayed, or simply confused by the controversy that surrounds the diagnosis, both within the privacy of his or her own thoughts, and in his or her professional community. Dell (1988) has studied the impact of professional skepticism about MPD on those who work with such patients. His distressing findings document "a very counterproductive and destructive emotional reactivity that all too frequently occurs when MPD patients and their therapists encounter disbelieving mental health professionals" (p. 530). Not infrequently clinicians avoid making the MPD diagnosis and/or decline to treat such patients out of concern for their professional reputation. Those who treat MPD may do so at the risk of the negative responses of colleagues; such apprehensions may color their therapeutic work.

Another pervasive background consideration relates to the traumatic pasts that MPD patients recount. Much remains unresolved with regard to what patients recount as memories. There remains considerable uncertainty about the historical accuracy of their allegations, and there is a sizeable scientific literature that attests to the malleability of human memory in response to post-event information and interventions. Such considerations are accentuated when hypnosis has been used in the retrieval of such information, or when the subject from whom information is received is highly hypnotizable. I have reviewed these controversies elsewhere (Kluft, 1992b). In summary, "Either to discount apparent recollections in a peremptory manner or to grant them automatic credence flies in the face of both clinical experience and the scientific literature" (p. 37). In work with MPD, "one must remain aware as well that material influenced by intrusive inquiry or iatrogenic dissociation (i.e., hypnosis) may be suspect to distortion. In a given patient, one may find episodes of photographic recall, confabulation, screen phenomena, confusion between dreams and fantasy and reality, irregular recollection, and willful misrepresentation. One awaits a goodness of fit among several forms of data, and often must be satisfied to remain uncertain" (Kluft, 1984b, pp. 13–14).

Therefore, the therapist working with MPD may have to contend with his or her own uncertainty about the historical veracity of what has been represented by the patient. Such uncertainty is very distressing to some clinicians; a minority become paralyzed by these concerns. This is usually not a major concern in the treatment of PTSD, in which the reality of the external stressor alleged to play an etiological role in the condition is rarely called into question. The more repugnant the patient's account, the greater is the pressure upon the therapist to disavow the allegations, and the greater the threat to the empathic connectedness within the therapist–patient dyad (Goodwin, 1985). A common outcome is the therapist's affective withdrawal from the patient (Kluft, 1991a).

Countertransference and MPD

I have (Kluft, 1984a) described the initial fascination and overinvestment that MPD patients often inspire and have observed that this often gives way to exasperation and exhaustion. Dealing with colleagues' skepticism frequently became a strain upon the therapist, and the variety of clinical skills required and the frequency of crises often caused the therapist to feel powerless and incapable—deskilled. I found that therapists were likely to experience MPD patients as demanding, intrusive, and manipulative, yet they found it difficult to set limits because they perceived the MPD patients as all too often alone, isolated, vulnerable, and overwhelmed by the materials that were emerging in therapy.

Furthermore, conscientious therapists found it hard to contend with patients whose personalities might abdicate or undermine the therapy, leaving the therapist to "carry" the treatment. My study indicated that MPD patients frequently tried to test, manipulate, and control the therapist, and, not infrequently, they behaved abusively toward him or her. An empathic strain is placed upon the therapist who must be empathic with the separate personalities' experiences of themselves, and retain an empathic connection across dissociative defenses in spite of the personalities' switching. I described the grueling pressure of empathizing with the experience of being brutalized, and discussed the frequency with which the confused and overwhelmed therapist may retreat to a skeptical and intellectual stance in which he or she, at a safe remove from the feelings of the patient, can ruminate over whether the personalities are real and their accounts of events are true.

In a later communication (Kluft, 1991a), I elaborated upon the ways that therapists retreat from optimal empathic involvement with MPD patients. There are four common patterns following upon the fascination and subsequent confusion and exasperation. In the first, there is withdrawal from empathic involvement to a detached, detective-like stance, in which the patient is overtly or covertly doubted or tested. In the second, the therapist comes to the conclusion that the MPD patient has been so badly harmed that nothing but tangible redress will cure him or her. The boundaries of therapy are abrogated in a rationalized attempt to "love the patient into health."

The third occurs when it seems clear (to the overwhelmed therapist, swamped by a sense of ineffectiveness that he or she may not be able to acknowledge and own) that action, rather than therapy, is in order. The therapist takes flight from the role in which he or she feels relatively powerless to assist the patient and becomes an advocate for the patient instead of the patient's healer. In the fourth, the transient trial identification of empathy is breached, and full counteridentification occurs. The therapist develops a variant of secondary PTSD and becomes devastated by his or her work with the patient's pain. If any of these stances appears in the therapist on more than a transient basis, consultation, supervision, and/or a return to therapy would be indicated.

I also (Kluft, 1989a) discussed the rehabilitation of therapists overwhelmed by their work with MPD, and addressed the plight of the "injured or wounded healers," the troubled therapists who may have had personal experiences of childhood mistreatment. Such therapists may, in treating MPD, be attempting to achieve a vicarious mastery of their own unresolved issues. Usually without conscious awareness, they project aspects of themselves upon the MPD patient, and they endeavor to treat themselves as well as the patient. They run the risk of becoming engulfed in the patient's pain, magnifying their own inner distress and turmoil. They may become symptomatic, or even decompensate.

Other works (Kluft, 1989b, 1990b) also explored the differential vulnerability of traumatized individuals with dissociative symptoms, including MPD, to seduction by their psychotherapists. In addition, I described behaviors by such patients that reenacted past sexualized scenarios in the treatment setting and noted their potential to lead to misadventures. In 1992, discussing a case of MPD in a special issue of *Psychoanalytic Inquiry* (Ross, 1992), I (Kluft, 1992a) elaborated the concept of selfobject countertransferences, in which the therapist perceives the MPD patient as a selfobject necessary to provide narcissistic equilibrium by responding to one's care and validating one's skill as a therapist (see also Putnam, 1989).

The collapse of such fantasies is nearly universal, and they damage patients and therapists alike. Also important are "scenario transferences," based not so much upon an object relationship as on a particular behavior during a traumatic scenario. This is similar to what Loewenstein (1993) has described in more detail as a "flashback transference."

Watkins and Watkins (1984) spoke of the hazards of treating MPD patients. They discussed the risks posed to the therapist by violent personalities, and noted "the more subtle possibilities by which an intelligent patient can frustrate the treatment and psychologically destroy the treating one" (p. 116). They described such patients' efforts to sexualize the treatment, their aggressive attacks on therapists, and their intense demandingness. They commented that therapists often had difficulty managing these situations.

Goodwin (1985) made a brilliant analysis of the tendency of psychotherapists to disbelieve their MPD patients: "Aspects of the physician's incredulity . . . are rooted in personal defenses against fear, guilt, and anger. Incredulity can be understood as an intellectualized variant of derealization; and, like the dissociative defenses, incredulity is an effective way to gain distance from terrifying realities" (p. 7). She argues that those who disbelieve such patients must do so in order to maintain their emotional homeostasis.

Coons (1986) surveyed 20 therapists, 19 of whom were treating their first patient with MPD. He found that the most frequent hindrances to therapy were overuse of repression and denial, excessive secrecy, and the production of numerous crises, to which the therapists responded with countertransferences of anger, exasperation, and emotional exhaustion.

Putnam (1989) noted and explored a number of situations that bespeak special countertransferential concerns. He described the confusion the therapist may encounter as he or she experiences different countertransferences to different personalities and the difficulty the therapist may have in responding to them. He found that many therapists struggle with concerns over "who is the patient?" They develop a loyalty to the personality that they identify as "the patient," and they have difficulty according equal consideration to the others. They may be confused, or feel betrayed, when the apparent usual personality proves to be a facade, disappears from the treatment, or is altered by the process of therapy. Such therapists implicitly are according particular personalities the status of real people. In fact, the real "personality" of an MPD patient is all of the personalities and their ways of interacting (Kluft, 1991a).

Putnam also described therapists' feeling of being overwhelmed by the sheer volume of the material and by their efforts to keep the accounts of the various personalities straight. They also feel profound pressures to be more "real" with MPD patients, and to abandon traditional, more technically neutral stances. There were pressures to violate the boundaries of the therapy. It often proves difficult both to be both more real and available and to preserve necessary boundaries.

Therapists also have difficulty with the flux and transitions in the personality systems of MPD. This is especially the case when therapists fail to perceive that the patient is the personality system as a whole rather than specific personalities. Furthermore, it is difficult to deal with the traumatic material. Not only is it difficult to hear and relate to, but when the patient experiences its pain anew in abreactions, the patient often berates the therapist for making him or her worse.

Putnam (1989) states that attempts to sexualize the therapy are not infrequent, and are usually undertaken by small groups of personalities that have particular motivations or are driven by unique experiences or concerns. Such efforts may be unwitting reenactments of past traumata, the testing of the therapist, attempts to control the therapist, or one of many other dynamics at work (reviewed by Dujovne, 1983; see also Kluft, 1989b, 1990b). Actual therapist–patient sexual exploitation is not uncommon in the histories of MPD patients (Kluft, 1990b; Putnam, 1989). Such events often follow in the wake of patients' requesting and being given (ostensibly) nonerotic touching and holding. These therapist behaviors are often associated with misguided attempts to reparent or provide a tangible corrective emotional experience to the patient. Putnam wisely suggests that all reparenting of MPD patients' personalities be undertaken within the system of personalities.

Putnam (1989) also observed that concern about colleagues' reactions was a major problem for those working with MPD patients. He discussed as well the problems posed for therapists when MPD patients treat their therapists in one or both of two polarized ways. In the first, the MPD patient pumps up the therapist's vanity in the service of his or her wish to have the perfect therapist, immune from all the failings of those who have hurt him or her in the past. The therapist may develop omnipotent grandiosity and believe he or she is as wondrous as the patient proposes.

In the second, the MPD patient "bad mouths" or publicly degrades the therapist, having projected upon him or her the negative polarized valences accorded to important transference objects, or to unfavorable aspects of self (either a split self representation or an alter whose characteristics other alters wish to disavow). The therapist's self-esteem may be deflated, and he or she may come to believe that he or she is indeed as faulty and lacking as the patient maintains. It is essential to bear in mind that both polarized attributions stem from split perceptions of crucial persons and of self representations in the patient's early life. When one such attitude is being voiced, the therapist can be sure that the other is also "in play."

Ross (1989) does not address the subject of countertransference explicitly. Instead he offers guidelines for approaching situations that other authors perceive as likely to provoke countertransferential responses.

Ogden (1992) encountered a number of experienced colleagues who had had severe difficulties maintaining appropriate boundaries in their work with MPD patients. In response, he wrote a passionate article warning colleagues against becoming entrapped in pathological relationships with them. He advises therapists to regard and respond to the personalities as constructions, rather than as actual persons. He points out that MPD patients have difficulty distinguishing between inner and outer reality, and this necessitates attention to and interpretation of their projective identifications. He describes "tyrannizing transferences" in which the patient expresses omnipotent wishes that the therapist respond to one or more particular personalities with "great deference and submission . . . due to the suffering it has endured. It is in the name of this self that these patients unconsciously impose tyranny upon their therapists" (p. 3). He warns against collusions with pressures toward transference enactments.

Recently Loewenstein (1993) has done an impressive review and extension of the literature on transference and countertransference with MPD patients. He describes the "traumatic transferences" of MPD patients, as earlier described by Kluft (1984a) and Spiegel (1986b), with their projection upon the therapist of hurtful intent, and he notes the difficulty therapists experience in being reacted to as if they were abusive and meant the patient ill. He also speaks of MPD patients' "flashback" perceptions of contemporary events, using the classifications proposed for PTSD by Blank (1985). He discusses the way they influence the perception of the therapist, leading to "flashback transferences" in which the therapist is perceived as a player in the reenactment of a particular abusive scenario. Furthermore, he discusses the implications of the MPD patient's high hypnotizability and dissociativity. A dissociative field develops between therapist and patient. The patient may experience trancelike and vividly enhanced phenomena that may lead to a very strong affective reactions in short order. Furthermore, the MPD patient is prone to processing materials with trance logic, that is, with the simultaneous acceptance and tolerance of mutually inconsistent and incompatible perceptions.

Materials

My observations are based on over 20 years of work with MPD patients, approximately 18 years of rendering consultations to therapists working with MPD patients, 11 years of directing a study group on MPD, extensive experience in addressing clinicians' concerns in workshops, and $4\frac{1}{2}$ years directing a specialized dissociative disorders program. In the course of acquiring this experience, I have talked to over a thousand clinicians about their experiences with and reactions to working with MPD patients. I have struggled successfully, with the help of Catherine G. Fine, PhD, David Fink, MD, and Eugene Boyd, RN, MSN, to recruit and retain a skilled staff for this program, mindful of the risks incurred of burnout and demoralization among staff members who spend many hours a day immersed in the complex, confusing, trauma-dominated, and the occasionally frankly "Twilight Zone-like" ambience of a dedicated dissociative disorders unit.

RECURRENT THEMES

I will try to offer a parsimonious classification of the types of countertransference issues that therapists recurrently encounter and express in their work with MPD patients. The following categories seem to encompass the predominant recurrent concerns:

1. Frustration/exasperation with the world of multiple reality disorder;
2. Frustration/exasperation with the patient's preoccupation with pain evasion;
3. Frustration/exasperation with the patient's preoccupation with controlling the therapist;
4. The price of empathy;
5. The rebuffing of the healer;
6. The loss of a sense of efficacy and the pressure to misguided repair;
7. The frequent absence of collegial appreciation for or validation of one's efforts; and
8. Feeling entrapped in reenactments of the patient's past with the discounting/invalidation of one's contemporary personal reality.

In sum, therapists frequently feel frustrated and/or exasperated by the patient's both conscious and unwitting efforts to recapitulate and repetitively reestablish the dissociative defenses in the therapy situation, are overwhelmed by the pain with which they must contend, and have a sense that their efforts are not appreciated by either their patients or their peers. In addition, they often feel powerless to bring about the desired therapeutic results.

Frustration/Exasperation with the World of Multiple Reality Disorder

A nurse new to work with MPD tried to set limits with a patient, only to have the patient switch into a lugubrious child personality that protested it should not be punished because another personality had committed the infraction. "What can I do?" the nurse asked. "That poor child doesn't seem to have been responsible."

A psychiatrist who was quite experienced with MPD struggled for months to help his depressed and highly suicidal patient abreact and work through her response to her murder of her abusive husband some decades before, only to find some time later that the man is alive and well. He barely can contain his aggravation and his feeling he has been duped. He wonders how to face the next session with his patient with some degree of professionalism and compassion for his patient.

A therapist finds that months of work to retrieve information across several reluctant personalities could have been saved had another personality been willing to share what it knew. However, that personality did not want the others to have the information and declined to involve itself in the therapy.

No sooner has one personality revealed abuse by the patient's mother, than another denies the abuse ever occurred and creates uncertainty in the first personality that made the revelation. As personalities refuse to work on any abuse recollections, maintaining they are not sure anything really occurred, therapy grinds to a halt.

Typical of severely abused populations are a fluid perception of reality and the willingness to supplant historical truth with more tolerable constructions that hold out the hope that one can ultimately have a positive view of the perpetuators of intrafamilial abuse and enjoy a good relationship with them (Shengold, 1979; Summit, 1983), and these characteristics are not restricted to MPD patients. However, MPD patients, with their dissociative and autohypnotic talents, can transmute intrapsychic defenses and wishes into simultaneously held, mutually exclusive versions or fantasies of events. The illusory versions may be perceived as equally compelling as those that actually transpired.

Not only will the "multiple realities" of the past, often with alternative scenarios encoded into the memory banks of different personalities, be brought into the therapy and projected into the transferences. The same defensive processes will be applied to the therapy and the relationship with the therapist. Unbeknownst to personality Maria, personality Joan had called and canceled a scheduled therapy session. When personality Maria arrived and found the session had been given to another patient, she was hurt. Personality Bill, who saw himself as the protector of Maria, became enraged and created a scene that disrupted the therapist's work with the patient then in his office. Furthermore, Bill declared the therapy was at an end. When Joan arrived at what she thought was her next appointment, a scene of equal complexity ensued. The therapist had great difficulty conveying that the patient was responsible for the actions of all parts of the mind.

Contending with such events once or twice usually will leave the therapist impressed with the power of dissociative defenses and the compelling nature of the alternate constructions of reality that the personalities embrace. It is easy to be empathic, or at least tolerant, due to the fascinating aspects of what is occurring.

However, as such events recur, the therapist may become upset, frustrated, angered, or exasperated, but may react with reaction formation or by accepting the patient's construction of reality and masochistically surrendering his or her own. More commonly, however, the anger reaches consciousness, and the therapist expresses his or her exasperation, irritation, or anger.

Clinical experience teaches that the therapist must remain outside of the patient's multiple reality disorder and maintain a more solid and stolid construction of events. The therapist must insist that the total human being, across all alters, accept responsibility for the actions of all alters, and he or she must build rules into the therapy that place the burden of maintaining alternate constructions upon the patient (Kluft, 1991a, 1993). Otherwise the therapist has allowed the patient to create within him or her the propensity for responding to stressors with alternative constructions of reality, or has given the patient implicit permission to make the therapist subject to endorsing such a situation. Such a therapist will be unable to help the patient extricate himself or herself from this type of morass.

The therapist must bear in mind that within the patient there are several ongoing threads of cognition, that what is unknown to the personality one is addressing is usually not completely unknown, but is an "elsewhere thought known," accessible through another aspect of the personality system. Therefore, the therapist may address the patient about what is alleged to be unknown, either asking the knowing parts to listen in, or attempting to access them—for example, saying "Let me talk to the part of the mind that brought the razor blades onto the unit."

Frustration/Exasperation with the Patient's Preoccupation with Pain Evasion

MPD patients are pain-phobic. The condition originates in the need to evade overwhelming pain, and this orientation continues to guide its function. Some personalities behave this way overtly, while other personalities are created that have vast powers of endurance, or who feel no pain. Some personalities are created just to serve as recipients of pain. In any case, the patient as a whole is usually involved in efforts to avoid allowing discomfort to be experienced by parts that are understood to require this type of protection. Profound autohypnotic maneuvers may be employed to effect this. Should those already in place be overwhelmed, a new personality may be formed to contain the overflow. Switching, virtual catatonia, flight (fugue), substance abuse, and self-inflicted injuries are aspects of this coping strategy. Manipulation, controlling behavior, lying, rationalizing strategic omissions of information, and telling misleading half-truths are also routinely encountered.

Most therapists react strongly to what appears to be an absence of motivation and a faulty work ethic. The MPD patient may appear unprincipled and irresponsible to the observer. Psychotherapy demands honesty in order to be successful. Psychotherapists' strengths reside in compassion and acceptance, not in skepticism and detective work. The therapeutic alliance is constructed upon candor, trust, hope, and identification with the work ego of the therapist. Therefore, we are often fooled and misled by our MPD patients, and we feel deeply betrayed and resentful when we realize that this has occurred. The patient often responds either by self-attack (designed to propitiate us by forestalling our anticipated attack), by attempts to represent the misrepresentation as essential and even wise in view of some other consideration, by further evasions, by counterattacks on what is perceived as the therapist's attack, or by portrayals of himself or herself as so piteous (usually accompanied by a switch to a terrified and/or weeping child alter) that only a sadist would press the confrontation. The therapist often feels a bewildering assortment of reactions and may find it difficult to remain focused on the therapeutic task. "Why," he or she may wonder (or mutter), "should I dedicate myself to the care of this impossible person who makes me work so hard, yet is unwilling to do his or her part in his or her own treatment?"

The therapist may struggle to contain his or her anger and exasperation, fearful lest therapy by disrupted by what might be said. The therapist may be unsure whether what occurs to him or her to say is a necessary confrontation or the venting of spleen. Very often the patient responds to the suppressed reactions, and the therapist must either deny his or her reaction, or concede. Neither is a useful position for the therapy. Conversely, the therapist may express exasperation, anger, and so forth, and the patient will often respond with a stance of wounded innocence or with a self-righteous counterattack.

Clinical experience suggests that it often is useful to track the sequence of what has been observed out loud to the patient and to indicate one's understanding of why the patient felt pressured to behave as he or she did. One then can reframe the patient's rationalized evasions as understandable in view of the universal human tendency to avoid experiencing pain, but as deleterious to the thrust of the therapy. Consultations and personal experience indicate that if such incidents are not identified and addressed, the therapist sooner or later will express his or her feeling state in a counterproductive manner. However, it is important not to "overdo" this injunction by such a repetitive focus on the patient's evasions that he or she feels incessantly criticized and that his or her efforts to contribute to the therapy are being repudiated. It is a rare MPD treatment that is not punctuated by episodes of mutual frustration and acrimony in connection with these types of situations.

Frustration/Exasperation with the Patient's Preoccupation with Controlling the Therapist

Many MPD patients survived by learning how to live "in the jaws of the tiger." Some parts of the mind identified with their abusers' behaviors. Some parts learned how to conduct themselves so as to control, as best they could, the behaviors of their actual and potential abusers. Furthermore, they have become accustomed, within their systems of personalities, to exploiting one another, punishing one another, shifting their pain to one another, and dominating and being dominated by one another. These three elements, which often are not mutually exclusive, predispose the MPD patient to enter the therapeutic dyad prepared to abuse, control (in any number of ways), or use the therapist (to fill a function or to serve as the receptacle of unwelcome or ego-dystonic feelings). The therapist recoils in response to such role assignments, attributions, and cycles of projective identification (see Ogden, 1979). He or she resents being misperceived, treated as an object, dealt with as if his or her feelings were of no consequence, and accorded only the reality that the patient is willing to assign. This may be tolerable when the patient accords the therapist an ego-syntonic designation—"You are a very special person. I don't think anyone could understand me/treat me as well as you do."—with implicit narcissistic aggrandizement. However, the patient giveth, and the patient taketh away—"You are completely insensitive and nasty. You keep saying it is transference, but you know, you really are a mean son of a bitch."

In essence, much as the relationship with the abuser was narcissistic, with the patient having been the extension of the abuser's desires and intentions, so may the patient experience himself or herself as being used by the therapist, and so may the patient treat the therapist in turn. Much as a trauma victim, the therapist comes to see that he or she has little or no impact upon the person who is acting upon him or her (Spiegel, 1991). When the therapist refuses to accept the role thrust upon him or her, the patient may redouble efforts to legitimize the attribution, usually by attributing to the therapist (by projective identification) some aspect of self or object representation, and then engaging in a provocative set of interpersonal behaviors that make therapist behavior consistent with the attribution more likely to occur. These are what Ogden (1992) referred to as the "tyrannizing transferences," each with its own tendency to promote in turn transference–countertransference reenactments.

The therapist almost inevitably is caught within some of these reenactments and the unconscious defenses and conscious coping strategies that are mobilized by the patient in connection with them. At times, so many constructions of the dyadic interaction are being experienced and reacted to by the patient, and their manifestations are impinging on the therapist with such complexity and rapidity, that some aspects, even the most crucial, may elude the recognition of the most alert and sapient clinician. While each is an extremely salient clinical communication and recounts important past experiences (an issue that will be discussed later), in the immediate moment the therapist may be deluged by an avalanche of material, all of which is valuable, but that, as an aggregate cognitive and affective overload, becomes confusing, assaultive, overwhelming, and unmanageable. Should he or she protest the misperception, misrepresentation, and/or the ablation of his or her self in the process of such activities, the therapist is seen as dishonest and deserving of further negative attributions. Had the therapist the patience of a saint, he or she would still react eventually. Most of us respond in shorter order to these attacks against the reality of our identities and selfhoods.

Clinical experience suggests that MPD patients respond unpredictably to confrontation, but that they do somewhat better when the therapist observes what the patient is doing, indicates the defensive purpose that is being served, and can state or reconstruct the pattern that is being reenacted. For example: "It might be that what I said earlier was so upsetting that you needed to convince yourself that it could not be true. By seeing me as a liar, a liar who means to hurt you, you can safely discount my earlier observations. You are reacting to me as if I were your father, who, you have said, would often make up false reasons to justify his beating you, and try to convince you that you had behaved as he said." Often the situation is best served by inviting the personalities to join the therapist in figuring out what incident or pattern is being recreated, but when the atmosphere has become tense and accusatory, such collaboration is unlikely. The therapist's ability to discern either the recurrence of a general pattern or the repetition of a specific scenario may be particularly difficult either early in the therapy, before the patient's trauma history has been elicited, or at any point in the treatment when a large number of alters is reacting simultaneously or in rapid succession.

The Price of Empathy

Vicki is a 37-year-old woman who was incested by her father and his three brothers, and by one of her own brothers. She was regularly beaten both by them and her mother. She was raped twice outside of her family, and she married an abusive, alcoholic man who mistreated her badly. She was sexually exploited by her employer and by a prior therapist.

The therapist pays a price for listening to this material empathically. Even with optimal transient trial identifications, the aggregate volume of the material is corrosive. Without appropriate distance, the therapist may become engulfed by the patient's misery and suffer vicarious or secondary post-traumatic stress. Even with appropriate distance, there will be moments at which the therapist may either suffer considerable pain, or beat an emotional retreat.

Should the therapist manage not to be swept up in the anguish of the patient's past, the patient's propensity for revictimization (Kluft, 1990a) may cause the therapist anguish. After the therapist has invested considerable effort in helping the patient find new ways of coping to avoid reincurring the hurts of the past, the patient's yearning to deny the abuse of the past and find happiness with someone who shares some qualities of the ambivalently perceived abusers from childhood will compel him or her to place himself or herself at risk again and again as the attempt to preserve or reinstate the multiple reality disorder proves too strong to resist.

At this point, however, the therapist may see the patient as the embodiment of his or her work, and thereby of his or her self. The therapist can be deeply affected by the patient's willingness to put what the therapist may perceive as an extension of the therapist's self at risk, and the therapist may experience severe distress, as if he or she had been traumatized. This experience of the patient as a selfobject has been discussed elsewhere (Kluft, 1992a).

In addition to suffering from the patient's suffering, the therapist may find it necessary to withdraw affectively from the patient, because the price of empathy is too intolerable. The therapist may disavow that this has occurred and provide unempathic therapy. However, the therapist may feel a sense of guilt, shame, and failure over his or her inability to "hang in there" with the patient. The shame may cause the therapist to avoid, misconstrue, or attack the patient, or to turn against himself or herself reproachfully (after Nathanson, 1992). Demoralization is not uncommon when the therapist begins to feel he or she has failed both the patient and his or her own ego-ideal.

Clinical experience suggests that the therapist who works in isolation is most vulnerable to such reactions. Conversely, those therapists who share their concerns and reactions with peers, who do not allow themselves to be alone with the traumatic material, and who engage in the gallows humor so common among those in the healing profession, tend to weather such storms.

The above remarks are relevant, but in the end less applicable to the recurrent crises and chronic suicidality that are characteristic of some MPD patients. It is difficult to remain empathically involved with that subgroup of MPD patients who recurrently place themselves at risk and in danger, and who flirt with self-destruction. Clinically, two stances seem to be held by successful therapists. In the first stance, crises and suicidality are responded to with vigor and alacrity, usually involving hospitalization or staying with a concerned other as alternatives. As is typical of all such preventively oriented interventions, the majority of them may prove, in retrospect, to have been unnecessary. In the second stance, the patient is given responsibility for his or her safety, and the therapist treats the patient in connection with whatever emerges.

These two stances both provide a predictable response to such episodes, and they both spare the therapist the prospect of recurrent agonizing over the possible consequences of the patient's behaviors. By building the response contingencies into the culture of the therapy, the therapist need not make anguishing decisions on an incident-by-incident basis and can better tolerate remaining connected to the patient. I myself favor the activist response. I will not be put in a position in which I will be overwhelmed by my concern for my patient's welfare or by my exasperation with his or her countertherapeutic activities. I and my patient know what action is to be taken under what circumstances, and I proceed accordingly. Putnam (1989) offers a useful discussion of the alternative stance, which is felt to be more empowering to the patient.

The Rebuffing of the Healer

One of the most frustrating aspects of treating MPD is the fact that one's efforts may not be appreciated throughout much of the therapy. Patients say such things as "I'm so miserable! Why don't you let me die?" "I was doing better before you messed things up by bringing up all of those traumas. Some therapist you are." A protector personality may say, "All you do is to cause her pain. You are as bad as her abusers!" One is often both overpraised and overcriticized, overinflated and deflated—at times one searches, often apparently in vain, for the patient's perception of the therapist's legitimate role, efforts, and accomplishments.

The patient continues to insist that the therapist is in fact abusive, or intends to be (the traumatic transference), and misperceives the therapist as if he or she were actually reabusing the patient as the patient (consciously or unconsciously) relives past events (the flashback transference). Furthermore such perceptions may be experienced as extremely vivid and compelling, and they may be processed by the patient without usual reality testing (aspects of the hypnotic or dissociative transference). For more detail, the reader may consult Kluft (1989b, 1990b, 1992a), Loewenstein (1993), and Spiegel (1991).

The therapist, who is prepared to face a considerable amount of negative transference in routine clinical work, still usually expects the patient to appreciate the "as if" nature of the transference, to understand that the therapist is trying his or her best to be helpful to the patient. All too often the therapist is confronted instead by an MPD patient's insisting loud, long, and to anyone who will listen that the therapist is indeed a nasty so and so. The therapist often will protest that he or she is being misperceived, only to be met by the patient's accusation that the therapist is attempting to deceive or gaslight the patient in a manner practiced by a past abuser. As Putnam (1989) has noted, the MPD patient's negative transferences may be played out on a very public stage, for example, "You said I am misinterpreting you, but I told my friends Trisha and Patti and Marie about what you said, and later Trisha told her therapist what you said and her therapist said that anyone who would say that should not be treating MPD."

Such events are often especially painful because the therapist may have extended himself or herself to a considerable extent to accommodate the treatment of the MPD patient. There is general consensus in the field that most therapists, sooner or later, will respond strongly to what must be considered the abuse and defamation of the therapist. Therefore, most therapists concur that it is useful to interdict excessive "therapist-bashing," acknowledging that many patients will respond by accusing the therapist of threatening them with adverse consequences for revealing the therapist's "abusive" behaviors.

Because so many MPD patients, especially those that are high functioning, appear to be so bright, perceptive, and sensitive to interpersonal nuances when such distortions of perception are not being held with ferocious tenacity, it is easy for even therapists quite experienced with MPD to be jarred and unsettled by such episodes. It is always useful to bear in mind that the MPD patient's reality-testing may be suspended or substantially impaired at certain points in time, notwithstanding the absence of a formal psychosis (Kluft, 1993).

I have found it helpful to demonstrate to the patient why the problematic behavior under consideration appears to be occurring at that particular point in time. Special attention is paid to the issues that this type of diversion may be protecting the patient from facing. I note experiences that the patient has had with being unfairly misrepresented and indicate that the repetition of this pattern toward me is unacceptable because it would tend to undermine the very treatment upon which the patient's safety and recovery so strongly depend.

For example, "You are accusing me of trying to humiliate you, and you feel you are entitled to humiliate me in turn. I suspect that something has come up that you cannot bring yourself to face, something that made you feel horrible about yourself. This flurry of accusations attempts to create in me the state of mind I suspect you are trying to avoid. It reminds me of how you said your mother kept shaming you to protect herself. I can't sit by and let you create an atmosphere between us that might harm our ability to work together. I won't help you shoot holes in your lifeboat. Can any part of the mind offer some insight into what you as a total person might be feeling a need to run away from?"

The Loss of a Sense of Efficacy and the Pressure to Misguided Repair

Often the therapist finds that his or her best efforts are ineffective and cannot attribute this to the patient's resistance. Some therapists suddenly find themselves confronted with MPD without having had adequate training in its management or treatment. Sometimes the therapist is strongly affiliated with a particular form of therapy or identified with a specific theoretical orientation. MPD does not conform to the ideas with which the therapist usually informs his or her practice, and it fails to respond to the types of interventions with which the therapist is familiar. The therapist may resent the patient for failing to respond in a way that validates the therapist's preferred modus operandi. Less frequently, therapists may become enraged at their training, their theories, and their discipline for "letting them down."

When the therapist goes to the literature on MPD, he or she may find that it is written in a strange vocabulary difficult to reconcile with the bulk of his or her knowledge, and that it advocates interventions involving unfamiliar techniques or modalities. It is easy to resent and to want to evade the apparent demands that one extend one's self to this degree. This reaction may be intensified if the MPD patient has begun to advise the therapist what to do to acquire the expertise necessary to treat MPD. This is an unfortunate tendency of a subgroup of MPD patients who have mastered the MPD literature in exhaustive detail, and who take it upon themselves to apprise the therapist of his or her shortcomings. The most distinguished and widely published experts in the field are not immune to the effects of such "helpful hints" upon their narcissistic vulnerabilities.

Even if the therapist makes efforts to acquire new knowledge and to master new techniques, the slow rate of improvement of MPD patients may make the therapist feel ineffective. In sum, it is not unusual for the person treating MPD to feel deskilled, impotent, and incompetent. It is not unusual for the MPD patient to "rub this in the therapist's face," either by overt insult or by what superficially appears to be solicitous empathy.

This may create an atmosphere in which the therapist may become masochistically self-effacing and/or angered at the patient. When confronted, the patient may protest with narcissistic entitlement that he/she deserves the best, and the therapist is derelict for not providing it. However, a large subgroup of MPD patients is protective of their neophyte therapists and is gratified that both therapist and patient are learning together. Unfortunately, this "togetherness" often leads to boundary difficulties. Under the aegis of "learning together," the therapist may forfeit his or her authority and therapeutic distance. For example, I have encountered many therapists who have brought their MPD patients with them to workshops and conferences.

Another group of countertransference errors is part of a large family of therapist misbehaviors in the face of their perceiving themselves to be therapeutically incompetent, or sensing that they lack the therapeutic tools with which to help the patient. Into the gap created by the self-perceived lack of skills and knowledge, the therapist may pour his or her person, attempting to love, gratify, support, and nurture against the day that he or she will be able to do an effective treatment. Numerous boundary violations are rationalized to defend the therapist against the perceived shame and guilt of being unable to offer effective psychotherapy. Such actions are never defensible, although for the overwhelmed therapist confronted with a desperate and voracious patient, they are all too easy to understand. Gestures made with the intention of offering comfort and support are all too easily subverted into the first steps toward a misalliance, a conspiracy to avoid the work of the treatment, or a seduction into the reenactment of a prior trauma, usually sexual exploitation.

There is a consensus in the field that if the neophyte acts promptly to acquire the necessary skills and expertises, it is possible to set the therapy back on course unless some egregious boundary violation has occurred. However, should the therapist spend more than a month or two in this type of quagmire, the therapy may come to a covert impasse that may not be appreciated for years. The therapist who finds that he or she is working or must work with an MPD patient should attempt to network with more experienced colleagues, seek out a workshop and/or a study group, obtain some relevant literature, and begin to learn about the disease and its treatment. I advise all who call me in such a state to obtain a good, recent review (Kluft, 1991a) and Putnam's (1989) classic text. I try to correct any fantasies that I will be able to convey the essence of the expertise necessary to treat MPD in a hurried telephone consultation or a casual interchange in the hospital cafeteria.

The literature is unanimous in stating that work with MPD is demanding and arduous, and that it requires the acquisition of specialized knowledge and skills. Therefore the therapist who holds to the stance that he or she can deal with MPD without such efforts is probably either threatened and/or terrified and trying to disavow this, or has been blessed with major narcissistic psychopathology.

The Frequent Absence of Collegial Appreciation for or Validation of the Therapist's Efforts

This discussion of common areas of countertransference difficulties would be incomplete without acknowledging that painful encounters with one's colleagues are often a significant aspect of the process of treating MPD. The therapist who becomes interested in MPD may not appreciate that in the early flush of his or her enthusiasm, he or she may try to interest other colleagues in MPD in a way that is likely to offend them or cause them concern. Even if this has not been a factor, one is likely to find colleagues inclined to warn one not to make too much of "this MPD thing," or prepared to make disparaging remarks when the patient must be hospitalized or engages in behaviors that draw the attention of the local mental health community. It is not uncommon for a few colleagues to distance themselves somewhat, to attenuate or interrupt their usual social discourse with the therapist.

The therapist may feel that his or her efforts on behalf of the patient are difficult and demanding, and that they should be respected if not admired. The therapist will understandably feel hurt, rejected, and angered when colleagues fail to accord such recognition. He or she may even make efforts to make it clear to such colleagues that they too may have such patients, unrecognized, in their practices. Also, such therapists may try to share their excitement and perplexity as a matter of clinical interest or in order to seek other's ideas and feedback. The outcome is usually ungratifying.

Clinical experience indicates that the therapist will only diminish his or her credibility by such endeavors. I have always found it useful to simply do good clinical work in silence, communicating about MPD only with those colleagues who clearly share (or at least tolerate) my interest.

The very fact of my working with such patients raises others' levels of awareness, and gradually more and more colleagues raise the subject themselves. This approach may be difficult or ungratifying for the professional who thrives upon or requires the positive feedback of his or her colleagues, but the pain of being rebuffed is a greater burden than the constraints advised above.

Feeling Entrapped in Reenactments of the Patient's Past with the Discounting/Invalidation of One's Contemporary Personal Reality

I have noted above that the intensity of the MPD patient's involvement in the recreation of the past in the present may so discount the therapist's genuine reality that the therapist responds to this threat to his or her identity with protest, hurt, and resentment. The MPD patient often has difficulty distinguishing inner and outer reality. Not only is the therapist the recipient of myriad transferences, he or she is the target of a variety of projective identifications (well discussed in Ogden, 1979, and Peebles-Kleiger, 1989). A unique subgroup of these projective identifications concerns the implicit acknowledgment of the presence of previously unsuspected alters, especially those that take a hostile stance toward those alters most characteristic of the patient, by attributing their qualities to the therapist. These can be among the most difficult types of distorted perception to address in treatment, because they are based upon information that has not yet entered the therapy. They often provide a troubling undercurrent in the treatment of the MPD patient and lead to an uneasy mistrust between therapist and patient. No matter what the therapist says or does, he or she always feels misperceived and invalidated, behaves defensively, tentatively, and at times with annoyance and irritability toward the patient, who is resented for his or her apparent unwillingness to see the therapist as he or she really is.

PREVENTION AND TREATMENT OF COUNTERTRANSFERENCE COMPLICATIONS

The treatment of MPD is difficult, but is not beyond the abilities of the competent clinician who is willing to grow and learn. The most consistent finding in my consultation experience is that it is the isolated therapist who has the most difficulties. The therapist who regularly discusses problems in patient care is likely to emerge from his or her work with MPD intact and enhanced. Because the field is still in its early stages of development, it is important to keep abreast of the literature. Most of the techniques widely discussed in the MPD field as of this writing were only published in the last 5 years. The therapist has to be willing to keep current. Recent findings have allowed the promulgation of several rules and principles of successful therapy with MPD patients (Kluft, 1991a, 1993). If these are followed scrupulously, it is likely that major countertransference difficulties can be recognized and addressed within a reasonable period of time, and the valuable lessons that countertransference manifestations have to teach the therapist will have a reasonable chance of being appreciated.

Equally if not more important is the importance of collegial discussion. In 1979, Bennett G. Braun, MD, and I were introduced by Cornelia B. Wilbur, MD, and Ralph Allison, MD. As we discussed our concerns about treatment we found that each had good advice to offer the other. We began an informal "buddy system" of ongoing telephone support and consultation that has lasted for over a decade. I strongly advise that therapists working with MPD patients find colleagues who are also involved, or at least interested, and get together to discuss treatment issues. One does not have to be an expert to sense that something is amiss. Often identifying the existence of the problem is the key to its resolution.

The proliferation of study groups throughout the United States makes it possible for therapists in many areas to get together for the purpose of learning about MPD. Participation is strongly advised. Once a therapist raises an issue in a study group and receives the feedback of peers, he or she has transmuted a problem into a communication and a request for help. It may be more possible to appreciate the nature of the communication from the patient to which the therapist is responding, and thus to comprehend the therapist's implicit understanding of the patient's communication that is implied by his or her countertransference responses.

Formal consultation or supervision may be quite useful, but due to the relatively small number of true experts, and the financial obligations that may be involved with obtaining their services, this option may not be available to many clinicians. On occasion, the therapist's responses to the MPD patient may be quite severe, difficult to understand, or unresponsive to the measures advocated above. In such instances, it may be necessary to consider therapy for the therapist or the transfer of the MPD patient.

Special circumstances surround the situation of nurses and psychiatric technicians who do intensive inpatient work with MPD patients in specialized units. Catherine G. Fine, PhD, has pioneered the use of weekly secondary PTSD prevention groups at the Dissociative Disorders Program at The Institute of Pennsylvania Hospital. Participation in these groups is voluntary. Ventilation and exploration of reactions to MPD patients' behaviors, memories, and concerns is encouraged. We have found that those staff members who attend these groups regularly have fewer countertransference difficulties, manifestations of fatigue, and periodic burnout than those who do not.

The Countertransference Response as an Unwitting Act of Reconstruction, or Countertransference as the Recovery of Implicit History

The patient is an attractive woman with a mercurial temperament and a quick, sarcastic tongue. She has been berating me for over 20 minutes. Her volume has slowly risen from unpleasantly loud to intolerable, and her tone from vitriolic to insufferable. My sin *du jour* appears to be that I did not immediately agree with and validate her account of an abusive experience some 35 years ago. The situation is complicated by the fact that another alter has given an account of the same event that is not compatible with what has been told to me in the current session. I find myself irritated, demoralized, wishing I were somewhere else, and wanting to tell a certain sympathetic person about this nightmare of a session and get a great deal of sympathy from her. Perhaps she will say something critical about the patient, which will be my invitation to unleash a tremendous amount of hurt and rage, which is increasing by the moment.

I pull back from my withdrawal and abandon this gratifying reverie. The patient is eulogizing a prior therapist in comparison to me. She rues the day that she entered my care. Somewhere in the back of my mind a thought is forming, but I cannot grasp it as of yet. The tirade continues. I find myself wondering what it would be like to trash the patient as she is trashing me. I sense the thought nearing.

"You are telling me something not only about how badly you feel I have betrayed you by not offering to believe you at once, but also about something else as well. Can we take a look across all parts of your mind and see what else might be behind the intensity of your response?" The patient protests vigorously, and sees my answer as evasive. However, in a few moments she looks shocked, and says she has heard, within her head, the voice of another personality, which said, "Kluft is right. We never trusted him so much that it would be a big shock if he let us down." She pauses, and then becomes tearful.

"I didn't want to remember this, but you know that doctor I always tell you you should be like? After I moved and began with another therapist, my mother called him for some reason. My talking about being abused as a child came up, and he said that he did not believe what I told him. I really was fond of him, and I couldn't handle hearing that. I blocked it out and I haven't thought about it since. I wonder how much else I don't remember, but I blame on you." I let that implicit apology slide by, and wondered aloud if the therapist and her mother had commiserated about how difficult they found it to believe her, to deal with her. She looked taken aback, but went on to say that they had, apparently at some length. The session continued, with her grieving the loss of the idealized image of the previous therapist and finally contacting her anger at him. She fulminated about her mother. I wondered if this hidden memory also could cast some light on her then inexplicable sense of having been betrayed by a female colleague to whom I had sent her in consultation, and her certainty that the two of us had ridiculed her behind her back. As she left, she smiled, and said, "That doesn't mean you are off the hook for being an insensitive, uncaring son of a bitch." In the next session she said that she thought her rage at the woman consultant might have some connection with the recovered incident, and we worked on this theme.

At times our countertransference responses reveal aspects of the patient's history and dynamics that have not yet become apparent. I wanted to betray my patient's confidentiality and call her veracity into question. Somehow, she had told me her story in a way that made me, without being aware of this experience, wish to reenact it with her. My countertransference constituted an unwitting reconstruction, an implicit recognition of her unspoken history. Luckily, I recognized it as a communication, and used it to inform my interventions. Unfortunately, however, all too often with MPD patients, such communications are so complex, coded, fragmentary, and obscure, that I only realize in retrospect that such a communication had been made, but that I had missed it or reacted in response to it rather than having been able to recognize it and use it in the patient's best interests.

The more the therapist is sensitized to the use of countertransference experiences as clues to events and scenarios in the patient's past, the more he or she will be able to welcome such experiences for their informational value.

GAINS AND LOSSES TO THE THERAPIST
FROM TREATING MPD

In numerous workshop settings, Bennett G. Braun, MD, has remarked, "After you treat MPD, you will never be the same." In general, those who work with MPD report a sense of a loss of innocence and a challenge to the benign and optimistic assumptions that had guided their lives and given them a sense of security. They become sensitized to the darker side of life, the appalling frequency of child abuse, and the ongoing pain of human life. Many find that they no longer can enjoy intense, serious drama, because it reminds them of being at work. I myself have noticed this and observed myself feeling compelled to select either comedy or action films for diversion. A small percentage of therapists appear to get "hooked" on trauma work and to find the treatment of other patient groups relatively uninteresting and unrewarding. One such colleague recently told me, "I'm sorry, but I have begun to find my other patients' problems trivial by comparison."

Conversely, many therapists report that their work with MPD has been a profound therapeutic education that has enriched their therapeutic expertise with other patient groups. This has been my experience. Specifically, they point to greater expertise at keeping therapy focused, making compassionate confrontations, offering necessary support, pacing treatment so that the patient is not overwhelmed, avoiding intellectualizations, managing abreactions, controlling flashbacks, halting regressions that are not in the service of the ego, identifying transference and countertransference manifestations, and, by using their countertransference feelings as a source of information, being better able to guide their understanding and their interventions.

Along with the negative awarenesses noted above, many therapists report that they feel they have attained an enhanced ability to cherish the positive and the good in life and to appreciate each moment with greater intensity and involvement, and they have come to have a greater understanding of the remarkable resilience of the human spirit. They state that they feel more confident that the traumatized can indeed improve, and that this allows them to approach all of their patients with more optimism and hope. Most believe that their increased optimism and hope is appreciated by their patients and has a positive impact upon their therapeutic progress.

REFERENCES

Blank, A. S. (1985). The unconscious flashback to the war in Viet Nam veterans: Clinical mystery, legal defense, and community problem. In S. M. Sonnenberg, A. S. Blank, & J. A. Talbott (Eds.), *The trauma of war: Stress and recovery in Viet Nam veterans* (pp. 293–308). Washington, DC: American Psychiatric Press.

Braun, B. G. (1986). Issues in the psychotherapy of multiple personality disorder. In B. G. Braun (Ed.), *Treatment of multiple personality disorder* (pp. 1–29). Washington, DC: American Psychiatric Press.

Braun, B. G. (1989). Iatrophilia and iatrophobia in the diagnosis and treatment of MPD. *Dissociation, 2,* 66–70.

Coons, P. M. (1986). Treatment progress in 20 patients with multiple personality disorder. *Journal of Nervous and Mental Disease, 174,* 715–721.

Coons, P. M. (1989). Iatrogenic factors in the misdiagnosis of MPD. *Dissociation, 2*, 70–76.

Coons, P. M., Bowman, L., & Milstein, V. (1989). Multiple personality disorder: A clinical investigation of 50 cases. *Journal of Nervous and Mental Disease, 176*, 519–527.

Dell, P. F. (1988). Professional skepticism about multiple personality. *Journal of Nervous and Mental Disease, 176*, 528–531.

Dujovne, B. (1983). Sexual feelings, fantasies, and acting-out in psychotherapy. *Psychotherapy: Theory, Research and Practice, 20*, 243–250.

Fine, C. G. (1988). Thoughts on the cognitive perceptual substrates of multiple personality disorder. *Dissociation, 1*(4), 5–11.

Fine, C. G. (1989). Therapeutic errors and iatrogenesis across therapeutic modalities in MPD and allied dissociative disorders. *Dissociation, 2*, 77–82.

Fine, C. G. (1990). The cognitive sequelae of incest. In R. P. Kluft (Ed.), *Incest-related syndromes of adult psychopathology* (pp. 161–182). Washington, DC: American Psychiatric Press.

Goodwin, J. M. (1985). Credibility problems in multiple personality disorder patients and abused children. In R. P. Kluft (Ed.), *Childhood antecedents of multiple personality* (pp. 1–19). Washington, DC: American Psychiatric Press.

Greaves, G. B. (1989). Observations on the claim of iatrogenesis in the promulgation of MPD: A discussion. *Dissociation, 2*, 99–104.

Kluft, R. P. (1984a). Aspects of the treatment of multiple personality disorder. *Psychiatric Annals, 14*, 51–55.

Kluft, R. P. (1984b). Treatment of multiple personality disorder: A study of 33 cases. *Psychiatric Clinics of North America, 7*, 9–29.

Kluft, R. P. (1985). The natural history of multiple personal disorder. In R. P. Kluft (Ed.), *Childhood antecedents of multiple personality* (pp. 197–238). Washington, DC: American Psychiatric Press.

Kluft, R. P. (1988a). On giving consultations to therapists treating MPD: Fifteen years' experience—Part 1. (Diagnosis and treatment). *Dissociation, 1*(3), 23–29.

Kluft, R. P. (1988b). On giving consultations to therapists treating MPD: Fifteen years' experience—Part 2. (The 'surround' of treatment, forensics, hypnosis, patient-initiated requests). *Dissociation, 1*(3), 30–35.

Kluft, R. P. (1989a). The rehabilitation of therapists overwhelmed by their work with multiple personality disorder patients. *Dissociation, 2*, 244–250.

Kluft, R. P. (1989b). Treating the patient who has been exploited by a previous psychotherapist. *Psychiatric Clinics of North America, 12*, 483–500.

Kluft, R. P. (1989c). Iatrogenic creation of new alter personalities. *Dissociation, 2*, 83–91.

Kluft, R. P. (1990a). Dissociation and subsequent vulnerability: A preliminary study. *Dissociation, 3*, 167–173.

Kluft, R. P. (1990b). Incest and subsequent revictimization: The case of therapist–patient sexual exploitation, with a description of the sitting-duck syndrome. In R. P. Kluft (Ed.), *Incest-related syndromes of adult psychopathology* (pp. 263–288). Washington, DC: American Psychiatric Press.

Kluft, R. P. (Ed.), (1990c). *Incest-related syndromes of adult psychopathology.* Washington, DC: American Psychiatric Press.

Kluft, R. P. (1991a). Multiple personality disorder. In A. Tasman & S. M. Goldfinger (Eds.), *American Psychiatric Press review of psychiatry* (Vol. 10, pp. 161–188). Washington, DC: American Psychiatric Press.

Kluft, R. P. (1991b). Clinical presentations of multiple personality disorder. *Psychiatric Clinics of North America, 14,* 605–630.

Kluft, R. P. (1992a). Discussion: A specialist's perspective on multiple personality disorder. *Psychoanalytic Inquiry, 12,* 139–172.

Kluft, R. P. (1992b). The use of hypnosis with dissociative disorders. *Psychiatric Medicine, 10,* 31–46.

Kluft, R. P. (1993). Basic principles in conducting the psychotherapy of multiple personality disorder. In R. P. Kluft & C. G. Fine (Eds.), *Clinical perspectives on multiple personality disorder* (pp. 19–50). Washington, DC: American Psychiatric Press.

Kluft, R. P. (1994). Dissociative disorders. In M. Herson, R. T. Ammerman, & L. Sisson (Eds.), *Handbook of aggressive and destructive behavior in psychiatric patients.* New York: Plenum Press.

Kluft, R. P., & Fine, C. G. (Eds.). (1993). *Clinical perspectives on multiple personality disorder.* Washington, DC: American Psychiatric Press.

Kluft, R. P., Steinberg, M., & Spitzer, R. L. (1988). DSM-III-R revisions in the dissociative disorders: An exploration of their derivation and rationale. *Dissociation, 1*(1), 39–47.

Loewenstein, R. J. (1991). An office mental status examination for complex chronic dissociative symptoms and multiple personality disorder. *Psychiatric Clinics of North America, 14,* 567–604.

Loewenstein, R. J. (1993). Posttraumatic and dissociative aspects of transference and countertransference in the treatment of multiple personality disorder. In R. P. Kluft & C. G. Fine (Eds.), *Clinical perspectives on multiple personality disorder* (pp. 51–85). Washington, DC: American Psychiatric Press.

Nathanson, D. L. (1992). *Shame and pride: Affect, sex, and the birth of the self.* New York: W. W. Norton.

Ogden, T. H. (1979). On projective identification. *International Journal of Psycho-Analysis, 61,* 439–451.

Ogden, T. H. (1992). Consultation is often needed when treating severe dissociative disorders. *Psychodynamic Letter, 1*(10), 1–4.

Peebles-Kleiger, M. J. (1989). Using countertransference in the hypnosis of trauma victims: A model for turning hazard into healing. *American Journal of Psychotherapy, 48,* 518–530.

Putnam, F. W. (1985). Dissociation as a response to extreme trauma. In R. P. Kluft (Ed.), *Childhood antecedents of multiple personality* (pp. 65–98). Washington, DC: American Psychiatric Press.

Putnam, F. W. (1989). *Diagnosis and treatment of multiple personality disorder.* New York: Guilford Press.

Putnam, F. W., Guroff, J. J., Silberman, E. K., Barban, L., & Post, R. M. (1986). The clinical phenomenology of multiple personality disorder: Review of 100 recent cases. *Journal of Clinical Psychiatry, 47,* 285–293.

Ross, C. A. (1989). *Multiple personality disorder: Diagnosis, clinical features, and treatment.* New York: Wiley.

Ross, D. R. (Ed.). (1992). Viewpoints on multiple personality disorder. *Psychoanalytic Inquiry, 12,* 1–171.

Ross, C. A., Norton, G. R., & Fraser, G. A. (1989). Evidence against the iatrogenesis of multiple personality disorder. *Dissociation, 2,* 61–65.

Ross, C. A., Norton, G. R., & Wozney, K. (1989). Multiple personality disorder: An analysis of 236 cases. *Canadian Journal of Psychiatry, 34,* 413–418.

Schultz, R., Braun, B. G., & Kluft, R. P. (1989). Multiple personality disorder: Phenomenology of selected variables in comparison with major depression. *Dissociation, 2,* 45–51.

Shengold, L. L. (1979). Child abuse and deprivation: Soul murder. *Journal of the American Psychiatric Association, 27,* 533–559.

Spiegel, D. (1986a). Dissociating damage. *American Journal of Clinical Hypnosis, 29,* 123–131.

Spiegel, D. (1986b). Dissociation, double binds, and posttraumatic stress in multiple personality disorder. In B. G. Braun (Ed.), *Treatment of multiple personality disorder* (pp. 1–29). Washington, DC: American Psychiatric Press.

Spiegel, D. (1991). Dissociation and trauma. In A. Tasman & S. M. Goldfinger (Eds.), *American Psychiatric Press review of psychiatry* (Vol. 10, pp. 261–276). Washington, DC: American Psychiatric Press.

Summit, R. C. (1983). The child sexual abuse accommodation syndrome. *Journal of Child Abuse and Neglect, 7,* 177–193.

Torem, M. (1989). Iatrogenic factors in the perpetuation of splitting and multiplicity. *Dissociation, 2,* 92–98.

Watkins, J. G., & Watkins, H. H. (1984). Hazards to the therapist in the treatment of multiple personalities. *Psychiatric Clinics of North America, 7,* 111–119.

6

Inner City Children of Trauma: Urban Violence Traumatic Stress Response Syndrome (U-VTS) and Therapists' Responses

ERWIN RANDOLPH PARSON

What happens to kids who learn as babies to dodge bullets and step over dead corpses on the way to school?
—Lois Timnick (1989)

VIOLENCE AND TRAUMA IN THE INNER CITY

From an early age, children living in the inner cities are exposed frequently to the use of drugs, guns, arson, and random violence. They witness injury, suffering, and death, and they respond to these events with fear and grief, often experiencing dramatic ruptures in their development. The list of psychological reactions is long and grim: hatred for self, profound loss of trust in the community and the world, tattered internalized moral values and ethics of caring, and a breaking down of the inner and outer sense of security and of reality. They are particularly vulnerable to traumatic stress illnesses and to related behavioral and academic abnormalities (Gardner, 1971; Parson, 1994; van der Kolk, 1987).

Two decades ago, Meers (1970, 1973; Meers & Gordon, 1975) spoke prophetically about the inner city child: "Since traumatization is endemic in the ghetto . . . this might produce in the child some equivalent of 'combat fatigue,' i.e., a further overloading of the ego because of the constancy of real dangers" (Meers & Gordon, 1975, p. 586). These socioenvironmentally induced stress reactions in urban children are what I refer to as *urban violence traumatic stress response syndrome* (U-VTS). Children's stress responses range from normal reactions (in response to an abnormal situation), to mild, moderate, and severe levels of distress and dysfunctions. When these children enter treatment, they present unusual challenges to therapists and often elicit powerful countertransference reactions (CTRs).

As of yet, no comprehensive studies exist on the traumatic sequelae of violence associated with "urban firefights" in ethnic minority children who live in the harsh brick and stone jungles of the inner city. Accounts of the experience of urban children have appeared in the media. Timnick (1989), in her *Los Angeles Times Magazine* article, "Children of Violence," highlighted the images of horror and traumatic effects of inner city-generated violence experienced by children of South Central Los Angeles. She presents the poignant verbal accounts by these children (pp. 6, 8, 10):

- "They shoot somebody everyday," "I go in and get under the bed and come out after the shooting stops."
- "My daddy got knifed when he got out of jail," and "My uncle got shot in a fight—there was a bucket of his blood. And I had two aunties killed—one of them was pushed off the free-way and there were maggots on her."
- "It's like the violence is coming down a little closer." "We don't come outside a lot now."
- "Just three people [in my family] died." "I been seein' two of them" (as haunting ghosts at night).
- "How about the cemetery?" (in response to teacher's request for ideas for a field trip).
- "Her eyeball was in her shoe" (boy witnessed woman's mutilated body).

The following are statements made by traumatized children served through my clinical practice in New York City:

- "At 5, in front of my own eyes I saw my dad and baby brother burn to death. They didn't get out. My dad had gone into the house to bring him out." (This adolescent was referred to me by a judge after he had shot a child he said had "hassled" him.)

- "I saw my mother stab my father with a knife and killed him. She was put in jail; he was dead. I had no one. I see a knife in my dreams every night."
- "They killed my dad as I watched, and I stayed with the body for a very long time, and all the time the killers threatened to kill me too."

Children who witnessed single extreme events or who suffer chronic exposure to aversive stimuli require interventions to repair cognitive, emotional, and physiological damages to the self to mobilize post-violence arrested development caused by violent acts. Interventions aim to create a climate in therapy that allows the child to learn how to cope and continue healthy growth (Winnicott, 1975). This is in part made possible by the presence and relationship of a benevolent authority—a therapist who understands children's unique reactions to traumatic experiences, and who is determined to empathically care for young victims by ensuring psychological continuity and integration of the trauma.

Working with children subjected to various forms of violence calls for sensitivity, maturity, and a stable sense of self in the therapist. The therapist needs to be the *symbolic representation of the safe, nonviolent world*. This work requires that therapist have the capacity and willingness to assist these children to decipher the riddle of their traumatic responses—a conundrum of mental confusion, of distorted moral values, of search for meaning, and of cognitive and emotional disruptions. In this regard, the issue of therapist countertransference takes on a special role and significance for psychotherapy outcome. Later in this chapter, the special role of countertransference in treatment will be discussed.

Most of the literature on inner city children of trauma identifies the problem young victims experience, but few highlight the nature of intervention with these children, and the role the therapist's personality and competence play in treatment outcome. Obviously, in the absence of outcome studies it is difficult to assess which interventions are most effective at this time.

This chapter highlights the reality of violent traumatic stress in the daily lives of urban children and explores the complexities of treating these children from the perspective of using therapists' human dynamic responses to promote healing in the child. Moreover, the chapter discusses the need for therapists to monitor and control negative responses toward the child's own response to the trauma-altered sense of self and his or her racioethnic heritage. Typical child reactions to the therapist include transference feelings directed toward the therapist who is perceived as an authority or parental figure, friend or foe, benevolent person or villain, rescuer or perpetrator, and similar transference projections. These transference projections have strong implications for countertransference processes in treatment that will also be discussed in this chapter.

Epidemic of Random Violence and Tragedy in the Presence of Children

Bell and Jenkins (1991) reviewed the literature on black children and youths living in violent communities, particularly those in South Central Los Angeles. They indicated that homicide will increase significantly in urban America. Compared to other Western nations, violent crime in the United States has climbed dramatically during the past two decades. Bell and Jenkins also noted that recent surveys found that the United States surpassed other industrialized nations in violent crimes, including homicides. Homicides have increased in black populations, and they are the *leading cause of death* among black men and women ages 15–34, a 39% increase since 1984.

The eyewitnessing of violence among children is also on the increase. Bell, Prothrow-Stith, Smallwood, and Murchison (1986) reported that 44% of murder victims were found in black populations, and that 84% of elementary school children had seen someone physically assaulted. Bell and Jenkins (1991) also reported that in 1982 in Los Angeles County, 10–20% of the 2,000 homicides were witnessed by dependent children, and that in 1985 one-half of the homicides cases were witnessed by 136 children 18 years and under. Dubrow and Garbarino (1989), in a small, uncontrolled sample, noted that "virtually all" of the inner city, ethnic minority children in South Central Los Angeles witnessed a homicide or a shooting of a person by age 5.

Case Example One: Toby

At age 11, a girl named Toby and her father were kidnapped from their inner city home in New York City. A child of African-American and Hispanic heritages, Toby watched as her kidnappers killed her father. They then continually threatened her with death for many hours.

The child was referred to an inner city, community mental health care facility for therapy. Toby was very close to her father, and the tragedy of that day had never left her mind. The vicious death of her father, and the accompanying loss and grief, made her feel very empty, bitter, and alone.

Though Toby's mother tried to care for her daughter the best she could, Toby was often abrasive and showed a lack of gratitude. The family felt sorry for her because of her ordeal, and they would overlook the girl's hostility, her moodiness, and her indiscretions such as visiting friends after school without first calling home to let family members know of her whereabouts.

Toby has a younger brother and two older sisters living in a squalid public housing building, where young children are recruited to "run" drugs, and where shootings and stabbings are daily expectations. Toby's mother describes her daughter as having been outgoing and a good student before the traumatic event. After the incident, the girl lost interest in school, and withdrew from friends and family, preferring solitude and isolation. She also showed a preoccupation with fantasy and with older boys.

At the time of the therapy, Toby presented with the symptoms of post-traumatic stress disorder (PTSD), depression, anxiety, phobic reactions, and hyperaggressive fantasies to destroy everyone around her. She suffered traumatic dreams and nightmares "almost every night," diminished interest, guilt, foreshortened future, irritability, hypervigilance, sleep disturbance, and general autonomic hyperreactivity. She was filled with rage toward the assailants, her mother, her brother and sisters, school teachers, and the world.

Toby was very cynical and distrustful of most people, and reportedly engaged in violent behavior in school against certain girls who she believed were attempting to humiliate her and steal her boyfriend, "Supreme." She would write him long letters cursing him for not loving her more, for going out with other girls, and for making her so lonely. The flavor of these letters manifested a psychotic or delusional quality. Toby often spoke of a sense of defilement, degradation, guilt, grief, sorrow, and death anxiety. She felt that life had dealt her a horrific blow, and she was determined to make everyone pay a high price for her misfortune. Toby usually gave the impression that people and reality were not worth relating to.

Case Example Two: Danny

At age 7, Danny, a 12-year-old boy of African-American background, witnessed his father and younger brother burn to death in a house fire in New York. His father had rescued him and his mother and three sisters. However, his father soon realized that the youngest child was still in the burning house. He ran into the house and upstairs to find the young child. As he and the baby descended the stairs, they were engulfed in flames and were burned alive as Danny watched in helpless horror and shocked disbelief.

At age 16, Danny was referred to me for psychotherapy by the juvenile court after shooting a 13-year-old boy who "had made me mad because he was calling me names." Part of the child wanted the world to pay dearly for what had happened to him: he had lost his best friend, his father, and still desperately missed him. Cocaine helped him kill the pain within and manage overwhelming affective turmoil and anxiety. Danny showed signs of PTSD, and, like Toby, suffered reenactments of the traumatic event in dreams, play, fantasies, and relationships with children and adults.

Prior to the traumatic event, Danny was described as a happy boy whose early developmental history was uneventful. There was no violence, and no alcohol and drug abuse in the family. Danny was his father's favorite child, and he knew this. Over the years Danny suffered traumatic dreams that reenacted the fire he had witnessed with horror 5 years before. His mother and older sisters mentioned how Danny's personality had changed after his father's death: he withdrew into a "shell of silence," and he became introverted, sad, angry, irritable, and defiant.

The child also suffered intense fears, annihilation anxiety, sleep disturbance, and what his mother described as "his depressed state." Danny's mother remarried and his stepfather tried to be a positive influence in the boy's life to help him forget his traumatic past. However, Danny was very rebellious and defiant. He felt he had only one father, and that *he* was dead. No one could replace his father. Danny's alcohol and cocaine abuse can be understood as attempts to manage inner tensions, depression, and post-traumatic memories through self-medication.

URBAN VIOLENCE TRAUMATIC STRESS RESPONSE SYNDROME (U-VTS)

Urban violence syndromes may involve psychic conflicts, central nervous system alterations, distorted images of social life, physical damage, and chronic stress. My experience in treating inner city children suggests that, though the PTSD criteria in the revised third edition of the *Diagnostic and Statistical Manual of Mental Disorders* (DSM-III-R; American Psychiatric Association, 1987) aid in the assessment process with violence-traumatized children, the DSM-III-R fails to address the clinical and socioenvironmental issues that children traumatized by violence bring to the clinical setting. It also fails to deal with most aspects of violence and the resulting self-altering biopsychic manifestations in behavior.

The concept of U-VTS is introduced to complement the DSM-III-R PTSD criteria and to offer a more comprehensive and realistic understanding of the responses of low socioeconomic status, ethnic minority and white youths living in the inner cities. Research is needed to better understand the common and unique properties of PTSD and the actual impact of violence upon the mind, body, and spirit of urban children of trauma.

The response to violence-driven stressors can occur after a single violent episode, after multiple episodes, or after ongoing prolonged exposure to overwhelming events of violence. Observation and experience suggest that these stressors can occur when the individual is either alone or in a group, and they affect very young children as well as older children and adolescents (Parson, 1994; Pynoos & Eth, 1985; Terr, 1979).

U-VTS features a number of component symptoms and reactions observed in child eyewitnesses to overwhelming events. In assessment and diagnostic work the relative weight given each of the following factors depends upon the developmental stage of the child; the specific kind, intensity, and duration of traumatic stimuli (Parson, 1994); the family structure; and the child's general experience in his or her community. The components of U-VTS are (1) damaged self syndrome; (2) trauma-specific transference paradigms; (3) adaptation to danger; (4) cognitive and emotional stress response; (5) impact on moral behavior; (6) post-traumatic play; (7) PTSD; and (8) post-traumatic health outcomes. Each of these has implications for CTRs that can either hinder or enhance the child's progress toward recovery.

Damaged Self Syndrome

Most, if not all, stressors leading to post-traumatic stress responses and U-VTS may be described as a violent intrusion into the self, its organization, integrity, and adaptive functioning. The concept of *damaged self syndrome* is an explanatory one, deriving from clinical observation of children's responses to extreme or chronic violence as seen in their behavior and interactions with others, and in analysis of dreams, nightmares, and spontaneous recall of events. Children with damaged selves appear to be in constant psychological distress.

The sense of powerlessness over the traumatizing environment creates within the child a sense of insecurity and an experienced sense of impotence. Chronic feelings of impotence harm the child's sense of self, which turns to a compensatory feeling of omnipotence to cope. With this sense of omnipotence, the child feels and behaves as if nothing can affect him or her, that the self is impregnable against further hurt and feelings of vulnerability. *Vendetta rage* is primitive, narcissistic rage against parental figures, other so-called protectors, and authorities and society. The damaged self, moreover, often maintains its organization and integrity by managing anxiety via the creation of defenses to protect inner vulnerability. This may be a partial explanation of why victims become victimizers.

Thus, traumatically damaged children appear disposed to impulsive actions that harm themselves (as in self-mutilations), and that defensively inflict damage to others, perhaps thus unconsciously "spreading the damage around." Violence, for many youngsters, is an issue of self-esteem regulation. This reflecting of self through violence against others is unconsciously geared to repair the experienced damage to self-esteem and to master the inner fragmentation, annihilation anxieties, and agonies in the child.

Referring to inner city children struggling with hyperaggressive impulses in a school-based therapy group, Dyson (1990) makes a similar observation: "Violence, for them, seemed the only way to repair their injured self-esteem" (p. 19). For some children, moral development becomes permanently fixated at the primitive vendetta or "pay-back" stage (Field, 1977, 1985; Garbarino, Kostelny, & Dubrow, 1991; Tapp, 1971).

This is often one of the most problematic issues for therapists, namely, the apparent transformation of the child from passive recipient to perpetrator of violence. This is because basic traumaphobia (fear of trauma repeating itself) in some children becomes traumatophilia (attraction to trauma) as a way to manage the internal effects of violence.

Like the survivors of psychological damage Krystal and Niederland (1968) saw in their clinical work with survivors of the Holocaust, many traumatized inner city children feel fragmented internally. Dissociative reactions in traumatized children represent a breakdown of internal systems of coordination of sensory, perceptual, affective, and conceptual functions. It implies that the child's synthetic and integrative ego functions are defective, and that there may be a blurring of self–environment boundaries. Dissociation accompanies psychological traumatization in inner city children, and it ranges in severity. Therapists can react to this with pity, an unhelpful Type II CTR (see Chapter 2, this volume). However, if they monitor their countertransference, they can instead offer an adaptive "containing function" (for the split-off, anxiety-driven defenses) for the child's ultimate benefit.

Meaning, purpose, and feelings of safety are the casualties of trauma, and they are replaced by cynicism, apathy, shattered values, and distrust. For many children these positive attributes have been stripped away from their lives as sequelae to traumatic witnessing. Toby (Case Example One) used this existential defensive strategy to cope with the murder of her father in her presence.

Tainted by death, loss, and a surfeit of sorrow and grief, children often suffer intense anxieties related to a sense of "death immersion" (Parson, 1988) or to what Lifton (1982) has identified in adult survivor groups as the "death imprint." Death-related anxiety comes from identification with the dead and the sense of being trapped in death with the deceased relative, friend, or other persons who died. Rage over physical and psychological injuries endured often prevents the working through of sadness, grief, and sorrow.

Both children discussed above in my case examples had grief and mourning reactions after their stressful experiences, particularly Toby. As the child's death imagery floods the treatment, the therapist's challenge is to begin to see how death invades the therapy and to monitor his or her defenses against it. Sustained empathic responses by the therapist may serve as a holding posture through which the child learns how to manage internal death stimuli and thus integrate the trauma.

There are many other expressions of narcissistic injury in children. Many of these themes have been discussed elsewhere (Parson, in press; Wilson & Raphael, 1993) but are important to identify here, despite the fact that space limitations preclude a full discussion of them. Among the indicators of damaged inner-self structure following urban violence are (1) cumulative grief and mourning, (2) feelings of hopelessness and powerlessness, (3) a sense of betrayal and defilement, (4) fears of recurring trauma and violence, (5) the expectation of danger and violence, (6) a loss of future orientation, (7) feelings of incompetence and an external locus of control over life events, (8) a disposition for self-abuse, (9) detachment and a loss of bonding capacity, and (10) dysfunctional socialization—a reversal of the normal, healthy patterns of interaction with abnormal and disruptive socialization.

Trauma-Specific Transference Paradigms and the Imprint of Violence

Stress associated with violence is often so toxic that a complex mental imprinting process occurs, which can alter the child's personality. This alteration sets up a number of response tendencies in the child that the therapist identifies and uses to enhance the efficacy of the treatment experience. For example, after trauma the child may experience self as both victim and perpetrator, as innocent and culpable, as passive and active, and as rescuer, benevolent authority, or malevolent authority.

Transference reactions occur in therapy when the unconscious dynamics of the child are activated in relation to the violence experience. The therapist is often seen in a distorted manner (e.g., as a perpetrator, a nonbenevolent authority that caused the trauma, etc.), and, depending upon the stability of the child's reality-testing and controls, he or she may act out psychological or physical violence in the course of therapy.

Children who were exposed to violence are often confused when they come for treatment, and so struggle between passivity and aggressivity. Although the latter may initially be avoided because it is too closely associated with the behavior of the aggressor, the former may be embraced as a way to distance self from internalized violent impulses. The child may later find the aggressive mode to offer an increased sense of inner stability and self-esteem management.

In violent trauma, the child internalizes self-images in relation to the traumatizing event, and self in relation to other people at the scene of the event. Thus, "trauma-engineered" identifications serve as the basis for transferential responses in therapy. These are (1) victim-self (identification with the victim[s]), (2) victimizer-self (identification with the aggressor), (3) rescuer-self (identification with constructive, competent behavior at the scene), and (4) authority-self (identification with culpable or responsible persons or government institutions).

Early in post-traumatic child therapy, Danny (Case Example Two), in the rescuer-self transference, saw the therapist as helpful but vulnerable, impotent, and self-destructive (his father had tried to help him but was killed in the fire). Seeing his father as self-destructive was an interesting distortion of the actual facts, but such distortions offer great opportunity for working through the child's traumatic responses and problems. The child's own self-destructive behavior was an identification with his dead father whom he perceived as "killing himself" in the fire. Later in the therapy, Danny realized that his father had not intentionally lost his life to hurt him.

A significant stressor (e.g., shooting) is therefore associated with co-occurring, multisensory immersion such as sirens from emergency vehicles (fire trucks and police cars), other loud noises, screams, confusion, shouting, smell, temperature, and other sensations. Transference reliving of trauma elements may be triggered or accompanied by any of these sensations. Socioenvironmental stimuli may trigger traumatic responses through one or more sensory channels, which may then be reenacted during treatment.

The therapist may be unconsciously seen as a benevolent and caring authority, as a victim or covictim, as a rescuer, or as a violent perpetrator from the traumatic scenario. These transferences should be addressed in most psychotherapy approaches with children. They are, after all, the other side of countertransference and constitute one whole unit.

CTRs may vary from time to time depending upon the specific identifications projected onto the therapist by the child. For example, if the child in the transference views the therapist as a violent perpetrator, he or she may invoke punitivity, violence attribution, or some other Type I CTR in the therapist.

Adaptation to danger may involve becoming "danger" itself: this may serve defensive ends, in that it spares the child the pain of experiencing the self as passive and vulnerable, or as different and separate from others in the socioecology. As such, these defenses can result in transference projections. The child's defenses against inner vulnerability may arouse latent fears and anxieties in the therapist that set CTRs into motion. However, by becoming the selfobject (Kohut, 1977), the therapist creates the climate in which violence-mitigating internalizations and a sense of internal safety can occur.

Cognitive and Emotional Stress Response

Cognitive development incrementally shapes and defines the child's view of the world. Piagetian theory of cognitive development is germane to understanding how in eyewitness trauma children's thinking and feeling are altered by the event(s). Traumatized children suffer a number of cognitive symptoms that include having trouble concentrating and attending to what is going on in the home, school, and community.

The *cognitive stress response* is a dematuring of the traumatized child's cognitive functioning. It is marked by regression from formal and post-formal operations thinking to more concrete operations as seen in (1) the deficits in cognitive controls and related loss of conservation and misalignment of emotion, time, and reality, (2) loss of once acquired language effectiveness in categorizing information, (3) disturbance in object constancy, and (4) a reactivation of sensorimotor functioning—focusing on less well-organized perceptual memories. Attention deficit disorder (American Psychiatric Association, 1987) is frequently found in cases of chronic exposure to violence stress. The existence of regressed states or attention deficit disorder causes a number of academic deficiencies in traumatized children. It may also be associated with the development of irrational omens.

The chief psychological reaction of children after trauma is an intolerance for strong affective tensions. Disturbing emotions include fears (e.g., fear of being alone), sadness, grief, guilt, depression, shame, anxiety, anger, belligerence, revulsion, despair, poor impulse control, and persistent, anticipatory fear of being overwhelmed by strong affects and losing control. The specific emotional symptoms and adaptive responses that children show after trauma are naturally dependent upon their developmental phase.

Emotional stress reactions reflect the disturbances in the reciprocal coordination of assimilation and accommodation that often accompany psychic trauma in children. Problems in this area produce serious impairments in self-regulation and in human relationships. Trauma-origin regression (from mature to immature developmental levels) is noted in the child's (1) reversion to intense psychophysiological symptomatology, irritability, and hypervigilance; (2) sleep problems; (3) annihilation anxiety; (4) separation anxiety; (5) panic attacks; (6) phobias (relates to specific places, persons, and structures in the physical environment); (7) enuresis or encopresis; and (8) the undoing of basic trust.

Stress Response Impact on Moral Behavior

Extreme or prolonged exposure to threat, danger, and violence may force a regression from advanced forms of moral reasoning to primitive levels of moral conviction and behavior. Changes in moral behavior may be sequelae to violence exposure—a shattering of pre-traumatic values, moral and ethical mental structures. In addition, the child may regress from a rational, beneficial, utilitarian stage (Tapp, 1971) to a morality of absolutist obedience, punitivity, and "a vendetta mentality" (Garbarino et al., 1991, p. 379; see also Flavell, 1983; Kohlberg, 1964).

It is important to keep in mind that strengths may also result from violence stress among urban children and youths, for social conflict and dangerous conditions may stimulate growth and moral development in many disadvantaged children (Coles, 1967; Garbarino et al., 1991), especially if there were opportunities for early "introjection of parental demands" (Mahler, Pine, & Bergman, 1975, p. 192) or the opportunity to transform traumatic experiences in more resilient ways.

Violence-based trauma often truncates human connectedness and breaks the "great chain of humanity" that connects us all. As a consequence of both psychic trauma and the failure of the post-violence milieu to restore confidence, trust, and function in children, many of them become hardened to other people's needs and points of view, adopting an interpersonal anesthetic in the form of a cold, tough, aloof, and intimidating street-wise demeanor.

In the aftermath of trauma, the child finds that painful, suppressed, repressed, and split-off feelings are difficult to express in words. Due to the relative reduction in the ability to use symbols, many children release tensions more through action than through thinking and reflecting. Many are unable to sit still for even a few minutes; they are unable to attend to details at home or at school. Post-traumatic behavioral abnormalities have a negative effect on these children's immediate social environments and result in rejection and hostility from others. Conduct disorders are significantly represented among traumatized children.

PTSD

Urban violence may result in PTSD, a psychiatric malady that manifests in the aftermath of overwhelming events (American Psychiatric Association, 1987). Frederick's (1985) research study on 150 children (50 survived disasters, 50 were victims of physical abuse, and 50 were sexually molested) found that 77% had PTSD. Arroyo and Eth (1985) found that 33% of children traumatized by Central American warfare had PTSD. Though the adequacy of the PTSD diagnosis for children has been documented (Parson, 1994), the DSM-III-R (American Psychiatric Association, 1987) included developmental issues that strengthened the diagnostic criteria for children. Thus, the following *child-sensitive criteria* have been added. These are (1) reliving via repetitive play, (2) loss of acquired developmental skills (e.g., bowel and bladder control, motility), (3) sense of foreshortened future, (4) omen cognition, (5) personality changes, and (6) regression in attachment security, resulting in separation anxiety and fear.

VULNERABILITY TO U-VTS

A child's vulnerability to toxic socioenvironmental stress involves several factors: the nature of the stressor, its severity and duration; the child's achieved developmental level, nature of family/community social support network, history of exposure to violence stress, previous psychic trauma (physical abuse, sexual abuse, etc.), and the child's personality organization before the episode (a critical factor, because urban children may have been exposed to many stressors). One or more of the following vulnerability factors may apply to a specific child.

1. Complete lack of parental care and absence of "good-enough parenting."
2. Paucity of credible and respected models, driving children toward identification with and emulation of the violent aggressor, the pimp, or the drug dealer.
3. Narcissistically traumatizing parental figures (those who wound the child's sense of self and safety by fostering chronic frustrations and disappointments).
4. Abuse by caretaking figures—the use of psychological means to abuse and devastate the child's sense of self and security.
5. Traumatizing parental behavior—inflicting physical and sexual trauma, such as brutalization, incest, rape, and the failure to provide a protective shield for the outside the home setting.

6. Lack of functional secondary family system (i.e., extended families, teachers, ecclesiastical figures, etc.).
7. Family aggression (e.g., wife-beating, husband abuse by wife).
8. Ineffectual ecclesiastical influences, eroding values, and lack of ethical and moral base.
9. Prevalence of drugs and pervasiveness of dependency/abuse.
10. Ineffectual educational institutions that kill hope in children.
11. Chronic cynicism and distrust of parents, teachers, elders, and other authority figures in the urban community (overtly disrespected, and covertly seen as "damaged models," too weak, too passively acquiescing to the racist status quo to inspire hope, confidence, and trust in youthful populations in trouble).
12. Breakdown of mutual trust and respect between law enforcement and youth and adults of inner city communities.
13. Instrumental violence (for power over adverse environmental contingencies, internal fears, learned helplessness, and low self-esteem).
14. Racism and its evil derivatives of systematic exclusion, leading to poverty, high infant morality, high rates of incarceration, especially among black males.

Realistic knowledge about vulnerability factors, U-VTS, PTSD offers the therapist an opportunity to cope with potentially harmful CTRs when intervening with the urban child in trouble.

PATTERNS OF THERAPISTS' RESPONSES AND COUNTERTRANSFERENCE MANAGEMENT

Therapists working with children and adolescents living in violent urban worlds face particular forms of CTRs—some beneficial and some potentially harmful to the child. My view is that countertransference is as important as transference, and that the ultimate success of the therapy depends upon the therapist's use of the "empathic tools" found in positive CTRs. Thus, in any intervention, "clinicians must come to believe that there is not only no place to hide, but also no reason to do so" (Maroda, 1991, p. 5).

Countertransference Considerations in U-VTS Treatment

Minimizing Response

Therapists who have this kind of Type I CTR may, for example, see the violence in urban areas as unusual but not clinically traumatic. They believe that no significant psychological scars and symptomatology should occur in these violence-exposed children, or they assume that the child will "grow out of it," and that such exposure is "normal for urban kids." These therapists often have great difficulty dealing with their own aggressive histories, impulsivity, passivity, sense of vulnerability, and they may feel overwhelmed by the child's stories of trauma. In Toby's case, for example, a therapist might have found it difficult to believe that the child had gone through such a horrific loss and traumatic ordeal.

Avoidance/Fear Response

When a therapist experiences avoidance it is usually a fear of reliving the child's traumatic past. This manifests in therapists who are confronted by intense reexperiencing symptoms by the child. In this instance, the therapist is unable to model the necessary courage and confidence the child needs to verbalize painful and "dangerous" emotions. A Type I CTR, avoidance is often too rigid to contain the child's fears and anxieties; to assist in achieving a sense of safety, freedom, and inner tranquility; and to efficiently process the trauma. Maneuvers to manage death imagery in the child's clinical dynamics may also be related to avoidance phenomena.

Racial Bias Response

This response derives from unresolved conflicts around racial prejudice, particularly unconscious racism (Butts, 1971). Views of urban children as "violent" and as "difficult patients" may find their source in racial or ethnic bias in the therapist.

Pitied Child Reaction

These therapists view the child as pitiful because of the tragic exposure to traumatizing violence. In this response, the therapist identifies with the helpless aspects of the child's experience and may fail to recognize and identify with the child's strengths and potential resiliency. If the therapist lacks self-confidence in alleviating the child's distress, he or she may vacillate between avoidance (or reluctance) to intervene and overidentifying with the child. In both case examples (Toby and Danny), therapists with these fears might see the children as hopelessly damaged and possibly too far beyond their professional capabilities and emotional stamina.

Passionate Parenting

This Type II CTR is found in therapists who are motivated to "right all wrongs" suffered by the child. They unconsciously desire to fulfill the child's total narcissistic and dependency needs as expeditiously as possible. However, though the therapist might be intent upon "spoiling the child," he or she actively avoids getting to know the child's own reality and "true self" (Winnicott, 1975) aspects of personality.

Raciocultural Countertransference

Some therapists are uncomfortable with racial issues in psychotherapy. *Race* refers to the historical legacy of a group of people whose phenotypic characteristics distinguish them from other groups; for example, the black race is ostensibly distinguished from the white race by skin color and other physical characteristics. *Cultural* means of or pertaining to culture, culture being the "shared creativities" (Hilliard, 1984) of a group of people, which include values, art, language, and other symbols of collective life. "Racio" is a combining form that refers to race. The term *raciocultural* thus refers to issues pertaining to racial differences and associated subjectivity in a context of a shared reality and customs. CTRs motivated by raciocultural issues are important to highlight in any discussion of therapists' responses to inner city children in therapy.

Some therapists, who may have been raised with strict discipline, negate the urban child's morality. They view the child's behavior as "loose" or "undisciplined," requiring reprimands and strict control in the therapeutic space. Often influenced by media reports, some therapists view urban children and families as basically immoral.

Additionally, many therapists, in different parts of the world, may view impoverished inner city children as inherently violent. This perception and bias may undermine the therapists' ability to interact therapeutically with the child. Holding such a view may create ambivalent feelings as to whether the child is a passive witnessing bystander or an active victimizer.

On the other hand, some therapists may be fearful of being the therapeutic target of intense transference reactions by children who have been exposed to violence. Children relive transferentially the various relationships associated with the violent event. When the child's transference feelings distort the therapist into being the perpetrator or victimizer, denial, avoidance, and other defensive mechanisms may be used in order to keep the child's feelings in check so they do not overrun the therapist's capacity for control.

The therapist may be concerned about the possibility of repeating the parental abuse, neglect, and abandonment suffered by the inner city child. As a result, the therapist may remain counterphobically aloof and avoid taking responsibility for the treatment enterprise. A Type I CTR abrogation of leadership is not uncommon in the treatment of trauma survivors (Parson, 1988), but does need to be managed for optimal beneficial effects.

Organizational Countertransference

Organizations have long been seen as living systems that may be understood by using dynamic principles borrowed from individual psychology. Organizations, like society as a whole, view certain racial or ethnocultural groups as inferior, deserving the harsh realities of crime, poverty, disease, and traumatic violence—of the life to which they are subjected. Similarly, emergency rooms, clinics, hospitals, and other health care facilities may allow the collective negative view (often stereotypes) of blacks, other ethnic minorities, and indigent white individuals to cloud their professional judgment in terms of offering equal or comparable quality of health care.

Countertransference management refers to the therapist's active coping with negative, treatment-destroying feelings and transforming these into empathic orientations that work on behalf of the child. Management efficacy may call for supervision, peer supervision, and training for therapists. It is important for therapists to explore and monitor their ethnocentrism and their feelings about race and about people who differ from themselves in economics, politics, race, religion, and gender.

POST-TRAUMATIC CHILD PSYCHOTHERAPY AND COUNTERTRANSFERENCE

Like dreams and traumatic dreams, play in child psychotherapy is perhaps the most direct way to access and influence the child's inner world of traumatic responses and illnesses. This is accomplished in part through the countertransference-controlled "archaeological work" of using cues from the child's trauma behavior that take "into account the nature of the . . . [traumatic] destruction in order to . . . make inferences about what has been destroyed . . . and its possible function" (Ekstein, 1966, pp. 134–135).

Empathic Resonance: Instrumental Countertransference

Integral to the practice of post-traumatic child therapy (PTCT) is the monitoring of negative CTRs and the applications of positive CTRs or "instrumental countertransference" to promote healing in the child. This response is one that places the child at the center of the therapy through empathic resonance. The term "resonance," as I use it here, comes from the fields of electronics and mechanical engineering. It is defined as "the enhancement . . . intensification and prolongation of a tone by sympathetic vibration" (*Concise American Heritage Dictionary*, 1980, p. 601). The child's "tone" is the traumatic anguish of sadism, brutality, and cruelty seen or endured. Empathic resonance enhances the strength of the therapeutic alliance.

The therapist's own positive regard affirms the tone, elaborates it, and by doing so makes the child's intrapsychic data materially present and real. It then becomes possible to reflect this back to the child in a "language" the child understands. The therapist may feel empathic horror, rage, outrage, contempt, shame, guilt, and fear of the child's trauma narrative and potential for violence transference. These reactions are "sympathetic vibrations" intuited through empathic channels of therapeutic communication in order to understand the child from within.

Owning the traumatized child's grief, hurt, anguish, anxiety, fears, guilt, and shame is the *sine qua non* of adaptive intervention with intrapsychically unstable, environmentally terrorized children. Unless the therapist can say of the urban child, "This part of you is I" and "This part of me is you" (Racker, 1968, pp. 134–135), the inferred emotional distance from the child endangers the efficacy of the intervention.

Basically, PTCT seeks to achieve empathic understanding, child-sensitive communication, reconstruction, and the filling in of missing events. PTCT incorporates three phases that integrally utilize the therapist's responses. These are (1) ego stabilization and development of trust, (2) "return to the scene," and (3) working through and completion.

Phase I: Ego Stabilization, Trust, and Attachment

The post-violence assessment is critical to realistic treatment planning. Parents may be seen alone and then with the affected child. Family and extended family members are considered in the assessment process, and the therapist's relationship with the child's family is seen as critical to efficacious outcome. After these two meetings the child is seen alone in a separate interview.

The formal assessment involves a structured interview to determine the following: (1) presenting complaints; (2) mental status (examining the child's orientation, motor and sensory functioning; mood, memory, judgment; and delusional or hallucinatory symptoms and behavior); (3) demographic information, medical history, developmental milestones and stress points, parental assessment, academic functioning, social behavior, the degree of impairment or disability, and the history of exposure to familial and community violence; (4) the specifics of the violent stressor event (e.g., shooting, stabbing); (5) post-violence psychological screening; (6) who was harmed and how the victim responded ("Children who witness injury to others and hear their cries for help appear to be especially vulnerable" [Pynoos & Nader, 1988, p. 447]); (7) the child's violence stress response symptoms; (8) the nature and cohesiveness of social supports (children recover with appropriate social support [Sander, 1967]); (9) the impact of parental trauma (Haley, 1987); (10) deleterious societal forces on the child's symptomatology; (11) the possible relationship between trauma and borderline personality disorder in the child (Parson, 1988); (12) "steeling qualities" (Rutter, 1987, p. 326) (used by some children to protect themselves from mental breakdown and from being overwhelmed); (13) problem formulation; and (14) recommendations.

The child's stabilization depends upon a psychologically stable and competent therapist who models trust and attachment behavior. Here, the child learns to internalize the safe, nonviolent, and stable environment. The therapist sets the tone for the treatment, strives to establish a working alliance with the child, and approaches the child in a positive, inviting manner.

It is important to remember that the child did not come to therapy on his or her own but was brought, and that therapy was probably considered as necessary only after previous strategies did not work. The therapist talks to the child: the child is reassured that the therapist feels deeply about the tragedy, cares about the child's welfare, and that the ordeal the child went through is of great interest to the therapist. Additionally, the child is told that the therapist can help because of interest and experience in helping children in similar circumstances feel less fearful, have fewer frightening dreams, and feel more relaxed and in control.

In the process of clinical management, the therapist takes a good clinical history of the traumatic event(s) in a systematic, step-by-step manner, investigating what happened (the cardinal behavior or event the child witnessed), and when, why, and how the child survived and is surviving. These data are later framed and structured to assist in achieving the cardinal task of Phase 2. The child is debriefed as a victim of violence by discussing the normality of violence stress responses and the ventilation of feelings, by detailing the fact about what happened, and by exploring and clarifying thoughts, sensory impressions, and emotional reactions.

In this phase the child is also given opportunity to release pent-up emotions, and to express fears, anxieties, phobic reactions, contents of nightmares, guilt feelings, grief over losses, blame, shame, punishment, and retaliation. These same issues will come up for exploration in Phases 2 and 3 as well. However, they are approached very differently. The emotionally immature child often expresses strong affect too soon and too intensely before sufficient ego maturation has occurred. For some children, this can be "retraumatizing" because the overwhelming nature of affectomotor responses bombard the sense of inner security and safety, resulting in hyperarousal and emotional constriction.

As the child's chief auxiliary ego or the person who will satisfy the child's post-trauma needs, the therapist provides an essential "affect-buffering function," by being a person who functions as protector against overstimulation. Children of trauma harbor strong aggressive feelings of retaliation or vendetta against people, things, objects, circumstances, and fate. Assisting the child early in therapy with feelings of guilt and vendetta rage can result in great psychosocial dividends of positive attitude and behavior change. Pynoos and Eth (1985) report that early in treatment children get the most benefit when drawings of their revenge fantasies are discussed.

As noted before, children with trauma bring to therapy intense fear, anxiety, feelings of inferiority, inner tensions, distrust, irritability, demanding and/or withdrawn behavior, low frustration tolerance, sleep problems, temper tantrums, fear of sleeping alone (in younger children), and a fear-based avoidance to becoming emotionally connected with the therapist.

The notion of therapy as an exclusively child-sensitive enterprise suggests that the child is accepted as he or she is, the child is offered freedom from inhibitions, the child is sufficiently understood to make identification and interpretation of feelings possible, and the therapist sustains empathic attunement over personal CTRs, keeping a focus on the child's needs and welfare, not on the therapist's unconscious feelings. Like other children, Toby in Case Example One was distrustful of adults because she had witnessed adults engage in kidnapping, stealing, cheating, lying, inflicting pain on children and adults, killing, and going to jail.

Denial of the trauma may still be present, and numbing may make it very difficult for traumatized children to get in touch with feelings in therapy. Such children are usually unable to express feelings directly. They are reluctant or unable to recall elements of the trauma and are intensely fearful of losing control over painful intrusive and repetitive images, ideation, affect, and memory. They also may fear "affective returning" and may have problems regulating their pessimism, depression, and inner world of confusion and chaos. This emotional chaos is in part caused by a "disturbance of affect" (Krystal, 1978) that makes it difficult for the child to know what he or she is feeling and to experience sharp, definite emotions. Associated with this disturbance of emotions are the underlying pathophysiological mechanisms and chronic family and community violence stress.

Some violence-stressed children may have a compulsion to move, and to keep moving to control hyperarousal, anxiety, and the associated fear of the "return of the dissociated" (Parson, 1984). A deep sense of insecurity (or defenses against it) is evident in these children: they never seem sure that the past will remain in the past. Therefore, like Toby, they anticipate new tragedies—new shootings and killings, new losses, new fears, and more disappointments—and they see life as short and their self as irreparably damaged.

Many indigent minority and white "multiple-problem" patients at first require concrete services as vital adjuncts to therapy. In Toby's case, therapeutic planning and implementation included local, community-based medical and social services organizations as an extension of her therapy. Food stamps and other social welfare services are essential for poor inner city families, particularly in those family systems where parents are not able to provide food and shelter for their children. An example of an external therapy-bolstering intervention (i.e., coming from sources outside the therapy relationship) is Friedlander's (1945) child guidance work in Great Britain after World War II. She found that the child's conflicts and difficulties were remarkably improved when she applied psychoanalytic theory to the entire child guidance process, and focused on prevention and on a program of education for parents, professionals, and the public.

Specific Treatment Techniques

Useful techniques for Phase 1 include stress management (particularly essential for entering Phase 2), therapeutic drawings and art, structured drawings, role-playing, and approaches that deal with desensitization of fear and cognitive restructuring. These latter approaches are utilized primarily to manage angry feelings to irrational thinking, which interfere with healing and recovery. As time progresses, psychological consolidation takes place as less internal fragmenting and dissociation are noted in the child's cognition, affect, and behavior. Reducing the child's sense of unpredictability and uncontrollability, both of which lead to "persistent arousal and increased generalized fear" in animal and human studies, contributes to the consolidation of intellectual, perceptual, emotional, and behavioral functions of the child (Foa, Zinbarg, & Rothbaum, 1992). Psychopharmacological agents for anxiety, depression, and other symptoms may be used as adjunctive therapy to the overall clinical strategy.

Phase 2: Return to the Scene

Returning the violence-stressed child to the scene of the incident (either physically or through memory work) is a necessary dimension of play therapy for severe cases of U-VTS. Accompanying U-VTS are "toxic memories," which trigger mechanisms of cognitive, affective, and physiological arousal that prove tormenting to every aspect of the child's life. Children suffering from the traumatic information embedded in these memories require the application of direct action techniques. Such direct techniques involve taking the child *in vivo* to the place where the incident occurred (through an affectophysical return), or guiding the child through post-violence reconstruction procedures (an affectocognitive return), in a "frame-by-frame, slow-motion reworking process" (Frederick, 1985, p. 92)—that is, "a controlled regressive pathway to the traumatic experience" (Parson, 1984, p. 35).

Frederick (1985) is correct when he points out that "merely talking will not suffice in undoing serious psychic trauma in either adults or children." Consistent with my own experience and previous theorizing (Brende & Parson, 1985; Parson, 1984, 1988), Frederick states that "trauma mastery must be incident-specific for specific resolution of the problem" (p. 93).

Undoing traumatic information, amnesias, and the related affective rigidity and constriction requires a return to the scene of the traumatic violence. Cognitive, behavioral, and stress management techniques designed for children and adolescents are most useful in preparing the patient for Phase 2's psychological return. Additionally, experience has shown that such temporal factors as the days of the week, time of the day, month and season of the year, anniversary dates, and holidays associated with the violence are integral to therapy with traumatized children. These are important markers for understanding the child's experience, aiding the regressive process, and ultimately achieving integration.

Specific approaches to achieve this goal include the post-violence, mutual story-telling technique (a modification of Gardner's [1975] interactive approach with resistant children), play, therapeutic color drawings, kinetic family drawings, and traumatic dream script rewriting (for adaptive outcomes). Some children and adolescents may benefit from "*in vitro* flooding," a behavioral approach understood in dynamic terms as a regressive therapeutic technique.

Because witnessing life-threatening events depletes mature internal resources and may replace them with dynamically less mature forms of functioning, it is clear that oral dynamics become pronounced after violent threat or traumatic witnessing. This therapeutic regression instigates responses geared to protect the self from intense stimulation and sensations of fear; of ravaging, devouring rage; and of reliving the scene of violent action through repetitive-intrusive responses. For this purpose, offering warm milk, hot chocolate, snacks, and other oral supplies can, in addition to the nurturing and encouraging presence of the therapist, motivate the child to persist in the very difficult task of reliving the painful event.

Phase 3: Working Through and Completion

In *Remembering, Repeating, and Working Through,* Freud (1914) spoke about the resistance against recollecting memories from childhood. He believed these memories lay at the root of his patients' neurotic illnesses. This process is also applicable to the treatment of U-VTS. Freud believed that, although uncovering, remembering, and repeating painful memories during the course of therapy were important objectives (as in Phases 1 and 2 of the present model), only working through them offered integration, long-term resolution, and positive lasting change.

In the working-through phase, many areas of Toby's life (Case Example One) were explored, including profound dependency, self-destructive propensities, impacted grief, bereavement, sadness, depression, accident-proneness, nightmares, stuttering, nervous tics, insomnia, and rage over her father's murder in her presence by cruel assailants. These data were often used to identify points of impasse and to gauge degree of ego integration.

Many of the transferential responses in therapy are tainted with violence, and it is usually violence and threat in the transference that induce Type I CTRs in some therapists. Though there has been a history of debate about the validity of the transference concept in work with children, the significant clinical evidence points to its utility and inevitability in moving the treatment forward (Parson, 1994; Trad, 1988, 1989, 1990; Trad, Rine, Chazan, & Greenblatt, 1992). Only when trust has been established, and the therapeutic alliance is solid, can the therapist interpret transference and share with the child the therapist's countertransference feelings.

Dyson (1990), an experienced therapist with inner city children of trauma, recommends "intensive psychotherapy programs . . . on a wide scale within the black community, as these children do, in fact, benefit from insight-oriented and supportive counseling" (p. 21). This is consistent with my observations and experience with inner city children. As both Toby and Danny continued their work in therapy, they manifested greater insight, sharper ethnocultural identity, and a greater capacity to see nonviolence as an alternative to violence in solving problems.

Children's traumatic experiences usually catapult them into "premature entrance into adulthood" (Pynoos & Eth, 1985, p. 243). Child-sensitive interventions allow the child to be a child again, to restore the broken link between self and others through forming new human attachments (Emde, 1982; Field, 1985), and thus to achieve growth and maturation beyond violence trauma. Working through sadness, grief, loss, bereavement, and other emotions of the post-traumatic affective response syndrome (Parson, 1988) is also a worthwhile achievement for the child.

Working through traumas with Toby and Danny called for some form of "socioenvironmental engineering"—that is, engaging public and private social agencies in the child's behalf (e.g., by getting specific information on what children and their families could do to remain safe on their way to school). Contacts with family members, the school, the church, and other persons and agencies are important aspects of PTCT. These contacts function to help reduce high levels of therapy-subverting stress from the home, community, and school.

During the working-through phase in the treatment of an inner city, African-American male child with dangerous levels of internalized rage and self-hate, Trad et al. (1992) found that assisting the child "to make connections between his behaviors and intentions . . . his actions and his feelings . . . his aggressive behavior and his anger" (p. 653) proved to be illuminating and integratively constructive in managing self-destructive behavior and violent propensities.

CONCLUSION

The concept of PTSD is inadequate to capture and describe the comprehensive nature of violence trauma in inner city children. U-VTS is a new term, which identifies a spectrum of violence-related responses in inner city children. Like PTSD, it occurs as a consequence of threats to a child's life and physical integrity, or of witnessing a person who was seriously harmed or in the process of being seriously injured. Unlike some forms of PTSD, U-VTS is totally "human-engineered." Violence trauma is injury to the self-structure of the child. Its consequences are often profound and severe.

In PTCT, the child succeeds in establishing a meaningful, supportive relationship in psychotherapy, so that the internalized violence structures of helplessness and vendetta rage may be transformed into structures of control and self-efficacy.

At this time, the effects of violence upon the minds of children are not well understood. Because of the impact of violence on behavioral adaptation, the child experiences internal disorganization and fragmentation. Therapy aims to restore a sense of organization and cohesion. The general goal of therapy, then, is to assist the child to integrate violence trauma, and to effectively cope with subsequent exposure to violence and its psychosocial impacts. As long as the child remains in the atmosphere of violence, the more psychotherapeutic and psychologic support he or she will need over time.

Violence continues to be a major public health problem in the United States and in many parts of Europe, the Middle East, and Asia. We need to understand more about the root causes of children's exposure to ongoing violence and a world that creates jackals and predators who say, "It's killing time."

This chapter has focused on children's problematic responses to witnessing violence, on therapists' responses and on the importance of understanding children's coping abilities (Parson, 1994). It has acknowledged "that the occurrence of the actual (traumatic) event . . . fundamentally skews ego formation, and distorts affective growth while casting a pall over object relations development" (Schaer, 1991, p. 15). However, the following is also true: "Clinical practice informs us that despite the existence of overwhelming, frightening events in the lives of inner-city children, they do not become marasmic, literally withering on the vine due to their submission to a hostile environment" (Schaer, 1991, p. 14).

Preventing violence from becoming a part of inner city children's life-style is an important social goal. For inner city children, preventing violence exposure means preventing violent behavior in the future. PTCT may reduce the power of internalized violence in the child through a living relationship with a therapist who commits to understanding U-VTS and PTSD, and who also commits to countertransference management during PTCT. The importance of addressing this issue of generational violence cannot be underestimated; left unchecked, violence will grow, with consequences yet to be realized. Effective social policy and interaction may not only save the lives of children, but also offer new paradigms of mental health service delivery structures. What is at stake is the well-being of the next generation of Americans, those subjugated to the perils of injustice, and often to the ills of economic and political inequity.

REFERENCES

American Psychiatric Association. (1987). *Diagnostic and statistical manual of mental disorders* (3rd ed., rev.). Washington, DC: Author.
Arroyo, W., & Eth, S. (1985). Children traumatized by Central American warfare.

In S. Eth & R. Pynoos (Eds.), *Post-traumatic stress disorder in children.* Washington, DC: American Psychiatric Press.

Bandura, A. (1973). *Aggression: A social learning approach.* Englewood Cliffs, NJ: Prentice-Hall.

Bell, C., & Jenkins, E. (1991). Traumatic stress and children. *Journal of Health Care for the Poor and Underserved, 2,* 175–188.

Bell, C., Prothrow-Stith, D., Smallwood, C., & Murchison, C. (1986). Black-on-black homicide: The National Medical Association's responsibilities. *Journal of the National Medical Association, 78,* 577–580.

Brende, J. O., & Parson, E. R. (1985). *Vietnam veterans: The road to recovery.* New York: Plenum Press.

Butts, H. (1971). Psychoanalysis and unconscious racism. *Journal of Contemporary Psychotherapy, 3,* 67–81.

Coles, R. (1967). *Children of crisis.* Boston: Little, Brown.

Concise American Heritage dictionary. (1980). Boston: Houghton Mifflin.

Dubrow, N., & Garbarino, J. (1989). Living in the war zone: Mothers and young children in a public housing development. *Journal of Child Welfare, 68,* 3–20.

Dyson, J. (1990). The effects of family violence on children's academic performance and behavior. *Journal of the National Medical Association, 82,* 17–22.

Ekstein, R. (1966). *Children of time and space, of action and impulse: Clinical studies on the psychoanalytic treatment of severely disturbed children.* New York: Appleton-Century-Crofts.

Emde, R. (1982). *The development of attachment and affiliative systems.* New York: Plenum Press.

Field, R. (1977). *Society under siege: A psychology of Northern Ireland.* Harmondsworth, England: Penguin.

Field, T. (1985). Attachment as psychobiological attunement: Being on the same wavelength. In M. Reite & T. Field (Eds.), *The psychobiology of attachment and separation.* Orlando, FL: Academic Press.

Flavell, J. (1983). *The developmental psychology of Jean Piaget.* New York: Van Nostrand Reinhold.

Foa, E., Zinbarg, R., & Rothbaum, B. (1992). Uncontrollability and unpredictability in post-traumatic stress disorder. *Psychological Bulletin, 112,* 218–238.

Frederick, C. (1985). Children traumatized by catastrophic situations. In S. Eth & R. Pynoos (Eds.), *Post-traumatic stress disorder in children.* Washington, DC: American Psychiatric Press.

Freud, S. (1914). Remembering, repeating, and working through. *Standard Edition, 12,* 145–156. London: Hogarth Press, 1958.

Garbarino, J., Kostelny, K., & Dubrow, N. (1991). What children can tell us about living in danger. *American Psychologist, 46,* 376–383.

Gardner, G. (1971). Aggression and violence—the enemies of precision learning in children. *American Journal of Psychiatry, 128,* 445–450.

Gardner, R. (1975). *Psychotherapeutic approaches to the resistant child.* New York: Jason Aronson.

Haley, S. A. (1987). The Vietnam veteran and his preschool child: Childrearing as a delayed stress in combat veterans. In W. Quaytman (Ed.), *The Vietnam veteran: Studies in post-traumatic stress disorder.* New York: Human Sciences Press.

Hilliard, A. (1984). IQ testing as the emperor's new clothes: A critique of Jensen's bias in mental testing. In C. Reynolds (Ed.), *Perspectives on bias in mental tests.* New York: Plenum Press.

Kohlberg, L. (1964). Development of moral character and moral ideology. In M. Hoffman & L. Hoffman (Eds.), *Review of child development.* New York: Russell Sage Foundation.

Kohut, H. (1977). *The restoration of the self.* New York: International Universities Press.

Krystal, H. (1978). Trauma and affects. *Psychoanalytic Study of the Child, 33,* 81–116.

Krystal, H., & Niederland, W. (1968). Clinical observations on the survivor syndrome. In H. Krystal (Ed.), *Massive psychic trauma.* New York: International Universities Press.

Lifton, R. J. (1982). The psychology of the survivor and the death imprint. *Psychiatric Annals, 12,* 1010–1017.

Mahler, M., Pine, R., & Bergman, A. (1975). *The psychological birth of the human infant.* New York: Basic Books.

Maroda, K. (1991). *The power of countertransference: Innovations in analytic technique.* New York: Wiley.

Meers, D. R. (1970). Contributions of a ghetto culture to symptom formation: Psychoanalytic studies of ego anomalies in childhood. *Psychoanalytic Study of the Child, 25,* 209–230.

Meers, D. R. (1973). Psychoanalytic research and intellectual functioning of ghetto-reared, black children. *Psychoanalytic Study of the Child, 28,* 230–246.

Meers, D. R., & Gordon, F. (1975). Traumatic and cultural distortions of psychoneurotic symptoms in a black ghetto. *Annual of Psychoanalysis, 20,* 580–592.

Parson, E. R. (1984). Clinical and theoretical dimensions in the treatment of Vietnam combat veterans. *Journal of Contemporary Psychotherapy, 14,* 4–56.

Parson, E. R. (1988). Post-traumatic self disorders (PTsfD). In J. Wilson, Z. Harel, & B. Kahana (Eds.), *Adaptation to extreme stress: From the Holocaust to Vietnam.* New York: Plenum Press.

Parson, E. R. (1994). Post-traumatic stress and coping in an inner city child: Traumatogenic witnessing of inter-parental violence and murder. *Psychoanalytic Study of the Child, 50.*

Pynoos, R., & Eth, S. (1985). Developmental perspectives on psychic trauma in childhood. In C. R. Figley (Ed.), *Trauma and its wake.* New York: Brunner/Mazel.

Pynoos, R., & Nader, K. (1988). Psychological first aid and treatment approach to community violence: Research implications. *Journal of Traumatic Stress, 1,* 445–474.

Racker, H. (1968). The meaning and uses of countertransference. In *Transference and countertransference.* New York: International Universities Press.

Roth, W. (1988). The role of medication in post-traumatic therapy. In F. Ochberg (Ed.), *Post-traumatic therapy and victims of violence.* New York: Brunner/Mazel.

Rutter, M. (1987). Psychosocial resilience and pretective mechanisms. *American Journal of Orthopsychiatry, 57,* 316–331.

Sandler, J. (1967). Trauma, strain, and development. In S. S. Furst (Ed.), *Psychic traumatization.* New York: Basic Books.

Schaer, I. (1991, August). A theoretical conceptualization of the multiply traumatized inner-city child of poverty. *Section II—Section on Childhood and Adolescence Newsletter, 1*(1), 12–22.

Tapp, C. (1971). Socialization, the law and society. *Journal of Social Issues, 27,* 21–33.

Terr, L. (1979). Children of Chowchilla: Study of psychic trauma. *Psychoanalytic Study of the Child, 34,* 547–623.

Timnick, L. (1989, September 3). Children of violence. *Los Angeles Times Magazine,* pp. 6–15.

Trad, P. V. (1988). *Developmental scenarios in pediatrics.* New York: Springer-Verlag.

Trad, P. V. (1989). *The preschool child: Assessment, diagnosis, and treatment.* New York: Wiley.

Trad, P. V. (1990). *Conversations with preschool children.* New York: W. W. Norton.

Trad, P. V., Raine, M., Chazan, S., & Greenblatt, E. (1992). Working through conflict with self destructive preschool children. *American Journal of Psychotherapy, 46,* 640–662.

van der Kolk, B. (1987). *Psychological trauma.* Washington, DC: American Psychiatric Press.

Wilson, J. P., & Raphael, B. (Eds.). (1993). *The international handbook of traumatic stress syndromes.* New York: Plenum Press.

Winnicott, D. W. (1975). *Through pediatrics to psychoanalysis.* New York: Basic Books.

7

Countertransference in the Treatment of Acutely Traumatized Children

KATHLEEN NADER

The Prevention Intervention Program in Trauma, Violence, and Sudden Bereavement at the University of California, Los Angeles (UCLA) has provided treatment and consultation nationally and internationally for child victims and their families exposed to natural disasters (e.g., earthquakes, tornadoes), violence (e.g., school and restaurant shootings, robberies), accidents (e.g., vehicle, shooting), and war (e.g., Kuwait, Croatia, and Central America). In addition to child victims, interventions have been provided for child witnesses of, for example, rape, suicide, and other injury or death (accidental, deliberate, disaster related). Children from a wide variety of backgrounds have been interviewed and treated; no socio-economic level is immune to traumatic experience.

Individual children and families in the Los Angeles area are seen in the UCLA Neuropsychiatric Institute (NPI) and Hospital and the NPI child outpatient clinic. Consultations are provided to groups such as schools, churches, and restaurants across the United States and, post-war or post-disaster, to other nations. Consultations include planning, triage, and the training of mental health and on-site personnel in methods of intervention for children exposed to traumatic events.

There has been considerable advancement in the understanding of post-traumatic stress and related symptoms in traumatized children as well as greater appreciation of the complexity of children's subjective reactions (Pynoos, Frederick, Nader, et al., 1987; Yule & Williams, 1990). There have now been several reports of different proposed methods of assessment and treatment (McNally, 1991; Nader & Pynoos,

1991; Pynoos & Nader, 1993). However, there has been corresponding attention paid to neither the difficulties encountered by the clinician engaged in this work nor the specific conceptualization of the counter-transference issues. We have supervised and trained child psychiatry fellows, clinical social workers, psychiatric residents, and psychologists in the screening and treatment of traumatized children. Training has been provided at UCLA through class lectures, ongoing supervision, and case conferences, and at other locations in the form of brief didactic (usually 1–2 days) or periodic on-site training sessions. The latter usually entails 1 week every 2–3 months for up to 2 years and has consisted of didactic sessions, observation of the trainer conducting treatment sessions, continued work with traumatized and grieving children, trainer's observation of trainees, and case presentations. This on-site training is supplemented by continued practice, local on-site supervision, and regular case presentations within the treatment group; the trainer remains available for phone consultations. This chapter discusses some of the countertransference difficulties encountered by trainees, primarily in mastering an active empathic inquiry during the acute phase of trauma treatment of children's post-traumatic stress disorder (PTSD).

SPECIALIZED CHILD TRAUMA INTERVENTION

The UCLA Trauma Program's assessment procedures for post-traumatic reactions involve two components: (1) the reliable measurement of children's distress and symptomatic responses (Pynoos et al., 1987; Nader, Pynoos, Fairbanks, & Frederick, 1990; Yule & Williams, 1990), and (2) the use of special interview techniques to explore children's subjective experiences (Pynoos & Eth, 1986; Nader & Pynoos, 1991; Pynoos & Nader, 1993). One of the first products of our program was an interview protocol that permits a thorough "debriefing" of the child.

The child interview is designed to elicit a thorough account from the child of her or his experience including affective, sensory, and physiological experiences; identifiable sources of traumatic anxiety; traumatic reminders; early coping processes; and trauma-related life stresses. In remembering life-threatening events, children's recall is not organized as a single episode, rather as multiple traumatic episodes within a single event. Spatial and temporal registration, affective and cognitive responses, sets of perceptions, intervention fantasies, and psychodynamic attributions differ for each moment and memory anchor point (Pynoos & Nader, 1989).

Imagined actions are incorporated into children's traumatic memory representations. Ongoing intervention fantasies are integral to children's reprocessing of traumatic events. They include the child's fantasies during and after the event of preventing or stopping harm, of challenging the assailant, or of repairing damage. Revenge fantasies, for example, rid the child of the external threat while answering the internal threat. When children's desires to act during an event go unresolved, the result can be a major change in behavior and personality. Lack of resolution of, for example, a revenge fantasy may result in increased aggression or inhibition (Nader & Pynoos, 1991).

Even one interview using specialized techniques to inquire about the subjective experiences of the trauma is helpful to children. The original model of traumatic neuroses as proposed by Kardiner (1941) described a constriction of both cognitive and emotional ego functioning. The goal of the initial interview is to begin ego restoration, which is demonstrated, for example, in the following ways:

1. Children become much less frightened of being overwhelmed by recalling their experiences and by identifying difficult moments;
2. They gain confidence in their ability to anticipate and manage traumatic reminders;
3. Their emotional range increases; and
4. They feel more competent in addressing some of the secondary changes that have resulted.

Moreover, the initial interview begins a process by which the child can engage in constructive intervention fantasies. It also identifies troubling moments that require more time to assimilate and assists children with their expectations about recovery. The clinician acts as advocate or involves others as advocate for the child in order to minimize secondary adversities. Attention is given to achieving the proper closure at the end of the interview to prevent leaving the child with renewed anxiety and an unnecessary avoidance of the therapeutic situation itself.

Children's memories are context specific. When children have initial difficulty in recall, rather than memory impairment, it is often because they lack an adequate retrieval strategy (Johnson & Foley, 1984; Pynoos & Nader, 1989). In this initial interview, the clinician is providing children with a strategy of recall. The result is an enhanced scaffolding for the children's descriptions of their subjective experiences.

The strategy of recall becomes a part of children's memory of the event. Giving children prohibiting or misleading recall instructions may limit memory and thereby introduce distortions. When a child either is told just to forget what happened or is taken only to a certain point in recalling the incident, future memories may be restricted (Pynoos & Nader, 1989). When this has occurred and we see a child years later, the child discusses only the limited portion of her or his experience. Therefore, the initial interview and the clinician's ability to explore the traumatic experience thoroughly may be key to the overall intervention with a traumatized child.

One key to intervention is ongoing attention to the reprocessing of both external and internal dangers (Freud, 1926). In addition to the external threat, children contend with a variety of threats from, for example, their physical and affective responses; a sense of helplessness and ineffectualness; disturbances to the emerging self-concept; intrapsychic dangers of abandonment, loss of love, anxiety about physical integrity, and superego condemnation; and disturbances in impulse control and processes of identification (Pynoos & Nader, 1993).

Treatment of PTSD in children can be both rewarding and trying for the clinician. Initially, the therapist takes an active role in addressing the impact of the traumatic experience. Although children may need assistance in understanding the influence of prior life experiences on current traumatic response, it is essential to maintain a primary focus on the child's full subjective experience and its impact. For example, a 12-year-old girl was taken hostage with a group of her peers, then witnessed the suicide of the assailant. She had previous ongoing issues related to early abandonment by her father. The primary focus of treatment remained upon traumatic issues including fears of being shot or having a friend shot while a hostage, seeing friends crying with fright, hearing an adult try to talk the assailant out of shooting or suicide, listening to the woman dictate her suicide note, seeing the assailant with blood spurting out of her head and mouth, other episodes of her experience and its aftermath, and primary and secondary symptoms. Specific moments of the event may bring up different issues in varying ways. For the 12-year-old girl, in trying to secure a greater sense of safety in examining particular traumatic moments, abandonment themes became a part of her processing and response.

On the other hand, during the course of long-term trauma work, earlier concerns may be addressed as they become enmeshed with trauma issues or become a necessary prelude to some aspect of trauma resolution. Approximately 1 year after treatment began, abandonment became a more central focus of attention for the 12-year-old girl. She was unable to focus on her traumatic rage until these abandonment issues had been addressed.

Expectations about recovery influence children's levels of ongoing distress. Because children may react adversely to the presence of symptoms, a major goal is to help them to understand that their reactions are expectable and normal. For example, adolescents may look on their posttraumatic stress reactions (e.g., the need for assistance or the need to be closer to parents) as childish. School-age children may feel they should be symptom free after a few months and may therefore attempt to hide or disavow their symptoms. For example, a 3rd-grade boy appeared to become more clumsy after the death of a classmate in a plane crash. He later admitted to the school nurse that he would hurt himself more frequently so that he would have a reason to cry. He felt that the other children were no longer sad and upset about their classmate's death and would think he was silly for continuing to cry.

COUNTERTRANSFERENCE AND EMPATHIC DISTRESS

The clinician's role often begins on the phone when parents, school personnel, or other individuals ask for advice. The trauma therapist may be asked, for example, what to tell children about a deceased individual or about the manner of death (e.g., "What should I tell Mary about her father's murder?"), what to do about relocation (e.g., "Should we move to a new apartment instead of staying here where my husband stabbed us?"; "Shouldn't they tear down the restaurant where the shootings happened? Every time we go near there, Randy gets upset."), or what changes to expect in the child (e.g., "How will I know if this has affected John?"). The clinician may respond to the demand (or perceived demand) to solve the impact of the trauma in all of its dimensions through quick decisions about specific family matters. The result may be the clinician's sense of being overwhelmed or ineffectual. Regaining an empathic, information-gathering stance about the children and the post-traumatic situation may enable clinicians to adequately apply their working knowledge of human and traumatic response to the current circumstances. For example, a guardian may not know that removing the traumatic reminder does not remove the traumatic response (e.g., moving away from home after her father was killed by a robber did not eliminate Laticia's bad dreams, intrusive thoughts, sense of estrangement, regressive behaviors, irritability, increased somatic complaints, rage, or new defiant behaviors). This principle may be relevant on the community level (e.g., tearing down the fast-food restaurant where the massacre occurred, in response to community outrage, did not reduce traumatic reactions and in fact was problematic when Randy was ready to return to the scene and walk through it as a part of his treatment). There may be social or political pressure to take some definitive action such as tearing down a building (e.g., after a sniper shot children from a second-story window, neighbors wanted to burn or tear the house down; painting the home a different color diminished their outcry). On the other hand, caretakers need to know that children may need protection from repeated exposure to specific, avoidable traumatic reminders (e.g., arranging school-site memorials so that viewing is optional) (Nader & Pynoos, 1993).

Vicarious Immersion in Trauma: Testing the Limits of Empathy

The anxiety is palpable in the treatment room with victims of trauma (e.g., the severely traumatized child may bring intense traumatic anxiety to the session; intense anxiety may be renewed as the child reenacts or reassembles the scene of the trauma). There are multiple components to the child's experience and response, and his or her sense of urgency and need for relief may be prominent. The clinician herself or himself may on multiple occasions experience the emotions common to trauma (e.g., helplessness, rage, confusion, desires to repair or retaliate) as well as personal emotional responses and anxieties surrounding what a "good clinician" should do. The clinician is confronted, on more than one occasion during the course of treatment, with the contagion of helplessness and the sense of being overwhelmed. She or he may feel that what happened to the child will always be too much to handle. It is essential to recognize helplessness as part of the traumatic response and as nonbinding on the clinician. As noted in Chapter 2 of this volume, all of these affective reactions are Type I and Type II countertransference reactions.

There are two immediate sources of empathic strain for the clinician: (1) listening to the threat to the child, and (2) listening to the child's distress at witnessing threat or injury to another, especially to a family member or friend. Interventions with traumatized children include their relating in depth, for example, (1) horrifying images, such as the sight of the man stabbing his victim, the assailant gouging out the eyes of the child's father, or blood streaming from all of the facial openings of the suicide victim; (2) extremely frightening moments, such as seeing the strange look on father's face before he lifts the knife to stab his child, looking into the barrel of the gun, seeing the man with the gun get angry, or bullets hitting the pavement to the right and left of the child; (3) extreme sensory moments, such as the knife pounding into the back of the child's head, or the smell and feel of the cigarette burning the child's skin; and (4) moments of intense helplessness, such as moments in which intervention is not available or is impossible (e.g., watching a mother die, seeing a father tortured, hearing a wounded child's cries for help when any attempt to assist would result in death or injury), moments of ineffectualness (e.g., attempting resuscitation of a schoolmate or parent, being unable to pull the assailant off of someone, being unable to pull the knife out of the father's hands), or the inability to tolerate the internal threat (e.g., not knowing when the gun will go off causing death or injury, murderous impulses toward the assailant or toward a sibling, feeling the heart will explode from pounding so hard and fast). Like others, the clinician may not want to believe that anyone would subject a child to such experiences.

TRANSFORMING EMPATHIC STRAIN INTO EFFECTUAL CLINICAL WORK

The desire on the part of mental health professionals and others to protect adult and child victims from further harm can be positive. Protectiveness may result in, for example, appropriate pacing, a sensitivity to the capacity to face specific trauma-related issues, and the imparting of protective information. The clinician's protectiveness is positive when the clinician acts as advocate for the child, when the protectiveness facilitates the development of a safe environment in which the patient can regress, express fantasies of intervention, and face the overwhelming moments of the experience. There are several common ways, however, in which individuals attempt to provide protection that are contraindicated, as they may interfere with the process of recovery. These countertransference tendencies of overprotection may result, for example, in delaying treatment, in participating in a conspiracy of silence, in avoiding upsetting issues or intense emotions, or in hesitating to push forward or review when looking for missing emotion-laden moments. Lack of protection may occur if, on the other hand, the clinician feels that she or he must remain neutral to the situation when, in fact, action is needed on behalf of the child.

Knowing When to Intervene: Traps and Pitfalls in Countertransference

Deciding when to intervene may elicit countertransference issues surrounding the clinician's need to rescue or protect, or it may elicit fears regarding doing harm to a child in fragile condition. Errors may occur in an attempt to protect the child from premature treatment. Especially with injured children, the inclination may be to delay treatment until the child has had some time to recover. Sometimes, the overzealous clinician may overprescribe treatment, feeling that every child must be treated rather than assessing the child's ability to recover within the family context. On the other hand, the clinician may minimize the effects of the experience and may underprescribe treatment. For years people argued that children were not affected by their traumatic experiences ("If you just leave them alone, they will be fine."). Even if ongoing treatment is not required following a traumatic event, it is helpful to see children to assist them to understand the event in the context of their lives. One interview can provide the child with a strategy of recall and thus be of assistance later. This is especially true if the child later seeks intervention after ongoing development or life experiences result in reassessment or renewed reaction to the traumatic experience.

Treatment can begin in the hospital. Identifying traumatic reminders in the hospital setting may reduce the child's distress and may reduce interferences to healing. For example, balloons were sent to cheer up a child who had been injured in a shooting. When one of them popped, the child's severe startle reaction disrupted intubation, which resulted in increased pain and bleeding in the wound. In the initial phases of recovery when injured children need to focus most of their energy on physical recuperation, they still need an opportunity to retell their experiences and may spontaneously do so. When this happens, a particular bond is formed with the listener. Making contact during the hospitalization is an opportunity to establish an initial rapport with the child, as well as to accommodate the child's need for recounting what happened and to ensure adequate recall.

Psychiatric interventions, especially with children, traditionally occur after the onset of significant emotional disturbance. It is both easier and less costly to intervene before disorders become fixed and severe. As is true for adult traumatic reactions (Kaltreider, Wallace, & Horowitz, 1979), treatment of traumatized children is most effective in the acute phase of response, when the intrusive phenomena are most apparent and the associated affect most available. There may in fact be a critical period in which to work with traumatized children (Nader & Pynoos, 1988). Traumatic material appeared to be less easily accessible after the first 3–6 months in working with groups of children after their exposure to a sniper attack, a tornado, and a murder.

The Willingness to Hear and the Need for Awareness of Countertransference

The goal of effective intervention is to hear everything, including the worst aspects of victimization. Like others, therapists may feel that the child has gone through something that is too horrible to talk about, or they may fear causing the child further harm by bringing up painful aspects of the event. The origin of the avoidance may be internal to the clinician rather than to the child. There may be an anxious need to contain affect in response to the child's experience. The clinician may not want to hear, for example, the viciousness of a child's revenge fantasy. Fear of not knowing what to do in the face of intense emotional pain may reinforce the avoidant bias.

If the clinician has had a previous traumatic or stressful experience, the child's story may reevoke the clinician's own previous symptoms or intense emotions (see Chapter 2, this volume, for a discussion). The reemergence of the clinician's symptomatic or emotional response may jeopardize her or his ability to take a therapeutic stance. For example, a school psychologist was unable to think about the traumatic deaths of two school children without remembering the traumatic death of her cousin when she was 12. She had difficulty sitting through training sessions regarding children's traumatic responses. She was also concerned when her anxiety and distress interfered with her ability to assist the deceased children's classmates and teachers with their reactions. In fact, some clinicians must eliminate themselves from treatment of the children altogether, because of their own experiences previous to or during the traumatic event. For example, the school psychologist who had been injured in war-related combat had to maintain a peripheral role in assisting children after a school shooting when he began to reexperience thoughts of the combat experience. After school children were killed, mutilated, and injured under the fallen bricks of a building, a psychologist who had been a part of the rescue effort found that hearing the children's descriptions of their experiences increased her own symptomatic response.

Countertransference as a Form of Therapist Resistance

Some clinicians have expressed concerns about questioning children regarding their traumatic experiences even for the purposes of diagnostic screening. For example, in one war-torn country where the threat continued, a few clinicians became concerned about our protocol, which called for directly questioning the children. They first focused on ethical issues, then the length of the interview, then on peripheral issues such as concerns about transportation to sites and availability of children, then on the potential harm in asking children about their pain. It became clear in observing the clinicians, before and during practice interviews, that they felt protective toward the children both from overidentification with their pain and horror and from discomfort at watching the children suffer. As they became comfortable with the interview, they were pleased with the results of administering it. In fact, although the children sometimes cried or expressed other intense emotions such as anger during the interview, they were relieved, unburdened, and more animated after the interview. They smiled, skipped away, and thanked us. They told their friends about the interview and the other children waited in line to talk with us. It can be a disservice to children to communicate, even nonverbally, (1) that it is too overwhelming to discuss the trauma, (2) that it is not okay to talk about their experiences, and/or (3) that they cannot discuss these intense experiences and still cope afterwards. It is therapeutic for children when the clinician recognizes the value of talking and recognizes in the child the strength and courage to endure and to process traumatic materials.

Moreover, especially during initial intervention interviews, any reluctance to directly discuss the child's experience may lead to disturbances in memory and cognition related to the event. It is essential to elicit the whole of the child's experience including her or his affective responses, rather than encouraging a journalistic retelling. It can be a countertransference to be unaware of affective constriction in the journalistic recounting, especially in latency age children. The child's journalistic review of aspects of the event, in fact, may diminish understanding of the event's meaning to the child and the particular way in which the child experienced traumatic helplessness.

Avoidance may occur in the form of collusion between the therapist, family, and child either not to address something that is important to the experience or to avoid or ignore clear links between the child's behavior and some aspect of the event. Responsible adults may hesitate to tell the truth (sometimes out of a sense of protection) or, to the contrary, may give the child information beyond her or his ability to understand. For example, misleading explanations, conspiracies of silence, or prohibitions against discussion of certain details of the event can all contribute to chronic difficulties in cognition or to an inability to accurately identify emotional responses (Pynoos & Nader, 1988b). Because of a desire to believe that the event had no real effect on the child, adults may avoid linking aspects of the child's behavior to a traumatic event. Effective clinicians recognize this avoidance in themselves and in the child's adult caretakers, for example, when a grandmother, now guardian, whose son killed the child's mother, finds it important to blame the mother and deny symptoms in the child. Moreover, the clinician may make the wrong link either in an attempt to make any link that presents itself or in order to avoid the more appropriate link, which might evoke an intense affective response.

Directiveness

Our specialized methods are directive in nature. The degree of directiveness is, of course, adjusted to the tolerance and needs of the child. Countertransference tendencies may contribute to uncertainty, leading clinicians either to pull back or to plunge forward. Hesitance leaves the child with the impression that aspects of the trauma are too horrible to face or that she or he is incapable of facing them. It lends inadequate support or energy to the child's reprocessing or resolution of specific aspects of the event.

Combining a sense of uncertainty with attempts to help children recount even difficult moments may result in counterphobically pushing forward into traumatic materials. Although pushing forward is essential in this method of trauma work, counterphobically doing so fails to respect the child's timing, limits, and needs. Failing to adjust the method to the child's needs may cause further resistance or avoidance in the child or cause a sense of failure in processing the event.

Out of their own needs to restore a sense of safety or normalcy or to avoid the intensity of traumatic emotions, clinicians may revert to less directive methods of inquiry and more traditional formulations. Interpretations of traumatic behaviors based on early childhood conflicts or on non-trauma-related symbolic formulations may both avoid traumatic issues and increase the traumatized individual's sense of aloneness and helplessness. For example, an adolescent patient reported to a psychiatrist that, in response to a traumatic reminder, she had been distressed and confused and had inadvertently entered the exit of the freeway. He looked for the symbolic meaning of entering the exit. This focus increased the girl's distress rather than leading to any resolution. It ignored the intensity of her trauma-related regression, concentration impairment, and confusion, and it failed to lead to protecting her from driving when symptoms might interfere with her ability to do so safely.

Intervention Fantasies during and after Traumatic Experience

Intervention fantasies are integral to the ongoing therapeutic processing of a child's traumatic experience (Pynoos & Nader, 1989). These include the child's or adolescent's fantasies during and after the traumatic experience of preventing or stopping the harm, of confronting the perpetrator, of effecting repair, or of revenge or retaliation. For example, a 5-year-old boy fantasized running for help when he saw the man on top of his stepmother but, after being slammed onto the floor, the boy followed the rapist's instructions to go back to sleep. A preadolescent imagined using his martial arts skills against the assailant. An adolescent ran for a knife to stab the attacker, was disarmed, and felt cowardly. Revenge fantasies against the trauma perpetrator may occur during or after the traumatic event as a desire to intervene or as a result of traumatic rage. Countertransference may result in seeing only the rage and in overlooking the revenge fantasy's specific link to the trauma. For example, a pre-adolescent boy witnessed the rape of his mother. He later entertained a fantasy of poking out the eyes of the rapist and putting a pencil up his penis. This fantasy of revenge was directly related to the visual insult of witnessing with horror while this man penetrated and ejaculated on his mother and to the boy's desire not only to injure the offender but to prevent him from ever again harming someone in this manner.

Countertransference as a Source of Insight

The clinician responds to the child's intervention fantasies with her or his own emotions of empathy or overempathy, identification or overiden-tification, and/or tolerance or worry about the intensity of the child's emotions. The clinician, too, follows the story of what happened, which evokes her or his own countertransference fantasies of intervention. The clinician imagines what could have been done to prevent or stop the harm, how someone could have intervened, or the appropriate actions to take during and after the traumatic event to mitigate pain or injury. If clinicians excessively relate, for example, to the rage or anger, their timing may be affected. For example, a young woman's closest surviving adolescent sister found her bloody body after the young woman shot herself in the head. The clinician who saw the surviving sister for treatment of her traumatic reaction felt drawn into an angry stance toward the deceased sister, in part, for traumatizing her patient (see case example later). She wanted to immediately address the patient's anger at her sister. The focus was ill-timed, as the patient needed first to address her strong desire to assist and to repair the damage.

    When a child's desires to act are unresolved, the result can be a major change in behavior and personality. For example, lack of resolution of a revenge fantasy may result in increased aggression or inhibition (Nader & Pynoos, 1991). A 12-year-old boy was under a table for nearly an hour and a half while a sniper walked around the restaurant massacring 21 people and injuring many others. The boy was shot in both arms. He spent a portion of the time he was immobilized under the table entertaining fantasies of beating up the sniper. When a SWAT member, wearing the same clothes and boots as the assailant, pulled him up by the arm, the boy tried to slug him thinking he was another assailant. Later the boy became violent any time anyone put their hand around his arm, when he wore boots like the sniper, or when anyone touched him in the way he had touched his dead friend in an attempt to awaken him. He provoked physical fights with his peers and carried a weapon into an area known to be frequented by other armed adolescents. If, as a result of their own countertransference fantasies or affective reactions, clinicians ignore or censor fantasies of intervention, or attend to them in a manner that is ill-timed or inappropriate to the child's needs, the child's resolution of these desires to act may be thwarted.

Anger and Impulse Control

Clinicians may oversympathize or overprotect when issues of anger and impulse control arise. Traumatic exposure challenges a child's sense of impulse control (Pynoos & Nader, 1988c). The oversympathetic clinician may find her or his own resolve undermined. For example, some children begin to wonder why they should bother to behave, if bad things can happen to you anyway. After a tornado killed nine children in one school, one teacher described that children acted as though they no longer knew the rules. When told that they had to behave appropriately some of the children asked, "Why should we?" Recognizing the child's (and others') need for structure, for a return to normalcy, and for a reduction in the post-trauma chaos, the clinician is able to assist adults in the child's world in responding.

Seeing an adult react violently during a violent event can make a child question her or his own ability to control herself or himself. Lapses in self-control may take the form of reenactment or traumatic play. One little boy whose father had strangled his stepmother began to play at strangling his peers, sometimes frightening them and causing them pain. Other than to prevent harm, both guardian and clinician in a countertransference may decide to overlook lapses in control because lapses are understandable after a traumatic experience or because the children should not be punished when they already feel so bad. Paradoxically the resultant absence of structure or control may be frightening to the child who, especially after the trauma, needs limits to regain self-control, a more normal sense of self, and a sense of safety.

Traumatic rage may further challenge a child's impulse control. When the lack of impulse control is amplified by the child's expression of traumatic rage, it may cause concern in the therapist. A clinician who already has difficulty with anger or rage may find the presence and expression of rage difficult to tolerate and may censor this effort of the child to manage the trauma. Even the clinician who tolerates anger may become concerned at the intensity and implications of its expression in a traumatized child, especially when there is repetitive aggressive play. A 10-year-old boy who had been injured twice by falling (once from his high chair; once from a second-story window) was referred for "strange" behaviors at school including head banging and poking himself with a pencil. He played regularly that toy soldiers, ninja turtles, and stuffed animals beat each other to death. When he told stories, the main character kept accidentally killing people. The therapist identified with the innocent victims in the play and thus failed to understand that it was the child who was the victim and that the accidental killer was the mother who had failed to prevent the boy's falls. The clinician became concerned that he was working with a budding serial murderer and had a desire to change the play and story endings so that the aggression was stopped or the aggressor transformed.

Censoring the child's expression of rage or revenge may create rather than solve the problem. On the other hand, the clinician wants to avoid desensitizing the child to causing pain or harm. The idea is to facilitate the expression of rage or revenge in the safe therapeutic setting while reinforcing the child's impulse control. When successfully accomplished, the result is a sense of relief, a reduced sense of helplessness, and freedom to examine the other aspects of the traumatic experience.

The Phasic Nature of Trauma Recovery and the Timing of Interventions

Trauma recovery is characterized by progress alternating with periodic exacerbation of symptoms. The child lends meaning to specific traumatic moments and puts them in the context of her or his life. The exacerbation of symptoms may elicit in the therapist guilt, a sense of self-doubt, or even a sense that the original assessment of progress was inaccurate. Fears of not helping the child or making her or him worse may result. These symptom exacerbations can be a dangerous time for the patients, who may also fear that they assessed their progress inaccurately or wrongly trusted the treatment and are not really getting better. Feelings of depression and sometimes suicidal ideation may increase at this time. Thus the patient's and the clinician's fears reinforce each other. Understanding the phasic nature of recovery and identifying the countertransference fear of harming prepares the clinician to appropriately label for the patient these predictable moments.

Also, during the course of recovery, there may be a reduction in numbing and a complementary exacerbation of intrusive symptoms. This increase in symptoms can be recognized as a sign of progress, rather than a failure of treatment, and as an indication that further exploration of specific moments is necessary. Unburdened of the countertransference fear of hurting the child, the clinician is able to respect the child's own timing. Initially, even though, for example, the clinician perceives that the child's first identified "worst moment" is less severe than other aspects of her or his experience, it may be more appropriate for the child to address the less trying moment first. For example, an 11-year-old girl was hit in the face by a flying table during a natural disaster. Her front teeth were knocked out, and she bled profusely. When asked about her worst moment she focused on a true moment of fear—calling for help after the injury, when the debris had stopped flying; the desperate need for rescue. Both initially and as numbing reduces and the child's confidence and ego strength improve, it is essential to push through difficult moments, to find the physiological, affective, and perceptual aspects of the experience, as well as any lost portions. Indeed, the aspects of the traumatic experience originally defined by the child as the worst moment may pale in comparison to what she or he is later able to face. On the other hand, the child's first identified worst moment may be psychodynamically more important to the child, and thus may be, for the child, the worst moment. For example, a school-age girl described being called by her nickname by her father before he shot her.

Moreover, each child establishes her or his own rhythms of trauma review. For example, Randy, the adolescent who was injured during a massacre in a fast-food restaurant, came late to trauma treatment. He engaged in trauma work only every other session in the initial phases of his trauma work. Early in his treatment this adolescent engaged in symbolic trauma-related activities for a portion of each trauma-focused session as well as in discussion of the trauma (e.g., waging war on the ants outside the therapy room door after discussing the death of his friend during the massacre). A girl who was the sole survivor of the kidnap and murders of her family needed to focus on the loss of her family about every fourth session, after she mastered specific traumatic moments and issues. Some children need periodically to stop and focus on secondary post-trauma changes to their lives or on the meaning of the trauma to previous or subsequent life experiences. The clinician's own comfort and confidence assists recognition of and attunement with the child's particular rhythm.

A child may redefine individual traumatic moments/experiences or her or his own response to them. As a result, trauma work involves re-review and/or a more thorough review of specific traumatic moments or moment complexes with thorough attention to the new issues, definitions, responses, and/or the deeper meanings of the experience. The clinician must be willing to re-review aspects of the event in search of the child's reprocessing. For example, a change in the child's intervention fantasies or resolution of specific issues may permit the child's deeper focus on certain details. For example, an adolescent girl, her mother, and brother were stabbed by her father. The girl was unable to recall the frightening look of intent on her father's face, his raising his arm to stab her, or his cutting her hands and face. She could not admit his murderous intent, her sense of betrayal, or her anger until she was certain that she would not lose him. The need for repetitive reexamination of aspects of the event may elicit the clinician's own avoidance of seeking their more difficult meanings for the child.

TRAUMA'S COMMON THEMES

Some level of emotion is naturally elicited in response to the child's story. Common traumatic emotions include helplessness, rage, revenge, hopelessness, horror, avoidance (especially with ongoing or repetitive trauma), regressive states, and fear. The therapist's own past experiences may have rendered her or him vulnerable to common traumatic emotions. Some traumatic emotions are contagious (e.g., fear), are common responses (e.g., anger that this could happen to a child or about issues of accountability), or are distressing because of their intensity (e.g., traumatic rage or helplessness). Even seasoned clinicians may feel ineffectual in response to a child's sense of helplessness or overwhelmed by a child's rage or the viciousness of the child's revenge fantasy. The clinician's knowledge that clinician and child are not helpless in this moment and observation of enough recovery from traumatic response to know that there is hope can aid both patient and clinician.

The therapist's own expectations and responses related to the event can interfere with the ability to facilitate the child's psychic integration of the event and/or of a traumatic loss. Specific attitudes may undermine the clinician's therapeutic stance or inhibit therapeutic action. We have different clinicians treating parents and children. The clinician treating the mother influences the care of the children. One resident felt that an injured mother would never be able to recover from the psychological wounds inflicted by her husband's attack. He was certain that the woman would never again be capable of a normal relationship with a man. This attitude left the resident with a sense of helplessness about the ability to effect healing after this trauma. One child psychiatry fellow reminisced about his own loss and had difficulty focusing on the child's loss of a parent. Attitudes toward dependence and rage, which are frequent components of traumatic response, must also be examined. The clinician may, for a limited time, encourage dependence and may find it important to facilitate the expression of rage and revenge fantasies while reinforcing impulse control and rational decision making.

The clinician engages in play with the traumatized child and may become the object of his traumatic emotions. One child who had undergone catastrophic treatment for cancer delighted in repeatedly mutilating and killing the clinician (Nader, Stuber & Pynoos, 1991). As discussed earlier, appropriately facilitating these fantasies of revenge becomes a part of the therapeutic process. Children take any of several roles in response to traumatic experience. The therapist must be comfortable being assigned by the child any of the several roles, for example, victim, aggressor, rescuer, witness, external conscience. Maricella became nurse to the clinician who acted as victim. Abdul punched the therapist in the cushion protecting his abdomen while pretending the clinician was the bad soldier who tried to rape him. Randy (injured in the fast-food restaurant massacre) carefully positioned the clinician to the side to silently watch as an external conscience while he played sniper in the wooded area near the hospital clinical rooms.

Children commonly exhibit changes in school behavior and cognitive performance. A child's fear of stigmatization or self-consciousness about physical or emotional symptoms may result in school avoidance. The clinician may need to respond to very complicated issues of reentry into school. The therapist may need to come to grips with her or his own sense of helplessness or revulsion with regard to the child's injuries, deformities, or disabilities. There may be a sense of guilt, a sense of helplessness or ineffectualness to repair the child or her or his damaged self-image, or a sense of distaste or fear at seeing that someone normal can be made handicapped. As a result, the clinician may be reluctant to push the child forward through review of difficult moments or may reinforce the child's own sense of damage.

The child or adult exposed to trauma may lose appropriate judgment about maintaining her or his own safety. This may be, for example, a result of trying to overcome traumatic fear, an indication of unresolved rage or revenge fantasies, or a form of reenactment behavior. After running from gunfire during a sniper attack, a 7-year-old girl began walking into alleys frequented by drunken men, misjudging when to step out into the street, or freezing in the street with a car coming. Recognizing this phenomena, it is important that the clinician avoid overidentification with the need to master fear and, thus, avoid pushing the child to overcome fears prematurely. Further, it can be trying for the clinician to be working with a child who is, for example, walking into alleys or carrying weapons into areas where there are other armed youths. It is essential for the clinician to maintain for herself or himself as well as for the child a realistic evaluation of danger and a need to protect from secondary harm.

Trauma victims often feel compelled to share their experience. For example, after a wartime experience, adults repetitively reviewed videos and pictures of the horrors and children repetitively replayed aspects of the event. The clinician may be asked to view pictures of mutilation and to see destruction. In one war-torn country, before dinner pictures were passed around of horrible mutilation, burned bodies, and rudely amputated body parts. The consultant was taken to see the instruments of torture and bloodied manikins depicting their use. The clinician may need to protect herself or himself as well as children from these secondary trauma.

Issues of Accountability

Issues of accountability may elicit a variety of countertransference responses in the clinician. Deaths during a disaster have been attributed, for example, to architectural defects, to caretakers ignoring the directive to evacuate, or to lack of proposed repair to at-risk buildings or bridges. In cases of violence, someone has intentionally threatened, endangered, or harmed others. Even with accidental death or injury, issues of culpability arise. The clinician may respond with anger, despair, or horror at the nature and results of the neglect, harmful intent, carelessness, or recklessness. Like others, in the absence of a clearly identified perpetrator of the harm, the clinician may consciously or unconsciously look for someone to blame for the victimization of children. These responses may jeopardize the clinician's therapeutic stance.

When the child has a preexisting relationship with the perpetrator of harm, a tension occurs between the need to facilitate traumatic response (e.g., rage, disappointment, fears related to identification) and the need to respect the child's relationship with the individual (e.g., issues of identification, attachment, loyalty). We have found it helpful to allow the child to begin to address traumatic issues as though from the third person ("If someone was angry at your father for what he did, what might they want to do to him?") or once removed ("If you were angry at your father . . . " or "If it was someone else who had done this, what do you think should happen to them for what they did?").

Different Agendas: The Traumatized Family System

The ability to remain neutral and to avoid overidentification with only one family member is essential to the trauma specialist. Following traumatic events, each family member may have different psychological agendas according to preexisting relationships, exposure, and subsequent impact. When there is work with individual children and parents after a traumatic event, these different agendas must be appreciated. In situations of mass trauma where there have been deaths, the intervention process can become complicated as there are those who are traumatized who did not know the deceased, those who are suffering traumatic grief without traumatic exposure, and those who are both grieving and traumatized. Each group has its own agendas and phases of recovery. Trauma therapists may find themselves caught between the need to protect the traumatized children from inundation with inescapable reminders of the event and the grieving parents' needs to have tributes to and reminders of their suddenly lost children. After a disaster at a school, there may be many proposals for memorials. Compassion for or identification with grieving parents may make it difficult to set appropriate limits on the number of memorials.

Clinicians may find it difficult to remain neutral or may overidentify with individual family members. In a family in which the father was unable to protect his wife and daughters from robbers, an 11-year-old girl weekly expressed, in her play, her anger and disappointment at her father's ineffectualness. The entire family's upset with the father kept the family divided and unable to provide adequate support for each other. Clinicians found it difficult to remain unaligned with the mother against the father, who was urging the cessation of treatment. The father was in an occupation in which he dealt with life and death situations. In his uneasy lack of ability to prevent this harm, the father insisted that no one was really badly hurt (there was a severe knife wound and a molestation that occurred during the robbery). Counterphobically, he left doors unlocked at night to the complete distress of his family and the empathic concern of the clinicians. The 11-year-old girl's clinician counteracted the temptation to align with the mother by searching for a method to restore family cohesion and mutual support. One of the goals of treatment was to help the child to understand that the father's behavior was rooted in his difficulty with accepting that he was unable to protect his family. With children especially, there is often ample opportunity to stay within or to facilitate the child's metaphor in addressing traumatic issues. With this family, it permitted constructive interventions that met the needs of the entire family. In a subsequent session, the child drew a picture of a sun with the measles (clearly a representation of the father) that could not be treated because it was too big and too sick and you could not get close to it or you would get burned or catch the illness. The discussion that followed permitted the child to first send medication to the sun (father) from afar via spaceship and then to recall what one might do to help someone sick to become well. The father began locking the doors shortly after this session and stopped asking the mother to cease bringing the child to treatment.

THE THERAPIST'S EXPANDED ROLE

In working with traumatic responses, the therapist's role expands from individual work to include assistance within the family and community

(Nader & Pynoos, 1988; Pynoos & Nader, 1988a). Clinician resistance or a sense of being overwhelmed may result or may increase in response to the number and locations of interventions needed. The therapist may need to relinquish ideas of treatment's confinement to the office, or she or he might need to make provision that other areas are given ample attention.

The therapist's role becomes that of advocate when dealing with some of the secondary stresses following a traumatic event. In the immediate aftermath of the event, children need protection from unnecessary reexposure to, for example, the sights of death, injury, or mutilation. Inappropriate media coverage, such as exhibiting corpses or mutilated bodies, or courtroom pictures taken in evidence may also have a harmful effect.

Family interventions may be necessary. Family members may be very unfamiliar with the nature of post-traumatic symptomatology, its appearance, course, and meaning. Parent education necessitated by exposure to adverse life events includes more than helping the parent to understand expectable emotional and behavioral changes. In addition, the clinician may need to assist the parent in creating an atmosphere conducive to open communication, to reinstate a sense of safety, to tolerate time-limited regressions, to identify and anticipate traumatic reminders, to observe traumatic behaviors, and to expect the phasic nature of recovery.

Providing a therapeutic atmosphere at home requires that parents, guardians, and siblings first work toward resolution of their own responses to the event and any loss of life or property. The clinician may provide brief interventions with other family members or make referrals for treatment. Randy's mother experienced intense guilt feelings for not keeping him from harm and later for not knowing that he needed early specialized intervention. As a result, she had difficulty holding Randy accountable for his behavior, which added to his difficulties with impulse control.

Loss of a sense of safety and issues about the lack or absence of adult protection are common to traumatic exposure. Lack of trust may be transferred to the clinician, especially by children with repetitive trauma or physical injury. It may be necessary to adjust pace and style for these children. Clinicians need to monitor a sense of disillusionment, irritability, or guilt in themselves resulting from the lack of an immediate connection with the child. The clinician may develop a sense of inadequacy with the trauma work or an attitude that the child is irreparable. Moreover, the clinician may become aware of her or his own issues about her or his ability to provide protection. Children with badly damaged trust will take longer to establish trust and will present differently than other children do in their initial trauma interviews.

It may be necessary to assist the child with changes in social interacting following traumatic experiences. Children can be helped to courteously decline to discuss the event with peers. Children have described renewed traumatic emotions when asked about the event. Some of the same children have felt stigmatized or disappointed in the lack of understanding when they have tried to share their experiences. Randy was called a liar and ridiculed when he said that he was in a massacre. Preoccupations with aspects of the trauma, changes in outlook, increased irritability, and other traumatic symptoms may affect peer relationships and may require assistance in maintaining peer support.

If the event occurred at the school, the school itself may become a traumatic reminder and its smooth functioning may be disrupted. Moreover, clinicians may be required to assist when the children are faced with teachers or other school personnel who react with upset to traumatic reminders. After a school shooting, one staff member began to confiscate toy guns or pictures and became frantic when there were bleeding children (the number of whom seemed to increase in the months following the event at the school). Because the alarm had been activated to get the children away from the site, most of the teachers and many of the students reacted the first few times it went off. School administrators can be helped to anticipate these reminders and to prepare the staff and children. The therapist may need to assist an injured child back into the classroom. A classroom visit and exercise, contracts with teachers and school counselors, preparation of the child and parent for the classroom discussion, and/or a graduated curriculum may be necessary.

If the child is a witness to the event, court testimony may be necessary. The child's emotional response during review of the event may incapacitate her or him as witness. It has been effective to work with children in reviewing the traumatic event prior to the testimony and to be present for the testimony. In addition to preparation for testimony, children are prepared for their subjective responses to recounting. In one kidnap and murder case, a special attorney was appointed on the child's behalf and he saw to it that the therapist was permitted to sit next to her when the child took the stand.

The clinician may feel confused or helpless at the hands of the court system or in attempting to understand the legalities of the case. It is essential but not always easy to gather the knowledge needed. In one case, a father stabbed his wife and two children. The mother became caught between wanting justice and protection for herself and her children and not wanting to do further harm to her suicidally depressed husband. Confusion about the legalities of providing this protection and a sense of needing to advise the mother left the clinician feeling ineffectual. The therapist's intense need to protect the mother from further harm resulted in overprotectiveness and overinvolvement in the woman's life. It interfered with the clinician's enabling the mother to handle these moments more independently and competently herself.

Ongoing Work with Trauma Cases

With a steady dose of trauma cases, the therapist requires ample debriefing and sufficient self-care to recover from the potential drain and to gain a sense of relief. A possible result of the therapist's inadequate self-care is premature termination of cases. This can occur, for example, because the therapist becomes less thorough in discovering and exploring the individual emotion-laden moments of the child's experience.

Fatigue from the intensity of trauma cases, the lack of thoroughness itself, overallowance of avoidance, and other concomitants of trauma work can produce an apparent boredom or a confusion over what is left to do. This attitude can affect the energy available from the child and the therapist to face, at a new level, the difficult traumatic moments. Like the child, the therapist may desire to step away from the impact on the child. The child and therapist no longer desire to bring the trauma and trauma-related emotions home with them.

Case Example: Sandy

In her first trauma therapy with an adolescent, Dr. J. found it difficult to listen to the following trauma story from her adolescent patient: Sandy returned home from a family gathering to find her sister, Rita, in the bathtub bleeding from head and nose, convulsing, and drooling bloody mucous from her nose and mouth. Sandy tried to talk to and comfort her. She agonized over where the wound was and what to do to stop the bleeding. Rita attempted futilely to communicate with one of her hands. Sandy telephoned the paramedics and returned to her sister's side, but Rita was dead on arrival at the local hospital.

Sandy described herself as "like her father, emotionally avoidant and the family caretaker" before Rita's suicide. After the suicide, these coping mechanisms became even more pronounced. In general, Dr. J. worked well with Sandy over a period of 1 year before Sandy relocated. Dr. J. established an excellent rapport and created a safe environment in which Sandy could review her horrible experience and could discuss what she thought were embarrassing fears and other emotions. The treatment was a challenging and stressful one for Dr. J. and its initial phase was difficult.

There were important parallels between Sandy's trauma and Dr. J.'s own life experience. At age 11, Dr. J. traumatically discovered her own mother "unconscious, limp, and eyes open" after a suicide attempt and saw her whisked to the hospital. She had concluded that living with her extremely rational, emotionally avoidant father was a toxic environment for her mother and an important source of her suicide attempt.

Partly because of her own experience, Dr. J. identified with Sandy's helplessness in the face of suicidal tragedy. She empathized with Sandy's feeling "stuck forever" with this traumatic memory and her loss of a sense of normalcy. "It [the traumatic experience] really is a loss of the illusion of safety." She was also quick to recognize Sandy's adaptive response: "What a good girl" Sandy was. "She never intrudes." Dr. J. worried that she was somehow prohibiting Sandy's expression of anger, as she had prohibited her own in order to cope with her mother's suicide attempt.

Recognizing the risk to Sandy because of her sister's suicide, Dr. J., as in childhood, would need to prevent a suicide attempt by Sandy. To add to her concern, Sandy's environment promoted an identification of Sandy with her dead sister. People called Sandy "Rita" or addressed her as "the sister of the girl who had killed herself." Her family members wanted her to wear her dead sister's old clothes and sometimes seemed to want her to replace her sister. Dr. J. felt that the emotionally avoidant, toxic atmosphere at home paralleled that of Dr. J.'s mother; Dr. J.'s countertransference tendency was to be protector. Dr. J. explained that craziness/suicidalness is inside all of us. Sandy's circumstances had made Sandy aware of her suicidal thoughts. Dr. J. next tried to intervene preventively. She called Sandy's father and told him to lock up his guns and separate the ammunition from the guns. Dr. J. wanted to show Sandy an article on the dangers of handguns. She wanted to reassure her that it was her family that was pathological for having handguns in the house, not that she was crazy. She was tempted to tell Sandy about her own mother's suicide. Talking it over in supervision, she decided that telling Sandy would focus attention upon Dr. J. and off Sandy, so she refrained.

Dr. J. continued to "reach out to her more and rescue her from her pain and sadness. Wanted just to whisk away her distress." Dr. J.'s protecting and rescuing impulses served a resistant function resulting in avoiding the details of the trauma. She wished to "leave this poor girl's trauma alone," and to work only on the mourning. She resisted facing the horror of what had happened. She preferred to calm Sandy and to "melt away" the sense of abnormality so "at least in the treatment session she could have felt normal." When Dr. J. could fully listen to an in-depth retelling of the trauma story, she was impressed with how powerful Sandy's imagery was. She discovered that the details were clarifying rather than horrifying.

In order to endure the trauma review, Dr. J. consciously said to herself, "It is not *my* mother who died. It isn't *me* experiencing these horrible symptoms." She did this "to protect [herself] from the intensity of [her] own frightening emotional responses." She initially resisted facing and re-reviewing with Sandy emotion-laden moments. She first seemed to use traditional listening and interpreting methods as an avoidance of pushing Sandy to thoroughly review her experience. Now, she wanted to hear everything and "recognized that this is where Sandy's environment [and her own as a child] had failed." She remembered having no one to talk to after her mother's suicide attempt—being frightened, lost, and alone. Her own father never talked with her or her mother. Dr. J. could now hear other differences from her own trauma.

Sandy's father had been a "provider—he lived at the office," but after the suicide her father put his arm around Sandy and said, "I've been a bad father." He began wearing his dead daughter's earring as a tie tack. Sandy was uncomfortable with this new display of affection and attachment from a man who previously was nonemotional.

Two weeks before the suicide, Rita had been lying on a table at a party with a knife saying she wanted to kill herself. No clinician was consulted because this was a good Catholic family with no mental health problems. Dr. J. saw Sandy's family as wealthy and hypocritical, as preferring to imagine they lived in a perfect world rather than to accept the fact that their daughter lying on a table with a knife indicated a troubled world. Had they really listened to their daughter and not maintained this false image, Dr. J. felt, they could have prevented the tragedy.

Rita had called Sandy at 2 A.M. to talk 3 or 4 days before the suicide. Sandy had been too tired to really talk at that time of night and remained unconsciously guilty that she failed to prevent the suicide. Listening to this preamble to the suicide, Dr. J. was annoyed that nothing was done to intervene and blamed it upon the family's value system. She imagined intervening at the party, where she would take Rita immediately to the emergency room, thereby obtaining intervention and averting the tragedy. She also entertained the intervention fantasy of going into the home after the initial warning and removing all of the guns. Dr. J.'s attitude toward the family initially interfered with her understanding Sandy's intervention fantasy, namely, that she prevent the suicide by listening differently to the 2:00 A.M. phone call.

Sandy was on a different emotional time schedule in her grieving and trauma resolution than her family. While she was attending to trauma issues, they were mourning their loss. Sandy's mother had been putting flowers on her daughter's grave many times per week. Sandy kept telling her mother, "Sis is dead, she's dead" in an attempt to stop this behavior.

Dr. J., in a fantasy, envisioned the two taking each other into the other's arms and comforting one another. She wished they could all reach the same phase so that they could return to being a normal, loving family and so that her patient could receive the familial support that she needed.

Soon Sandy's increased risk-taking and other reenactment behaviors put Dr. J.'s intervention fantasies to the test. Sandy reported driving fast down mountains and jumping over cliffs during hiking. She wondered out loud what it must have felt like for Rita to die. Unconsciously identifying with her suicidal sister, she placed Dr. J. in her own role of trying to prevent Rita's death. At one point, she "slashed her wrist" (Sandy's words) accidentally when she dropped some industrial-strength plastic wrap while waitressing. She bled profusely but remained totally calm while everyone else became hysterical and rushed around. She, in fact, calmly took control of the situation to see the accident did *not* become a tragedy. She gave her fellow workers instructions on how to stop the bleeding and to get her to the hospital for stitches. Unlike Rita, Sandy chose a course of survival. Dr. J. said that Sandy chose to be competent in the face of the trauma even though Dr. J. remained concerned that "she had to slash her wrist in order to do it." Sandy now realized that she had tried her best with her sister, although she felt very guilty at her lack of success. Dr. J. noted that the treatment was moving to a new level. She felt both empathic and competent.

Sandy underwent a reduction in numbing and an exacerbation of symptoms following attending a play about suicide. She graphically described to Dr. J. her experience. Her leg began to shake as it had during the attempt to comfort and get help for her sister. While she watched the fake blood on the suicide victim in the play, she recalled the stickiness of her sister's blood and felt stickiness on her perspiring hands. She felt a renewal of traumatic anxiety and revulsion and experienced flashback imagery. Her heart was racing, and her respirations quickened. After viewing this play, these and other symptoms increased. It helped a great deal to tell Sandy what was normal so that she could tolerate her symptoms. Dr. J. used the increase in symptoms successfully to enhance Sandy's ability to explore the symptoms and traumatic material.

After successfully facing some of the traumatic issues, Sandy began to grieve the loss of her sister. She felt sorrow over things her sister would never experience. While on a water mattress on the ocean, she felt the warmth of the water droplets on her skin. She realized her sister would never experience this again. Dr. J. empathized with the sense of loss and found herself regretting this with her patient. She focused on the fact that Sandy had more sympathy and appreciation for life now that she had successfully processed much of her traumatic response.

RECOMMENDATIONS

Trauma work can be both stressful and rewarding. The following are several ways in which clinicians can prepare themselves for the difficulties of trauma work:

1. Become well informed about the trauma.
2. Engage in debriefing regarding the event.
3. Engage in ongoing, adequate self-care (e.g., rest, recreation, support, debriefing, reprocessing, self-pampering).
4. Regularly examine responses, resistances, and tensions related to trauma materials.
5. Develop a willingness to hear anything.
6. Be prepared to move a child forward through a review of horrible moments and emotions with a sensitivity to the child's timing and tolerance and a recognition of and respect for the child's ability to face and cope with the trying aspects of her or his experience.
7. Recognize the phasic nature of trauma recovery and the need for occasional "time-outs" from direct traumatic focus.

Countertransference issues change with the type and duration of treatment (e.g., consultations; individual or group interventions; brief or long-term treatment). This chapter has focused primarily on issues of acute phase and brief individual interventions. Over time, issues become focused in the transference.

ACKNOWLEDGMENT

Many thanks to Dr. Robert Pynoos, Director of the UCLA Trauma, Violence, and Sudden Bereavement Program, under whose directorship many of the consultations and interventions represented in this chapter were provided.

REFERENCES

Freud, S. (1926). Inhibitions, symptoms and anxiety. *Standard Edition, 20,* 77–175. London: Hogarth Press, 1968.

Johnson, M. K., & Foley, M. A. (1984). Differentiating fact from fantasy: The reliability of children's memory. *Journal of Social Issues, 40,* 33–50.

Kaltreider, N. B., Wallace, A., & Horowitz, M. J. (1979). A field of study of the stress response syndrome: Young women after hysterectomy. *Journal of the American Medical Association, 242,* 1499–1503.

Kardiner, A. (1941). *Traumatic neurosis of war.* New York: Hoeber.

McNally, R. J. (1991). Assessment of PTSD in children. *Psychological Assessment,* 3(4), 1–7.

Nader, K., & Pynoos, R. S. (1988, May 12). *Treatment issues: Post-traumatic stress disorder in children.* Paper presented at a symposium sponsored by the UCLA Prevention Intervention Program at the annual meeting of the American Psychiatric Association, Montreal, Quebec, Canada.

Nader, K., & Pynoos, R. S. (1991). Drawing and play in the diagnosis and assessment of childhood post-traumatic stress syndromes. In C. Schaefer, K. Gitlan, & A. Sandgrun (Eds.), *Play, diagnosis and assessment.* New York: Wiley.

Nader, K., & Pynoos, R. S. (1993). School disaster: Planning and initial intervention. *Journal of Social Behavior and Personality,* 8(5), 299–320.

Nader, K., Pynoos, R. S., Fairbanks, L., & Frederick, C. (1990). Childhood PTSD reactions one year after a sniper attach. *American Journal of Psychiatry, 147,* 1526–1530.

Nader, K., Stuber, M., & Pynoos, R. S. (1991). Posttraumatic stress reaction in preschool children with catastrophic illness: Assessment needs. *Comprehensive Mental Health Care, 1*(3), 223–239.

Pynoos, R. S., & Eth, S. (1986). Witness to violence: The child interview. *Journal of the American Academy of Child Psychiatry, 25*(3), 306–319.

Pynoos, R. S., Frederick, C., Nader, K., Arroyo, W., Steinberg, A., Eth, S., Nunez, F., & Fairbanks, L. (1987). Life threat and posttraumatic stress in school age children. *Archives of General Psychiatry, 44,* 1157–1063).

Pynoos, R. S., & Nader, K. (1988a). Psychological first aid and treatment approach for children exposed to community violence: Research implications. *Journal of Traumatic Stress, 1,* 445–473.

Pynoos, R., & Nader, K. (1988b, October). *Responding to children traumatized in the school setting: A workshop for service providers.* Presented at the Society for Traumatic Stress Studies Annual Meeting, Dallas, TX.

Pynoos, R. S., & Nader, K. (1988c). Children who witness the sexual assaults of their mothers. *Journal of the American Academy of Child and Adolescent Psychiatry, 27*(5), 567–572.

Pynoos, R. S., & Nader, K. (1989). Children's memory and proximity to violence. *Journal of the American Academy of Child and Adolescent Psychiatry, 9,* 236–241.

Pynoos, R. S., & Nader, K. (1993). Issues in the treatment of post-traumatic stress in children and adolescents. In J. P. Wilson & B. Raphael (Eds.), *The international handbook of traumatic stress syndromes.* New York: Plenum Press.

Yule, W., & Williams, R. M. (1990). Post-traumatic stress reactions in children. *Journal of Traumatic Stress, 3,* 279–295.

8

Rape and the Phenomena
of Countertransference

CAROL R. HARTMAN
HELENE JACKSON

"How come they didn't believe her?" The question came from a member of the audience listening to a case presentation on the treatment of trauma. The patient had been hospitalized following a rape she stated had occurred in a parking lot of a major shopping center. She reported she had been held at knife point by a man who was hiding in the rear of her car. Neither the doctors nor her family believed her story. It was only when she revealed the details of the rape during a sodium amytal interview that she was believed.

Sexual assault, or its legal term, "rape," is a personal event. It usually occurs out of the awareness of others and rarely presents clear physical evidence. Because it is only the word of the victim against the word of the perpetrator, the perception of others becomes critical in the response *to* the victim and in turn the response *of* the victim. Although victims of many types of trauma are suspect and/or prematurely blamed for their misfortune, in no other situation is this attitude manifested with such devastating consequences as with rape. The degree of individual and institutional biases is apparent in both the clinical consideration of the treatment of rape victims and the lack of protection and justice found in the courts.

Case Example One: The Crime Is in the Eyes of the Jury

It was evening when the therapist received the call. In a monotone Jane said, "I was raped!" The therapist responded, "When? Where? Are you with someone?" Jane said, "I've been to the hospital. I'm home now. Can I see you tomorrow?" The therapist answered, "Of course." Details were not discussed over the phone. An appointment was set up for early next morning. The unemotional, monotonous style was characteristic of Jane. However, it seemed to her therapist that even for Jane, her current lack of affect was extreme. The message had been conveyed with even more deadness than when Jane, in the past, had spoken of other traumatic aspects of her early life and their painful consequences.

The next morning, Jane detailed the grim, terrifying aspects of being held captive and brutally raped for over 3 hours. When she finished, she told of her experience in the emergency room at the local hospital where a female physician had responded to her disclosure coldly and unemotionally. The therapist listened to Jane with pangs of anguish. She could imagine the two extremely controlled women, trying to communicate with one another, only to find themselves in a state of frozen isolation. In contrast, soon after the incident, the district attorney's office assigned an advocate to Jane whom Jane experienced as warm and supportive.

The day Jane was to testify, she asked her therapist to attend. Jane took the stand. She recounted to the jury, in an honest, straightforward, nonemotional manner, how she had met the defendant at a party given by her artist friends. She spoke of how, for the first time after several years of difficulty in social situations, she had enjoyed herself. She recalled when the defendant, a young black man, asked her if she wanted some "coke," she had said yes.

Jane told how she followed the defendant out of the building and down the vacant street. It was about 2 A.M. Suddenly, she testified, she felt vulnerable. Before she could change her course, a knife was at her throat. He dragged her into an abandoned building, through a dark basement, to a back room where she felt cut off from the outside world. She remembered there was a single overhead light. He threw her to the floor and removed her clothes. For 3 hours he sodomized her, vaginally penetrated her, forced her into oral sex, and inserted a "pick comb" into her vagina and her rectum. The investigating officer testified it had been one of the worst rapes that had ever been described to him.

The jury found the man not guilty. When the verdict was announced, Jane was devastated. She went to the judge, who was black also, and asked how such a verdict could come about. He said he could not explain it to her or to himself. However, he told Jane he believed the man was guilty because he had recently been convicted of another vicious rape that had occurred less than a week after Jane's. Jane concluded that the reasons the other woman was believed were that the other victim was younger and had not gone with him for drugs.

The therapist found herself pondering a moral and therapeutic dilemma. To what extent, she wondered, did the fact that Jane was a white woman, a mother, older than the rapist, and alone in a high-risk neighborhood affect how the jury interpreted blame and responsibility? To what extent were Jane's blunted expression and her monotone misperceived as casual or distorted, and thus interpreted as a sign that she was lying? To what extent, despite the physical evidence of a brutal rape, did the jury hold her responsible for her own misfortune? And, to what extent would it be therapeutic to address these issues with Jane?

Jane's therapist, familiar with Jane's lifestyle and her defensive emotional blunting prior to the rape, had suspected that her nonconventional, artistic style might be used in court to challenge her veracity. She asked herself how, and to what extent, should she have raised these issues with Jane at a time when Jane had been emotionally traumatized and at the height of her reaction? Should she have told Jane that she must go to court and be "convincing"? In brief, how and in what way does the therapist inform the victim of the possibility that she, as much as the rapist, is on trial? How does the therapist prepare the rape victim for the expectable countertransference of crucial others?

The above example reflects common individual and institutional countertransference reactions (CTRs) to rape that are evident in our society. Manifestations of these reactions set the stage for a variety of potential therapeutic mishaps. For example, immediately following the patient's disclosure of rape and the simultaneous confusion, the clinician may press for facts and clarification like an adversarial attorney, contributing to a climate of disbelief and adding further terror to the victim. At a time when the victim has a critical need to be protected from further social judgment, she may interpret the clinician's questions as reflecting disbelief and censure.

Wilson and Lindy (Chapter 1, this volume) propose a framework for the analysis of countertransference in cases of trauma. They present five interacting factors that determine the nature, quality, and dynamics of CTRs: (1) the nature of the stressor, (2) the clinician's personal factors, (3) the client factors, (4) institutional/organizational factors, and (5) factors indicative of CTRs in the clinician.

From these factors, Wilson and Lindy develop a typology that describes two different modes of empathic strain found in CTRs Type I, "avoidance," is marked by empathic withdrawal and empathic repression. Type II, "overidentification," is marked by empathic disequilibrium and/or empathic enmeshment. In the extreme, each typology and its respective modes represents an excessive state of personalization. That is, the clinician is responsive to her or his own self-generated information, to the exclusion of that of the victim. Separated from a sensitivity to the flow of information between herself or himself and the victim, the empathic connection between self and other is broken.

Implicit in Wilson and Lindy's model is a dynamic process in which clinicians have the capacity to move alternately from a state of self-orientation to a state of "other" orientation. They can identify with the victim while sustaining an active, observing sense of self, separate from the victim. The case of Jane demonstrates the additional disequilibrium (reinforcing blame and disbelief of the victim) that occurs in the therapist when society's "countertransference" to rape interacts with the five factors outlined in the Wilson and Lindy model.

In this chapter we consider what we know about the phenomenon of rape. We discuss its social interpretation, its impact on the victim, and its unique countertransference phenomena. We present clinical material gathered from our personal accounts and those of other clinicians participating in this study, which demonstrate the five-factor framework and dual typology of empathic strain proposed by Wilson and Lindy (see Chapter 1, this volume). Among the 10 male and female clinicians who participated in this project are nurses, social workers, and psychologists. They represent front-line workers, as well as those in long-term therapy relationships with rape victims. Their generosity and honesty is attested to in the material they have provided.

They join us as colleagues in the effort to shed light on countertransference and trauma. These serious and dedicated professionals were open and eager to participate in contributing to the chapter. We randomly selected them from a health service directory, called them, and introduced ourselves and the aim of our efforts. They made time available and agreed to having our conversations recorded. We used an open-ended set of questions we had devised and a list of behaviors that indicated both countertransference and signs of trauma preoccupation, such as dreams, images, or thoughts about the trauma material presented to them by their clients. Every effort was made by the interviewers not to turn the interview into a supervisory session but, rather, to let the thoughts and presentations of the interviewees enlighten us as to the layers of complexity and struggle manifested in countertransference. We strived to stay with them and use their interpretations rather than ours. After their interviews, we shared with them the preliminary developments of the conceptual framework for exploring countertransference. They also told us that it was important to them to discuss their thoughts and feelings about their work with another professional, and that the experience underscored how isolated they felt in their work. They also made comments and recommendations regarding the basic preparation of professionals with regard to dealing with trauma victims.

THE FIVE FACTORS AND THE UNIQUE FEATURES OF RAPE

Factor I: The Stressor

According to the combined figures reported by the *Boston Globe* (1992) in its account of Dr. Kilpatrick's analysis of the National Women's Study, and the FBI Uniform Crime Report (1990), there were 683,000 rapes in 1990. These data show that the majority of rape victims are raped by family members and acquaintances (29% by an acquaintance, 22% by a stranger, 16% by another relative, 11% by a father/stepfather, 10% by a boyfriend/ex-boyfriend, 9% by a husband/ex-husband, and 3% unsure/refused to answer). More startling are the ages at which rapes occur. Among women who were raped, 33% were raped between the ages of 11 and 17, 38% at the age of 18 or over, and 29% at age 11 or younger.

It is generally agreed that obtaining incidence rates of rape is difficult because many women fear the consequences of having their names released and their subsequent humiliation. Although the majority (70%) of rape victims are not physically harmed beyond the damage of the rape itself, a large number (24%) suffer minor injuries, and 4% are severely injured (this does not include statistics of sexual murders) (*Boston Globe,* 1992).

Rape is a legal term. In the United States, each state has its own statutory definitions and criteria for the phenomenon of rape. Although old laws viewed rape as an act of illicit sex, more recent legislation defines rape as a type of assault. As defined by the FBI Uniform Crime Report (1988), forcible rape is the ". . . carnal knowledge of a female forcibly and against her will . . ." (p. 15). Assaults or attempts to commit rape by force or threat of force are also included. However, *statutory rape,* without force or threat of force, and other sex offenses are excluded (FBI Uniform Crime Report, 1988). Although there is variation among states, rape, as legally defined, generally refers to the forced sexual penetration of a victim by an offender who is not the victim's spouse.

Because the legal definition of forcible rape is so restrictive, *sexual assault* has been used to cover a wider range of sexual crimes including attested rape, indecent assault and battery, and sodomy. *Sexual assault* has been defined as manual, genital, or oral contact with the victim's genitals without consent and obtained by force, threat, or fraud. In these definitions the perpetrator and the victim can be of either gender.

Most statutes define as illegal any type of sexual behavior with a child, irrespective of the use of force, threat of force, or victim's consent. *Statutory rape* may also be charged in cases where the victim is legally unable to give consent by virtue of mental deficiency, psychosis, or altered state of consciousness induced by sleep, drugs, illness, or intoxication. *Molestation* has been defined as noncoital sexual assault, and *incest* as coitus between a blood relative or caregiver (e.g., stepfather) and a young victim.

Another area of sexual misconduct that has statutory support at the national and state levels is sexual harassment. This behavior frequently occurs in the workplace where sexualized verbal and behavioral actions are directed toward a coworker who has requested that the other person cease his or her activities. Often concomitant with the sexualized behavior are threats of reprisal, particularly with regard to work stability and status. Consequently, the work environment becomes extremely uncomfortable and stressful. Often, to escape the tyrannical behavior, the victim is forced to give up a valued and/or needed position. Although both genders have been identified as perpetrators of sexual harassment, more often than not the victim is a woman. The perpetrator is usually a man who holds a real or perceived position of power over the victim. Power and domination are the important dynamics in this phenomenon.

The term "rape" implies a host of complex social issues regarding aggressive sexual acts. Whether or not a sexual assault is defined as a violation and a trauma is not based solely on the victim's perceptions. Rather, specifics of the act, such as the amount of physical trauma, the relationship of the victim and the accused, and the context in which the act takes place become potent definers. These are such powerful determinants, as documented in the case of Jane, that despite overwhelming physical evidence, the actions of the perpetrator are secondary to the behavior of the victim.

Societal values and attitudes impact on those who provide services to rape victims. These social forces may be internalized as fundamental, often unconscious, beliefs about female psychology, female sexuality, and victimization. Although the number of false accusations is small compared to the total number of sexual assaults perpetrated, the seriousness of the act and its sequelae, as well as its believability, is constantly challenged. The following examples underscore the relationship of believability to rape myths.

Case Example Two: Why in Harm's Way?

A young married, male nurse working in the emergency room of a major city hospital spoke about this dimension in describing his experience working with rape victims.

"We see a lot of victims on the evening and night shift. I really didn't expect to be working with them. I thought a female should work with them. Almost didn't take the job when I knew I had to work with them. But now, it's sort of second nature now. *(pause)* You know, we get a lot of women off the street here, lots on drugs, alcohol when they come in. We have a good protocol and I do what I can do, but, I do think to myself, 'How come they put themselves in such dangerous or risky situations?' I guess this is what makes me the most irritable and mad at them."

He went on to explain that he was very glad that his work began and ended with the emergency room examination and referral for follow-up. He was aware of his limited patience with many of the victims who came in. However, he was dismayed when others in the system operated on their biases. He reported the following memorable experience in which he was not only visibly shaken, but more aware of how he almost succumbed to the prejudice of the treatment group.

"One night, this guy came in . . . said he had a table leg in him. Ugh . . . nobody listened to him. Yeah, he said a table leg, uh, had been shoved in him. Nobody paid attention. They were yelling at him to move from the table to the gurney. I noticed he seemed in pain. Finally, I couldn't stand it. I got one of the docs to look at him. I didn't like the guy, but he was in pain. She examined him. There it was *(shows length with his hands)* . . . able to take it out of him. It was about nine inches . . . had a nail in it."

Although this had happened some years before, the nurse was still visibly shaken by the incident. He explained that the young man had been loud, with flamboyant and effeminate characteristics, which put him off. However, he was in psychic pain as he watched the young man tell people what was wrong only to find that they did not believe him or ignored him. The nurse himself, he said, had been a victim of sexual abuse. In part it was his own experience and his sense of outrage at the young man's not being believed and listened to that had motivated him to seek out a physician who he thought would be more reasonable and agree to do an examination.

When the victim of rape and sexual assault has a prior connection with the perpetrator as in the Case Example One, it is hard for the general public and even clinicians to believe that a sexual violation has occurred. Consequently, assumptions about rape that "blame the victim" have developed. These are referred to as *rape myths*. Couched in theories of female and male sexuality, they are often used to justify or rationalize sexual assault (Scully & Marolla, 1984).

About women, these myths (Burt, 1980) include, but are not limited to:

Women want to be raped;
Women falsely accuse innocent men of rape;
Women provoke rape by their physical appearance and dress;
Women secretly enjoy being raped;
Nice girls do not get raped; and
Women ask for it by being in certain places, by drinking, and so forth.

About men, myths includes:

Men by nature are attracted to beautiful women;
Men by nature have a stronger sex drive and need for sexual activity;
Physical damage can occur if a man is aroused and cannot complete
the sex act; and
Men cannot stop themselves once they are sexually aroused.

These biased explanations of rape were presented as fact in the earliest literature on rape. Their continued use reflects how deeply ingrained these beliefs are and that contextual factors still dominate the interpretation of sexual assault (Benedek, 1984; Brownmiller, 1975; Burgess & Holmstrom, 1974; Gold, Fultz. Burke, Priscol, & Willett, 1992). The remnants of these myths are internalized in clinicians and the cases they describe as they debate with themselves their reactions and responses to sexually assaulted clients (Best, Dansky, & Kilpatrick, 1992).

Factor 2: Clinician's Personal Factors

Beliefs, values, defensive styles, personal history, training and experience, motivation to work with trauma victims, and theoretical orientation (Jackson & Nuttall, 1993) play a role in CTRs to rape victims.

We are just beginning to investigate the extent to which professionals have trauma backgrounds and how they impact on clinical practice (Howe, Herzberger, & Tennen, 1988; Jackson & Nuttall, 1993; Kelley, 1990; Kendell-Tackett & Watson, 1991; Nuttall & Jackson, 1992). Approximately half the therapists interviewed in our study were victims of sexual abuse. The remainder reported physical abuse or alcoholism in their family or origin. Abuse and trauma histories were major determinants in the countertransference with the rape victim.

As suggested by Wilson and Lindy, these factors may play a role in either overidentification or avoidance. Thus, a trauma history may not predict the direction of countertransference interference, but it plays a critical part. It is reflected in the defensive style of the therapist and her or his general level of stress.

Those most involved in therapy efforts struggle in an ongoing way with their own assessment of the manner and extent to which their abuse/trauma history colors the relationship with the client and their interventions. The following excerpts from several interviews helps us examine this important factor in the helper's countertransference reactions to the victim.

Case Example Three: It Happened to Me!

The young therapist interviewed here had completed her doctoral program and had been in private practice for approximately 2 years. She views herself as psychodynamically oriented and adheres to the concepts of transference and countertransference. She presents the impact of her personal history on her work with an individual client. Countertransference themes of theoretical confusion, guilt and responsibility, lack of clarity of boundaries, and biases are underscored in her straightforward presentation.

INTERVIEWER: In practice now, how many of the clients you see have been victims of interpersonal violence?
THERAPIST: How many? What percentage? Probably eighty percent. It might be more than that . . . to be more specific, almost everybody I work with has a history, between seventy and eighty percent.
I: So, through the years, how successful do you feel you've been with these clients. You have one or two rape victims. How successful do you feel in your work with victims?
T: It's interesting. [In one case] we are about to terminate. She moved out of the Boston area but we're still in contact. I guess there is some sort of sadness with not continuing with her. I feel it's been hard work, very hard work. She was raped March of this year and we've had a lot of contact, twice-a-week therapy and a lot of telephone contact. Especially right after the rape, we would speak three and five times a week and there were times I felt more on track than at other times, at times, zero. It is complicated by the fact that we both think she has a sexual experience that is not conscious to her, which is what we were working on in the treatment before she got raped. So it's hard to know how much of what she is experiencing is post-traumatic from the rape and how much it is from the earlier experience or abuse and how the rape might have retraumatized or traumatized her anew, and a lot of her symptoms were present before the rape in some version.
I: So this is not a planned termination in terms of your therapy. What has prompted the termination?

T: It was actually [unplanned]. It would not have happened had the rape not happened. She had a very strong reaction to Boston as the perpetrator and the Boston area—also she needed to get out of the area. So we tried to talk that through, sort it through, and how much of it was the wish to be invulnerable. The violence sort of dichotomized it as 'Boston is all bad' and the area to which she would move to would be all good and safe and that she still thought it would be healthier for her to be out of the area. So that's what prompted her to move and now she has finally opened up treatment out there. So that's what's prompting her termination out there. We have had telephone treatment out there about twice a week in the interim and that has been since July.

I: Now, I know [from what you said earlier in the interview] that you have been referring to a patient of yours who was raped and who terminated prematurely. How much did you experience or reflect on what happened to her both in the sessions and outside of the sessions?

T: How much?

I: Well, let's go from zero, nothing, to twenty, a lot.

T: I would say eight.

I: Jumping to conclusions as to what was going on with the victim?

T: I would say it was more not knowing where she was at in terms of her past history and the acute aspects of the rape.

I: Premature interpretations?

T: No . . . don't feel I did that.

I: Overdirectedness?

T: She was craving for any structure, so I don't think it was too much. I worked with her in working out plans for the day, structuring her days. This is what she wanted to function.

I: Overreacting?

T: In the sessions? Not sure.

I: Confrontive?

T: Yeah, I remember one session. I . . . it was really interesting. I was really impacted upon by this woman in general, but also her rape. I took notes after the rape because it was so powerful to me. I was trying to keep on top of what was happening to me and what was happening in treatment and I . . . and one of the things that most surprised me was when I was able to continue to do the [her] analytic piece of work, dynamic work, while helping her to function day by day, post-rape, and that surprised me, that we were still able to do the work, and the confrontation, it might not have been such a confrontation. She came in in such a rage. All men, all men are rapists, all men take power of her, her reaction to her boyfriend, and I remember in that session, maybe it was such a confrontation, but I remember saying to her, I felt she had an absolute right to be enraged, enraged over what happened, but at the same time I hoped that she wouldn't let her anger toward men override her own conflict and anger over being female, that her rage and outrage toward men not overshadow her earlier conflict of being angry over being female . . . that predated her rape. But she was feeling that her femaleness was leaving her open to be raped over and over in many different ways by men and the way she was talking about it—"Men are rapists"—and I was saying her work was around femaleness and what it means to her to be rapable. From my end of it, it seemed confrontive.

I: How did she respond to what you said?

T: She took it in, actually [she would say,] "Yeah, yeah, you are right I know what you're saying." She was able to work with the response.

I: So you are saying that she was angry at the rape, but she had been angry earlier over her feelings of being female?

T: Yeah.

I: What were your concerns that prompted you to say what you did to her?

T: I think I was worried that she would get herself into a dichotomized world that . . . no escape from it . . . once men are evil and women are victims. Where do you go with that? And I remember a question in my mind at that session, the question was, "Where is the conflict?" . . . and then, "What's the conflict?" . . . and wanting to respect the part that this is a woman who has been raped and that . . . and a man did it and men rape and women are raped and ugh . . . that's all really, and that there was simply more there than the rape. I think that she would be immobilized by that construction and, in a way, victimize herself, whereas maybe [I was saying those things to her] out of my sense of helplessness, that there was nothing I could do about men raping. What I could do as a therapist, was help her look at what could help her. She was stuck in a female body. That's what she's got. She said she would much rather have a penis. She said that. So, I think it might have been out of my sense of helplessness. It was my sense that she could get stuck.

I: You said this woman had a profound impact on you. Could you explain this?

T: Yeah, I felt completely devastated. I felt like it had happened to me. Uhm . . . I felt, I remembered, I was dazed. I had trouble getting through the sessions with other patients. The day I found out she had called my voice mail . . . and I had called into my messages between session, and . . . and . . . I called my messages. She had called at three-thirty in the morning, "Hello, this is so and so. I just wanted to tell you I was raped tonight on the way home from my session." Again, a helpless barometer goes up, but she said, "I'm okay. I'm going to sleep late, so give me a call later tomorrow." She was completely dissociated, you know, "I have been raped but I'm okay," you know. I was just . . . I didn't want to see the next patient. I didn't think I could get through the day. I didn't know how I would get through the day. I wanted to talk to people.

I: Did you talk to anybody?

T: Yeah, I did. I was very preoccupied, talked to a colleague . . . and I felt I could not listen to anything she was saying. I was just . . . needed for her to know. I called a friend of mine. She had the T.V. on. I said a patient of mine was raped, and she said, "Oh, my god, I just saw it on T.V.," and I thought, "Oh, people knew," but the connection to me wasn't on the news and I felt they should know this happened to me. I was very . . . I felt like it happened to me and talking to her was reassuring to me . . . that she was still there. She was alive.

I: Like you were there and she was there, and you were okay, but separate?

T: Yeah, I think, I came across [it] in my notes before you came . . . the feeling that I had that there was something that I could not know about this experience. I couldn't bear, or I couldn't live through with her or within myself, that I couldn't live through it . . . even something too horrible to know even what to do with her or within myself. And then it was sort of reassuring to me to have contact with her and to see that she was still alive, still functioning. That she had people around her. Then it began to feel that we would really get through this together. One of the things that I felt was, I felt my style as a therapist was to be straight out, to be real. I don't think of myself as a technical doer, but one of the things that I found in my notes, I was even more real with her, and it was strange because I always thought that she and I had a real connection . . . and that we could laugh together. She is very intellectual, and we could come up on intellectual twists and we could congratulate ourselves. We had a nice camaraderie. . . . Anyway, there was something that happened after the rape where she was devastated and I was devastated and she . . . we got through it together . . . and I felt so much closer to her and honest and she also sensed that I had really been there through this. It was scary, she knew it had impacted me, she said that each time she disclosed [the events of the rape] to a friend she would see the impact on them . . . and it was as though they had been raped, raped by the knowledge that she had been raped. And she expected that was true for me as well, and wanted assurance at some point that I was okay.

I: Taking care of yourself.

T: And I was actually, and I actually confronted her. It was one of those moments, I didn't know who was sitting on which shoulder . . . but what I ended up saying to her was that it had impacted upon me and that I had a support system as well. And felt that wouldn't preclude me being available . . . but that I was . . . I let her know that it was right, that she was picking it up [that her rape impacted me] and it was true. And later when she said to me, she said that she had mixed feelings about it. Mostly she said she felt like I was really there, I was really feeling it and that was reassuring to her, but it was also reminiscent of her mother, of her fear of how her mother reacts, which is, things are so devastating that her mother freaks out and she ends up taking care of her mother.

I: So in the context of your disclosure she brought up the transference.

T: Um hmm.

I: Her fear that she has to take care of you.

T: Right, right.

I: How have you worked with that?

T: Well, I think what she will say, and she will say it with a smile, knowing that she doesn't tend to bring up what she is thinking or feeling about, either something I say or something that I'm not saying or her fears about . . . I will say to her . . . wondering if there is something in this about the two of us.

I: Does that mean you have brought it up in the context of the termination?

T: Her needing to take care of me? No, uhuh . . . what were you thinking of?

I: You were talking earlier about this whole complex issue of the rape and the countertransference and how you deal with other issues of countertransference and how you laughed together, worked together. That she was very bright and being a real good sister. Does she get mad at you?

T: That's something we talked about, her fear of getting angry. But had she never gotten outright angry with me I think that would have been the goal of the treatment. So I'm sure there's a lot that has been enacted between us and I'm sure would be useful to deal with.

I: And the rape revealed another aspect of the transference, her fear that her experiences will impact on the mother and she has to take care of her.

T: Yes.

In these excerpts a young therapist is deeply moved and pained by the client's rape experience. The rape occurred on the way home from a session with the therapist. The therapist feels as if she has been raped when the client informs her of the event. The therapist is temporarily overwhelmed. Initially, the therapist is unaware of how her vicarious traumatization and her resultant compassion and pain are impacting on the client.

For the client, the stress in the therapist is interpreted in light of her [client's] experiences with her own mother. For the client, when something serious happens, her mother "freaks out." This is a burdensome experience for the client and she reveals to the therapist her pattern of feeling responsible for and needing to "care for" her mother. The therapist's sense of "impact" activitates the client's transference. When asked by the client, the therapist openly affirms that she is affected by knowledge of the rape. The therapist believes she has reassured the client that she [therapist] is all right and can take care of herself. In part, this blocks the therapist from recognizing the transference and her ensuing CTR of irritability toward the client's neediness. Both become angry and begin to pull away from one another. The therapist becomes more fixed in overidentification with the rape experience, assuming that the positive transference has been reinstated. Both remain fearful for their own safety, because the rape occurred near the office and the rapist is still at large. Thus the powerful issues set into motion by the therapist's overidentification contribute to the premature termination, as much as the common need of the rape victims to leave the area of the assault.

I: At any point were you irritable with the client?

T: *(silence)* I don't know if I was irritable. It's sort of true with what was kept outside of the treatment. I don't know if I was irritable with her. I may have been. There was a point I felt irritable because I was getting so many phone calls from her and had to be so available to her ... and actually ... there was a time when she was describing it in terms of her social network ... that people were forgetting. After a certain point they were reconstituting in terms of themselves and forgetting that she was in a crisis, where she couldn't. And I was feeling that I wanted to reconstitute myself and move on and didn't want to be in her crisis anymore.

I: There are times when someone is within the crisis and you want to back off. How did you handle that?

T: That's a good question. I remember it gave me some sense of what her friends were going through, when she was saying people weren't hearing her. And I remember talking with her about, you know, the whole issue. You know, her ... that other peoples' denial was still ... they still had access to their denial. You know, or their capacity to move on with their assumptions that the world can be a safe place and controllable and predictable place, whereas hers ... she was raped and shattered and she is now struggling to be safe in this world where others believe they are ...

I: What did that type of interpretation do for you? Her?

T: For me, it probably intellectualized my irritation with her ... sort of ...

I: What was happening to your world?

T: Yeah, well, I was probably struggling to put it back together. That's another thing I had almost forgotten this. After she was raped, I was very anxious going outside. There was a rapist out there, so I was trying to get back into my role of thinking of a safe place.

I: How long did that last?

T: Probably six weeks . . . two months . . . it began to fade over time, but initially I was very anxious. And I had dreams and nightmares about her being raped . . . or it might have been about me being raped. You know, it was ambiguous as to whether it was her or me.

I: So you went through a period of being overwhelmed then. Did you have any sexual fantasies about the rapist?

T: That's interesting, I don't remember any.

I: Then there were no dreams or anything involving the rapist?

T: No . . . also the way she was raped. She was attacked from behind. He instructed her not to look at his face . . . and, uh, he anally penetrated her with his finger. And there is some of that replayed for me . . . my own abuse. So I think of the rapist . . . I think it ties in with some of the specifics that happened to her and that happened to me.

I: Were you restless during these sessions? You weren't avoidant?

T: Of her, you mean?

I: Did you ever have feelings that you wanted to get out of the room?

T: Oh no, I don't think so. I also felt invigorated around some aspects of the work. As she pulled herself together around certain aspects of the rape, I saw her functioning better than she had before the rape. I even kept a file on this, notes on my computer. I thought, "maybe I'll write this up," or maybe she and I would write this up these fantasies.

I: We will get through this . . . we will write it up . . . we will have a story here.

T: Right, right. We will understand this together.

I: When you say, "understand this together," what did you think had to be understood?

T: *(silence)* Hum . . . I guess when I said that I was thinking more about the process between her and me . . . how this interfaced. What I called the title of the file was . . . ugh . . . "Incest History and the Rape." The interface between the unknown incest history and some of what she was experiencing during the rape, during the rape and post-rape. Part of what she had been struggling with . . . how she could trust her memories . . . how could she trust she was an incest victim when she doesn't have memories or vague memories, except her reactions to things. And yet, after the rape she was clearly raped. She went to the emergency room. She called 911. The police believed her and she did have specific memories. She was a little amnesic about experiencing exactly where the rape had taken place. And when she returned to the scene of the crime with the police, she had these same sense of feelings that . . . like she had for the incest of her childhood. And she would say, "I think it happened here," and the police were able to say, "We found your shoe," or "I think something's there," and they would say they found blood there. And they validated her hunches that weren't visual memories and she made the connection between that. And she said, "At least I'm not crazy. My memories mean something. My hunches mean something." So she was making her connections between her memories and the rape.

I: So what you had were her kinesthetic memories, but not visual memories that she could tap into and therefore confirm that the event existed. She could remember feelings and they would say, "Yes, there is blood." Was she blindfolded during the rape?

T: No.

I: Was it dark?

T: Oh, you mean when she was raped? Oh, yeah, it was dark. It was around seven thirty . . . it was dark.

Further exploration of the therapist's experience allows our understanding of the role of personal factors in the deepening levels of countertransference. Indeed, the therapist had traumatic dreams of rape following her client's trauma. Anal penetration in the rape had reactivated the therapist's experiences as a child and threatened her fragile view that the world was a controllable, predictable, and safe place. Burdened by the enmeshment, the therapist wanted distance. Stimulated by the enmeshment, she fantasized an omnipotent and altruistic union between the client and herself in which the two could be safe and help others by writing how they "got through this together." She buttressed her client's efforts to reconstruct the details of the trauma and shifted the negative constructs of self-blame harbored by the client. The client had validation of her experience and this was most helpful and supportive. However, the ferment of the underlying transference issues persisted and dominated the direction of the early termination.

This example demonstrates the interaction between the dynamic forces within the client and the therapist. Those with more experience might note the struggle and remember how they learned from their own self-discoveries and those shared with the client. Most therapists are midway in the journey toward understanding the complex layers that exist in their responses to the client.

Factor 3: Client Factors

Age, gender, ethnic and cultural dimensions, response to the traumatic event itself, personality characteristics, defensive and coping styles, level of traumatization and injuries, family dynamics, type of traumatic event, and cognitive styles are a few notable aspects of the client that bear on the countertransference. It is not that these features elicit a specific reaction. Rather, they are sources of behavior that may arouse strong reactions in the therapist. If the context is not understood, the client may be blamed, ignored, or responded to with avoidance, overidentification, and/or intensive rescue efforts.

Rape and sexual assault clients demonstrate special responses consequential to the trauma which may be confusing to the therapist. Although most crimes have an impact on victims (Kilpatrick, Veronen, Amick, Villeponteaux, & Ruff, 1985), sexual assault can be particularly damaging (Burgess & Holmstrom, 1974; Herman, Perry, & van der Kolk, 1989; Kilpatrick, Veronen, & Best, 1988). Of critical importance are the characterological defenses manifested in self-defeating traits, a loss of self-protective functions, hypersexuality, numbing, and dissociative reactions (Foa & Kozak, 1986; Putnam, 1989; Teicher, Glod, Swett, Surrey, & Brasher, 1989). Although these reactions are part of the general syndrome of post-traumatic stress responses, they are particularly important with victims of rape and sexual assault. As noted elsewhere, youthful victims of rape acquire a propensity for the repetition of victimization. Sexual assault at a later age is, in part, a sequel to the original rape trauma. Although the connection is often out of awareness, exploration of the victim's experience of rape in later life often reveals a prior sexual trauma. The stigma and shame of the experience reinforce the victim's secrecy and denial. When coupled with the biological consequences of trauma (Giller, 1990), it is understandable that the client's adaptive efforts to defend against a full-blown trauma reaction elicit strong reactions in the therapist. The following example of a hidden rape demonstrates the client's confusing defensive styles and the therapist's CTR.

Case Example Four: The Twittering Client

The therapist has been working in the area of family violence and sexual abuse for over 5 years, prior to which she had extensive clinical experience. She is consciously aware that her history of family alcoholism might play a part in her work with clients. She also expresses her awareness that since she has been working with survivors of sexual assault, she notes many symptoms of overload, such as dreaming about clients, experiencing vivid images of their abuse, being preoccupied with clinical material when not involved in work, and being hypervigilant about safety factors while in public. She is not a novice to supervision or consultation. She tells of her struggle with her strong negative countertransference feelings elicited by the client's interpersonal traits. Despite personal work, supervision, and consultation, her therapeutic dilemma remains unresolved.

When asked to recount her experiences with a client who had been raped, she relates the following:

THERAPIST: What keeps coming up is one woman. I'll try to tell you about it quickly. There was a woman who felt so disjointed to me. She was this lovely, cutsie, perky lady toward whom I developed this strong dislike, at times hatred. I just couldn't bear it. And as far as I knew, she had denied all sexual abuse or trauma history. Finally I had to terminate the relationship, the therapy was not moving, and in the last three minutes of the last session she told me she had been lying through her whole treatment. She had been raped almost nightly by her boyfriend [Phil]. It was this intrusion into me. It felt like . . . it was this stressed, intense reaction I had, as if we weren't getting anywhere. It was like identifying with her self-hatred. When I get mad at people, I get mad at them and it's about something and we work it out, but with her . . . there was just nothing that accounted for the strong reaction toward her. When I get mad at people it's for a reason. This was outside of anything I had experienced before. It did feel like the stuff was there for me to be mad at her for.

INTERVIEWER: Did you ever bring up your intense feelings with her?

T: Some, but not to the degree I was feeling them. It was such a strong feeling it verged on hate at some points. And I didn't think I could bring this up with her.

I: Did you talk to anyone about it?

T: Yes. I went to a supervisor and she suggested that I terminate with her. Eventually I did.

I: Did you know her reasons for terminating?

T: Ah . . . it was disguised. She said it was a place for short-term treatment and she wasn't a candidate for sort-term treatment, that she wouldn't be eligible for any more services.

I: What brought her into treatment?

T: She was living at home with her parents. It had been a very angry, tough divorce. She had been married to an Arabic guy, and her family wasn't sure he wouldn't try and take the child away. She didn't know what she wanted to do with her life. She was . . . she had a pretty good job. She was in a relationship with a guy named Phil and she wasn't sure that everything he told her was true. He told her that she was not pretty, but she was beautiful. She was a very narcissistic women who had no sense of self and all she did was . . . she fixed her hair, she fixed her nails. Everything was perfect except she was empty. And she came in and told all of this stuff and she went to assertiveness training classes. She did everything she was supposed to do. She wouldn't come in. She would be late . . . cancel sessions.

I: Did you suspect she was abused?

T: Yes, initially. I went over it several times . . . went over her early history. It did occur to me that it [abuse] was going on in the present in an ongoing way. It was her boy [son] that kept dragging on me. I kept asking about that. Was he [son] being abused [by boyfriend, Phil], when she denied it. So I didn't go back . . . but it was the last session that she said she had been lying the whole time [and that it was she who was being abused].

I: Why do you think she told you?

T: I called her over a year later. She had split up with the boyfriend at the time of the termination . . . she was going to a group. She didn't go to the group and she went back to him and then split up with him again on her own terms. And now she was living with her son. She was living peacefully. She was always ashamed of everything. She was ashamed that this was going on.

I: Was she afraid you would ridicule her?

T: She admired me a great deal. She thought of me as strong . . . that I would think badly of her. She saw me as strong throughout the treatment.

I: And you knew that throughout . . . do you think that had anything to do with your reaction?

T: Hmm . . . *(silence)*

I: It's sometimes a burden to carry those expectations. How was it for you hearing those things at the same time feeling [interviewer's thought— "not effective"] . . .

T: *(interrupts)* And she wasn't getting better! It was miserable. I think it was the hardest time for me. It was one of my most uncomfortable, unhappy treatments. And it wasn't that, because I had other good people that on the surface were tougher to deal with.

I: What thoughts did you have about this woman who was so self-centered on one hand and then, on the other, viewed you as so powerful?

T: And then she wasn't getting better and I would present her as powerless. But we . . . I think, have you ever been with anyone who just seems to psychologically cower? It was like being with someone who was cowering all of the time, and if you're with someone all of the time who cowers like that . . . you start to feel like an abuser . . . and this I have been through. Have you ever been with people who have been abused and cover and cowering people? I have a lot of trouble being with them.

I: How did this fit in with what you knew about her family?

T: It didn't. I knew she was shielded, that her father was tough, that he shamed her but . . . father was a Marine Reserve. Her mother had been mentally ill. She had gone to her mother's appointments with her for years. Her mother was a drunker. Her mother would get hysterical if any needs were there for the client. There was more cowering in her behavior than fit with background . . . than feeling like an equal.

I: How did you handle that with her? Did you ever talk to her about them?

T: I remember talking to her about this . . . but for some reason it went nowhere.

I: Did your supervisor ever meet with both of you?

T: No. It would have been helpful. I did get consultation.

I: What was your reaction after she told you everything in the last session?

T: I went around and told everyone because now I could understand. I had been talking about this case with people because I had been so stymied by it, you know, I went to people on the team. I was trying to pull it together, using the people I knew. I was talking with other clinicians, talking in supervision and it wasn't getting anywhere.

I: I know this is doing some mind-reading, but what do you think blocked the supervisor?

T: We don't do consultations that way, around strong reactions. And we have to fight for supervision. The only thing I can think of as consultation is the one I did on her [supervisor's] case— the only stuck case [was this one]. I think the case had her stymied too. She knew what I was doing most of the time. She knew I was a pretty good clinician. I remember when I brought the case up to the team and they told me, "Quit worrying about the child, give the child over to us and focus on her, just focus on her need for ego building." I knew it was interfering with my work. It was something about her behavior. She got a new job, then she failed. It was something about her behavior—"tee-hee-hee, I screwed up again." It would bring out such hate in me. She wanted me to tell her she was fine, she wanted my approval.

I: You say her profound helplessness and her twittering drove you up a wall!

T: At the time I analyzed it she reminded me of my mother. I was in therapy and I was working on my mother. It wasn't just that she was being beaten and raped that I was responding to.

I: You were doing a lot of work trying to straighten this out. You were working on your own roots within the countertransference, but it wasn't resolving, so you brought it up and rather than work it through, others said, "Terminate." The issues of shame, cowering were never looked at in terms of what might be going on [now] or how they [issues] might be stopping inquiry.

This example provides clues to how the client's underlying defensive behavior (twittering in the face of abuse, hiding the abuse) impacts on the therapist. The countertransference evoked in the therapist is contempt and identification with the aggressor. Although the client's defensive strategies are maladaptive they are consistent with her early childhood traumas (surviving in an abusive home) and her subsequent accommodation to an abusive partner. Her shame, cowering, and self-defeating efforts coexist with compensatory narcissistic grandiosity. Although self-destructive, her idealization of the therapist and her fear of exposure are efforts to assert control over the therapeutic process. The therapist's dilemma is compounded by the clinic's goal of limiting its services to short-term therapy. Further, the therapist is vulnerable to her own self-hatred, which originates from her background (contempt at mother's cowering). She recognizes this tendency in part and attempts to deal with her own conflicts. However, it is not enough to restore a neutral, curious tone regarding what must be under the client's facade. Although the need to somehow address the overt behavior is recognized, the strong emotion of "hatred" prevents exploration of the evasive interactive style.

The level of support the therapist receives its insufficient to attenuate her intense emotions and conflicts. Unlike what was available to the male nurse in the emergency room, there is neither clarity of goals nor a protocol. The fragmentation in the consultation functions to protect the therapist. When the supervising and consulting staff feel stymied, they present themselves as if they know what to do (terminate the case). The dynamics between the therapist and client ("If you won't help me, I'll leave") are recreated between the therapist and the staff.

The client's defenses and coping styles trigger the therapist's defensive and coping mechanisms. Distancing occurs to ward off expression of strong emotions. However, the countertransference anger remains. Others in the system respond in a similar manner. What we witness is the client's negative projective identification onto the therapist. The client's split-off rage at the abuse is felt by the therapist but directed inappropriately to the behavior of "twittering." The client's defensive cowering and self-defeating behavior add to the therapeutic difficulties. The therapist struggles with what she knows to be the core of her own conflict and her difficulty in responding to this type of behavior. Unfortunately, she is not supported or encouraged to step back. Consequently, she is unable to explore with the client the nature of her obsequious behavior or its relationship to the stated therapeutic failure. Clues were given by the client that her boyfriend, Phil, was verbally abusive to her, thus providing an opportunity to override her secrecy. The confusion, misery, and discomfort experienced by the therapist created a fertile field for the emergence of numerous agency issues. It is not unusual for the client to be sacrificed under these circumstances.

Another client factor is gender. The majority of rape victims who come to treatment are female. In the past, male rape victims were considered rare and more often than not associated with homosexuality. Current research suggests that among male children there is a higher rate of rape outside the family compared to girls and that, in general, early male molestation is underreported (Hunter, 1990). There are large numbers of male-upon-male sexual assaults that are not associated with homosexual lifestyle. Rather, the male victim is often raped and accused of being homosexual by the dominant male gang (Hunter, 1990). An increasing number of cases are being reported in high schools where this practice is occurring among adolescent males. At the core of sexual assault and rape are issues of gender identity. The specific attack on the genitals of the victim by the genitals of the offender underscores the issues of sexual aggression and dominance.

Case Example Five: To Shoot or Not to Shoot?
That Is the Question

The therapist is a male who has worked in the area of community and domestic violence. He presents his work with a female client who had been raped by a stranger.

THERAPIST: I find it frustrating, that it seems that when I work with women who have had sexual assault, there seems to be a barrier. They tell me there is a barrier with everyone. With my male patients, well, it's like they don't know what a feeling is so it's hard to see this strictly as transference. There was this client who, in the process of therapy, recovered a memory of being raped. I sent her to a rape recovery group and she really became hard to contain. She became most emotional over an idea that she had that her father had arranged the rape, which in reality he hadn't. The group leaders were angry at me for sending her to the group, but I had no idea. She was calm with me.

INTERVIEWER: What is that like for you that she and some of the other women you have worked with seem to get more emotion out in a group?

T: There seems to be something about a group of women that allows them to express themselves. I would like to be a fly on the wall to observe what is going on.

I: Have you ever worked with a male who was raped?

T: No, but I was at a meeting when a nice-looking, attractive man got up and talked about being raped. I was startled at my reactions. First, I was taken by his graphic story of being threatened with a club, then raped and an ashtray forced into his rectum. A part of me thought, "Why didn't he do something?" I was aware of this when he told of how he was treated by the police when he went and told them. They kept asking him why he didn't do something . . . and I found myself having the same thoughts as these asshole macho policemen. I had the same thoughts as the police and their questions, but I think I had better answers. Could it not be that he somehow enjoyed the risk he was under? Could it be that, that, he had misrepresented the risks he was under? Those were more thoughts. I did admit it to the group, at great risk . . . and I said it is very hard for most men to think that this sort of thing can happen to them.

I: So there is some sort of guilt that rape happens to females, but not to men, some distress over the distancing.

T: Yeah, for me rape happens to females, not to me, not to males. It's something outside of me. You know, I do a lot of community crisis work. I do go into a lot of places where there is violence, so it isn't like I don't know. But the first time I really felt traumatized was, I heard this guy tell of his rape . . . but I notice that things are impacting on me more. We did a big debriefing of a murder in a family-owned company. It was bloody. A place that was safe that had been violated. There was blood all over, and here were these macho guys . . . scared, upset, and I carried it to my home, getting mad at my wife when she was dying some red cloth.

I: How is it that until recently you haven't been afraid of men?

T: Well, I lived in the suburbs growing up and you live your whole life knowing that you are one of those that live their life in bars . . . being macho. Or you choose a different life, somewhat isolated until you find more like you. In your mind you make this distinction. I was jumped a lot by other gangs of kids going to and from school and my older brother picked on me.

I: So, it's been hard to recognize that men are terrorized as well as women.

T: Sort of. It's like the question I get in working with women victims: "What do you do with the guilt since it's your gender that perpetuates the assault?" I answer, "I don't have guilt because I don't identify with those men," and I don't have much problem with guilt because I don't see myself as part of that group. I am as angry as the women because they [men] terrorize me. But I wonder if sometimes I don't push with women around those feelings . . . because I have backed away from that terror and rage so much. Maybe that [fear of male behavior] backs me off.

I: Can you give me an example of someone where you think that has happened.

T: Well, the woman we were talking about. She was hitchhiking with another girl, they were going across country. While there was risk to this, I didn't raise it because that was the sort of thing her father did that made her furious, but she was picked up by a guy, and he drove the girls to a remote area. He had a gun. He raped her in front of her friend for a considerable length of time.

I: Well, what were your thoughts about the hitchhiking?

T: Well, here's that kind of counterphobic response. During the '70s I had hitched across the country, you know, nothing would happen to me. I spent several days, I remember, in Spearfish, South Dakota . . . no one picking me up. When I finally arrived in a little town, I found out someone had picked up a hitchhiker and killed him.

I: So, her situation triggered some memories.

T: Yeah, but the weird part of the situation for her was that after he had raped her for some time, he went to sleep with the gun on his forehead. She kept looking at it and then she grabbed it, aimed, and pulled the trigger. But the safety lock was on. He woke up and took it away from her and made fun of her. I think he was suicidal in some way to take that risk. My image was . . . what she said was that by the end of the ordeal, she felt tenderness toward him.

I: How do you understand her reaction? How does she?

T: Well, she was close to being a perpetrator. I recognize that she is capable of extreme rage. She has expressed extreme embarrassment that she had failed at doing something. My efforts have been to help resolve this rage. Yet, here are two people pushed to the brink . . . something they shared.

I: And she seemed blocked in her expression of emotions. They were partners in crime.

T: Yes . . . and then she went to the group and just exploded.

I: Did you ever suggest in fantasy that she pull the trigger on the gun?

T: God, no!

I: How come?

T: It would be worse to know that you have killed someone.

I: How do you know that?

T: When I was a little boy, my older brother used to beat up on me and tease me all of the time. One time I fought back and he played dead. I thought I had killed him and he let me believe I had killed him. It was terrible.

I: So she raises the existential fear that the line between the good guys and bad guys is not that clear. It is sort of horrifying.

T: It's a crucial moment when one of her actions would have resulted in crossing a line.

The gender issues related to vulnerability, perpetration, and aggression are evident in this young therapist's struggle to work with the terror and revengeful rage of victims. His own struggles with masculinity play a role in his tolerance and capacity to tap into the strong emotions of his female clients. Yet, he is perplexed when his women clients respond emotionally within their group. The case he cites demonstrates his fears of aggression and identification with a potential killer. His own tender childhood experiences result in a precipitous awareness of his homicidal potential. The client mirrors his own defensive style (controlled emotional expression) and they share an identification with the aggressor.

Defensive styles of sexual assault victims are most often expressive of avoidant strategies, such as passive compliance in the face of threat. As in the example, the emotional avoidance of the client parallels the nonemotional, nonaggressive style of the therapist. When the client was in the therapeutic context of a group of women, some full of rage, her rage and intense emotions were expressed.

The second set of issues that is highly associated with sexual assault and rape are issues of gender and male/female identity, which are linked with aggression.

Case Example Six: Is Every Man a Rapist?

This is an example of a female therapist working with a couple. Prior to the couple coming together, the female partner had a history of rape.

THERAPIST: A couple I'm working with now . . . the woman has an abuse history and the husband wants to know . . . is he the rapist because, when they get into sex, and he has no experience sexually, and where she is experiencing him as raping her. She cannot say you are raping and doesn't necessarily feel he is a rapist. Nevertheless she experiences him as the perpetrator. So is that rape or isn't that rape?

INTERVIEWER: How is that for you as you try to figure it out?

T: It's very difficult. Well, the other night we really got into it [in therapy session]. He asked the question, "Am I really a rapist?"

I: What did you do with his question?

T: Initially, it was very tough. Initially, I felt taken aback. What I did was sort of talk through that she has an experience of no will at the time she is having sex with him. Nonetheless, as we can see in the sessions with him, she is an adult with a will and very much using her sense of boundaries in important ways. But when she is into sex she loses her voice, she feels mute. But she isn't, she really is not. We're making that distinction, that she experiences him as the rapist, she experiences herself as helpless, but she really isn't helpless. We never got to whether he really was the rapist and I got to telling him he really has to get to asking her, as well, as to whether she believes he is the rapist. She was able to say to him, "You're not the rapist, I know you are not," but she has been raped. And I hadn't thought about it . . . also has a childhood history of sexual abuse. And she said, "I am going to feel like you are [raping me] because sex for me is . . . that's the experience of sex for me," that it's something that gets done to her, and that she loses her own sense of her own volition and desire, and her participation. So, she was able to reassure him but I felt stuck. I wanted to say [to the husband], "You are not a rapist," but I don't know what happens in their bed at night, if he was forcing himself on her. And I didn't have that information. So I might respond . . . I had the impulse to say he's not a rapist. But you don't know what he does. Is he causing her sense of it . . . or is she . . . ? What we did talk about is that he does not want his sexuality to be that of a rapist. We just now . . . that's not a part of his self-perception or his wish.

I: What was the specific reason the couple came to see you?

T: She was wondering whether or not she wanted to remain married to him. It was a couple that in a million years I would have never thought would break through to communicate with one another. They came in as two individuals . . . coexisting, with a several-year history of no communication, no collaboration, no partnership. I think she felt the pain of that more than he did. He also comes from another culture, where the male identity in that culture doesn't involve the dialoging and processing that relationships here that we have . . . to be empathetic to both the process and content. I'm not sure. I don't know whether I am doubtful or feeling I have to be cautious. I have to play both sides. I feel like in his heart this is not about sex, violence for him, but there may be a certain amount of naïveté on his part or obliviousness on his part toward her, signals which I know are nonverbal largely. I wonder does he pick up on that and is nonresponsive . . . or if I am in a stronger alliance or protective position with her. I think my struggle was feeling more of an alliance with him and protective of him. Yet in that moment . . . I think she is too tough on him, it's hard at times. She has a significant trauma history that is being played out and she does not take time out for a certain type of perspective on him . . . that is for him.

I: How have you handled the disclosure of her trauma history with him?

T: It's been early in the couple's work. It's been about three months and they actually started with this as an issue and then allowed it to submerge for awhile, while I . . . we talked about it the other night that they were building the groundwork to become partners in the marriage, and just the other night they were opening this up again. So I really allowed her to pace it, and actually, he initiated it, with a question to how much of this is due to her past history projecting itself onto the relationship and how much of it is her responding to him as the perpetrator. So I feel that it is more appropriate for her and them to pace it more . . . (*silence*).

I: Where does that leave you as far as your work with the couple?

T: She has an individual therapist and I haven't felt the strong pull to take care of that. I'm in contact somewhat with her individual therapist.

I: If this were a situation where a couple came in to see you and this came up, what might you do?

T: If there weren't an individual therapy and I felt like there hadn't been or there needed to be, I would make a referral to an individual therapist, as well as continuing with them as a couple. If it hadn't been touched . . . I'm not sure. One impulse I had the other night of wanting to look into this more. I wanted to suggest that he go to some groups for partners of abuse victims. I'm thinking of recommending this for him around this particular issue.

I: So . . .

T: If they came asking for couples therapy, I wouldn't feel uncomfortable using support groups or psychoeducational groups around sexual trauma. I recommended a book for him by the author of *Courage to Heal*. I haven't read it, but by the same author, for partners. I'd read her chapter in the other book and told him I had read it, but not the book. I'm comfortable doing that sort of thing, you know.

I: How does that fit up with your notions of transference and countertransference?

T: Uh, how does that . . . you mean with the concepts . . . ? That's a good question. I haven't yet come to some understanding about the transference in the couples work for me. I think it would be very different for me in individual therapy, how I would. I don't know how much of this is due to transference as a couple, or where I am in my work. Because I find myself doing it a lot more in my work, offering books to clients. It has to be very powerful to people, that you think of a particular book in response to them.

I: Did you feel someone was going to catch you at doing this?

T: At first . . . did I feel guilty? Oh did I do it. I struggle with my emerging role as a therapist and the guilt of being a therapist. God forbid that you should be a gratifying human being . . . questions and struggles with the upbringing . . . to deal with something so concretely as giving a book. And so, how much do I forfeit? . . . the analysis of that impulse . . . and how much do I gain? So, what is the tradeoff? But with a couple, I feel less responsible you know, less responsible. I feel less guilty. My analyst jokingly says I have a Freudian superego. *(laughs)* He says, "Where did you get that stuff?" *(laughs)* Where did you get that stuff . . . to feel guilty for giving a book to a client, for suggestion? What I shifted is that the guilt of five years ago would have precluded me giving the book. Now I give the book and feel the guilt, or the struggle.

I: Your working with survivors of sexual abuse and trauma is forcing the change.

T: Yes, I feel I have to be more really real, more there.

I: What is it that's behind that desire to be really, really there?

T: Something about respecting that someone's reality has been abusive. That makes me feel like I don't want to toy too much within the realm of fantasy and conflict to the exclusion of really getting at it with them. I don't know. There is something about that, that their sense of reality needs to be acknowledged, that you don't go for fantasy or for the weights and balances. Yeah, one thing that . . . I don't think that I don't go for unconscious process. I think that I do. But I . . . the first step is in validating the concrete reality of it. It feels potentially abusive not to do that. Maybe in terms of my countertransference, I feel I could continue to run the abuse by not acknowledging the reality of the abuse.

I: How did you come to that insight?

T: I am a survivor. I was wondering if you would ask it directly?

I: It depends whether it is asked in the beginning, or becomes a natural expression during the interview, or if it is avoided. But it does become an important point in understanding reactions to victims by therapists. Now were you physically and sexually abused or . . . ?

T: Not violent physical abuse . . . sexual abuse within the family. And there was more than one person.

I: Were you ever raped?

T: No, but how I came to terms with it was through my own therapy, which was very analytic. When I began to tell my story, not as it was, but how I came to experience it . . . as if I was seductive, participatory. And he stopped me and said, "You need to be thinking about this as sexual abuse and it's worth it [thinking about having been sexually abused]." And that was a nonanalytic thing for him to have done. There were many ways for him to process the issue without him saying, "This is it, this is a trauma for you." I initially did believe him. I became very anxious. And the phrase that I used . . . and I remember, this was ten years ago. And the phrase that I used since then . . . that one comment turned my entire world around upside down, how I related. Completely inverted my role in the world, my role in relationships, my self-worth, in a way that was pretty unnerving initially. And then, ultimately, I was able to pull in the parts of myself that I didn't like, hated and pushed away, by assuming that I was the perpetrator, in a way that I would never have known. So it is something like being reassured that I was a kid and a victim has allowed me to do the work.

I: It sort of helped you deal with how to process it, but you were a little ambivalent.

T: Well, while I had mixed feelings in my experience of the confrontation, I don't feel ambivalent about the confrontation. If he hadn't said something and I went on talking about it for months, he would have been remiss. What he said to me was . . . I told him a story, one of my stories, and he said to me, "Had you ever thought of yourself as being a victim of sexual abuse?" And I said, "No, this is a crazy question, why are you asking it?" It was more of a question but I felt it as a declarative. He had influence, power. I respected him.

The young therapist became lost in her identification with the victim wife and her confusion over the trusthworthiness of the husband. Her countertransference confusion is manifested in her ability to help the couple talk more directly about their sexual encounters with one another. Rather, she feels she must be protective of the wife and yet becomes annoyed and wishes to defend the husband when he is told by his wife that having sex is equivalent to being raped. The therapist is enmeshed with the wife as well as the husband. The lack of boundary differentiation is prompted not only by the childhood history of incest in the wife but in the therapist's own background of sexual abuse. The cultural differences with the husband make the therapist's concerns about sexual propriety even more confused. The childhood need for secrecy by incest survivors is manifested in the therapist's avoidance of direct discussion of the marital relationship, plus there is a fear of the male. The therapist is afraid to confront him with regard to his sexual behavior and yet she wishes that he not be a "rapist." She just cannot be sure.

The honesty displayed by this therapist and the struggle to clarify therapeutic boundaries are also evident in the stories of other contributors. Examples of countertransference dynamics are articulated. Again, there is a clear lack of support, guidance, and resources, which therapists need to assist them in the complex work with rape and trauma victims.

Particular characteristics of the client, the rape, and the client's lifestyle often trigger some of the unique CTRs found in therapists treating rape victims. For example, rape victims present a range of behaviors, each depending on how close they are to the time of the traumatic experience. Different client reactions to the event place different demands on clinicians, which can move them either toward or away from the client. Victims of rape, like many individuals, often have complex life-styles, which may interfere with the clinician's capacity to believe and/or accept the client. The impact of rape on the client can result in defensive patterns that are problematic for the professional. For example, the projection of negative images upon the therapist (you are reacting just like my mother) may tap into the clinician's own vulnerabilities (I never could feel anything but contempt for my mother's weakness), confounding the therapeutic relationship and inhibiting any examination of the function of the client's maladaptive behavior. Further, many therapists find it difficult to understand or believe disclosures from those who are often most vulnerable and specifically targeted for rape and sexual assault, for example, developmentally disabled, brain-damaged, and mentally ill individuals.

Rape of psychotic patients is not a new phenomenon. Part of the reason psychotic individuals, retarded individuals, or brain-damaged children and adults are subjected to sexual assault, is that the disability almost assures that the incident will not be reported, and if it is, the victim can be easily discredited.

Case Example Seven: Psychotic Women Are Victims of Rape

A nurse with years of experience in emergency rooms explains that many people in the emergency medical service have little patience with rape victims, and often find rape victims to be some of their least favorite patients. She points out that many women who come in and tell their story confront the staff with seemingly impossible lives, full of pain, deprivation, and continuous abuse. She sees nurses under her charge become overwhelmed and unable to do anything to help. She tells of a woman who came in saying she had been picked up on the street, dragged into a car, raped, and thrown back out on the street.

NURSE: When she came into the emergency room I knew she looked different. The others were impatient with her. When I talked with her, it was clear that her agitation was more unusual than most. She was just hanging on. It took considerable tact and persuasion to get a psychiatrist down to see her and give her some tranquilizers before the rape examination took place.

INTERVIEWER: How were you able to manage this?

N: It was difficult. There were things to consider, such as the police report. But it was clear that her emotional disintegration had to be addressed first. I remember another woman who had come in. She seemed to go through the whole examination with calm and control. She was discharged, and three hours later, she returned to the emergency room flagrantly psychotic and manic. I was so shocked . . . and for a period of time blamed myself for not assessing her more carefully.

Case Example Eight: I Want a Friend

A similar situation emerged when a young, retarded woman was talked into going over to a neighbor boy's house. At the house she was sexually abused by the neighbor and a number of his male friends. They put a plastic baseball bat into her vagina and when she began to cry, one of the boys made them stop. She ran from the house to her home and told her parents. Criminal charges were brought against the males. Their defense was that it was consensual. The young woman desperately wanted friends and was told by the boys that if she told she would not have their friendship. She was reluctant for fear she would "get the boys in trouble." She wanted them to be her friends. She was seen by several physicians who claimed she was all right and had suffered no harm. Yet when examined by a consultant, she had classic symptoms of post-traumatic stress disorder mixed with exhibitionist behavior, that is, exposing herself in public. Her symptomatic sexualized behavior became the basis for the conclusion that she was not harmed.

This error in clinical judgment and understanding of the normal developmental needs of the mentally disabled is all too prevalent. Rapes in mental hospitals and institutions for the mentally impaired are all too frequent an occurrence. The countertransference is realized in the dehumanizing attitudes and behaviors of staff toward the patients, who have deficits in reality testing. It takes time to get to know people with limited capacities, to understand their struggle to live in and adjust to the world. The very real needs for companionship, friendship, and expression of sexual needs and interests are not altered by being retarded—nor is the consequential hurt and damage from rape.

Factor 4: Institutional/Organizational Factors

The fundamental and pervasive social, cultural, and value biases about rape and sexual assault, impact the victim and the perpetrator. They may cause frustration and feelings of powerlessness in the clinician working with rape victims. At no time does the therapist experience more frustration in confronting these biases than when working with children and adolescents whose parents adopt these negative views of children and fail to protect them.

Case Example Nine: When the Therapist Hears the Truth/ When the Family Hears the Truth

A male therapist with many years of experience working in both institutions and private practice tells of his increasing despair over his efforts to reach out and treat adolescents. He began his professional life working in the criminal justice system, in the prisons. There, he encountered rapists, child molesters, and murderers. Later he made the transition into individual practice and work with children and adolescents with hopes that he could make a difference. In part, this move was precipitated by an experience he had in treating a rapist.

THERAPIST: For about a year, I had been working with this very bright, appealing young man. He was a model prisoner. He not only progressed in therapy, but he had been assigned to work with us within the clinic. One day, he asked me if I wanted to hear about the crime that had brought him in. I agreed to listen to him. I couldn't believe what he told me. It was horrible. I was stunned.
INTERVIEWER: It was a violent rape?
T: Yes. *(face contorted)*
I: He mutilated the person?
T: Yes . . . he bit her all over.
I: So, when you hear a rape story, do you get an image of the rapist?
T: Yes, and there is anger. But perhaps my greatest frustration is with the families of the adolescents I see. These kids are just neglected, without love. I'm working with a young girl who was raped by a boy in her high school class.
I: Is there a court action?
T: No, that's the problem. She's afraid to report him.
I: How come?
T: Well, she's threatened by the gang in the high school. But more than that, her parents are not supportive. Her parents accuse her of being responsible for the rape. She went out after hours to be with her friends and it was in that context that she was brutally raped. What even makes it worse is that when she was twelve, she went to visit with her grandparents in Maine. They had arranged for her to go to a local dance with a high school boy of seventeen. He raped her, bit her labia and vagina, causing profuse bleeding. When she went to her grandparents, they told her not to tell anyone. And they kept her at home and away from medical

treatment because they didn't want people in the community to know. Now, I feel my hands are tied in trying to help her. There is no safe place.

The therapist talked at length about the loneliness of being in private practice, and how the frustration of not being able to do the work his clients need leads him to seek other ways of expressing his professional interests. This therapist demonstrates how the reactions of rage and disgust are manifested outside of the office in a sense of futility regarding his ability to mobilize the environment to protect "his kids." The overgeneralization to the total society of the problems of each child begins to paralyze this seasoned therapist. His sense of efficacy is challenged. If the belief of ineffectiveness dominates, we see the terminal stage of countertransference—"burnout."

Another private therapist was clear that work with victims did not overwhelm her. What bothered her was dealing with the larger bureaucratic structures. She is a therapist who works with children, parents, and families. Her most recent rape client had been raped by her ex-husband. She had left an abusive relationship with him. However, the restraining order she was able to obtain did nothing to prevent him from raping her. Prior to the rape, he had tried to run her over with his car. Despite all of his violence and repeated threats, she received no help from the police. The therapist's fury was apparent and striking in her otherwise controlled presentation. The denial of her feelings about the victim's experiences was supplanted by her rage toward the larger system. When queried about the intense frustration, she revealed that she was a first-generation child of Holocaust survivors. Although she said she could put the terrible things that happened to clients out of her mind once she left the office, she confided that she had daily images of her parents' concentration camp experience. The social system's support of the violence and nonprotection of the women and children she attempted to help was intensified by her knowledge that a whole society had sanctioned the destruction of a specified group of people.

The difficult work with victims is intensified by institutional/organizational refusals to take rape and sexual assault seriously. Levels of fear, disgust, and emotional confusion seem the most immediate factors that contribute to this avoidance.

Case Example Ten: Not Me!

A group of emergency room nurses told of their efforts to set up rape services in an upper-class, urban hospital. They found that most doctors and nurses did not view the rape patient as a serious medical problem. In addition, these doctors and nurses felt overwhelmed by the life stories of rape victims. They had neither the inclination nor the time to become involved, because the protocol for collecting evidence is tedious and time consuming, and the possibility of going to court to testify discourages them from working with sexual assault victims.

As noted before, those dedicated to work with victims direct their energies toward consulting, badgering, and manipulating reluctant people in the system to help. In time, however, they are worn out. Despite extensive educational programs within these institutions, only a small number of professionals are motivated or prepared to deal with the emergencies inherent in rape cases.

Case Example Eleven: Adding Pain and Confusion

Institutional denial was evident when several mentally ill, hospitalized women revealed in their semi-delusional chatter that a technician was drugging and forcing oral sex on them when he was supposed to be doing EEG recordings. Prosecuting attorneys called a consultant to determine if the women were telling the truth. When questioned, one woman said the voices told her that she had to do whatever the man asked her to do. Another thought that because the other women had gone through it, it was part of her treatment. One woman was more articulate and was "appropriately" aggrieved by the action. She became the witness. It is noteworthy that all of the women manifested symptom changes and signs of trauma even though there was, in some cases, a mental accommodation of the event because of either their delusional thinking or their expectations of long-term institutionalization. In this instance, the hospital responded to the complaints, but the legal system presented challenges to the credibility of the women even though the hospital made it clear that their [clients'] symptoms and statements were specific to the recent events.

In the various examples, the institutional factors (e.g., lack of clear policies about rape and/or encouragement of staff members who have difficulty working with rape victims) interact with the dynamic factors of client and therapist. Within traditional mental health centers, there are instances in which, despite therapists' efforts to obtain supervision and consultation, the impact of sexual assault and victimization becomes clouded by other institutional dynamics (e.g., power and control of staff, status within an organization) and the therapists are abandoned in their struggle.

Limited resources, institutional conflicts, and the impact of the trauma—all coalesce to compromise the therapist/helper within institutions. Their status in the institution is perceived through the minimizing attitudes directed toward the rape victims themselves. These realities play a large role in the eventual disillusionment and withdrawal of those who work with rape victims.

Factor 5: Factors Indicative of CTRs in Clinicians

The foregoing examples of Factors 1, 2, 3, and 4 relate to many of the dynamic aspects of the victims' behaviors and conflicts associated with the rape and their lives, which impact and interact with the therapists' responses. The sensory bombardment that occurs in the revealing of the trauma story has to be considered as a primary source of CTRs when working with rape victims. Every one of the interviewed professionals expressed strong emotions when talking about their experiences with victims. All but one affirmed that at points they themselves had manifested symptoms and behaviors indicative of personal trauma, because of the information they had integrated from the victims. They were aware of hyperarousal, sleep disturbances, nightmares, depression, and altered responses to the opposite sex. None of the therapists interviewed thought they had an adequate arena for the expression and exploration of their reactions. Most had therapy experiences that helped them recognize what was going on. Those that did not make use of past or present therapy tended to restrict the nature of their involvement with rape victims. The continuous nature of some of the therapists' personal responses suggests that there is an impact on the therapists similar to the victim (Hartman & Burgess, 1991). The last example addresses this point.

Case Example Twelve: Which One Hurts the Most?

NURSE: It's so hard. You remember the cases when someone comes in beaten up, stabbed, bite marks all over her body, but it's the hidden damage that you note in her eyes. When this is followed by a car accident case, a shooting, and someone burned, by the end of the shift, you've had it. It's the cumulative stress that assaults you in one day.

INTERVIEWER: How do you cope with it?

N: I don't know. At the city hospital, we all used to go out after work.

I: And drink?

N: Yeah, lots of drinking. It was intense. But part of what makes it work is the intensity and then the fast action that something is done. I balance it with a private practice where I don't see any trauma patients. Actually, after seven years I left to work in a general clinic. Before that, the hospital gave me a leave for four months. I traveled. That was important . . . to see something else . . . something pretty. That sustains me. I know that the world has beautiful aspects to it. It's not all that I see day by day.

CONCLUSIONS

Citing our clinical work and that of others, we have reviewed the unique aspects of rape and sexual assault in the context of Wilson and Lindy's five factors of empathic strain and their respective modes (see Chapter 1, this volume). The therapists who contributed to this chapter demonstrate a strong commitment to understanding their reactions in the context of the therapeutic process. The sensory bombardment they experience when listening to a rape story is a primary source of their CTRs. Denial of the power of this factor precludes a productive treatment effort and can cause serious harm to the clinician.

In our sample of 10 professionals, more than 75% revealed they were having, or had had, acute symptoms of post-traumatic stress. Many reported unrelenting levels of hyperarousal and sleep disturbance. Although some of the stress was attributable to reactions to specific clients, most was a reflection of a more generalized response. Signs of countertransference and secondary traumatization were reflected in the therapists' images and dreams of violence. Many felt isolated and frustrated. They reported a sense of futility and a need to change to a different kind of work.

The case examples presented in this chapter reveal an alternation between the avoidant and overidentification poles of countertransference phenomena. Therapists eloquently describe the fears and struggles associated with personalizing their experiences with their clients. Their own ambivalence about rape victims is parallel to their clients' attempts to protect, yet reveal, themselves. They acknowledge how the rape victims' defensive styles and acute symptomatology may resonate with their own, thus stimulating transference–countertransference reactions.

Clients, submerged in their own terror and pain, demonstrate a type of sympathy for and protection of their therapists. Embarrassed and humiliated, they fear their rape experience is too intense and shameful for another person to share or bear. Yet, their need for affirmation is constant. It is the rare therapist who finds ways to be attuned and objective at the same time.

We find it helpful to expand the usual therapeutic contract to a discussion of transference and countertransference issues. With rape victims this can initially be addressed when the client experiences strong fear responses to behaviors and cues emanating from the therapist that appear threatening to the client. When sexual abuse is hidden, as in Case Example Four, the "Twittering Client," ongoing patterns of behavior can be directly discussed through an explanation of how behaviors and reactions between the therapist and client become an important context in which to learn much about how people express and protect themselves based on past experiences. This becomes increasingly necessary when therapists are confronted with time limits. Also, this initial explanation serves as a basis for dialogue when, later in treatment, the manifestations of the transference–countertransference reactions may threaten the working alliance. Using lay language, we acknowledge the feelings of betrayal, shame, mistrust, and stigma associated with rape. We anticipate with the client the fragmenting and damaging defenses she or he may employ to cope with the profound emotions and memories attached to the rape and sexual assault.

The need for networking with others who work with victims of trauma is compelling. Professionals who treat rape and sexual assault victims are often subject to discrimination and stigma, which may compromise the safe context in which effective services can be rendered. Those who become symptomatic in response to their own and their clients' defensive strategies need special attention so that the therapist dropout rate can be decreased. Private practitioners, as well as clinic and crisis center staff, require supervision and consultation that focuses on self-awareness and the transference–countertransference reactions unique to rape victims. Professional education and training programs need to include more content on rape and sexual assault.

The sociocultural values, myths, and biases about gender and gender roles are fundamental to countertransference phenomena with rape and sexual assault victims. Despite recent efforts to alter these prejudices, they remain pervasive in our society. Inevitably, they contribute to the therapist's avoidance and/or overidentification reactions to the rape victim. The institutional denial of the traumatic sequelae of rape continues, as does the backlash against educational and legal attempts to convince the public that sexual domination of either gender is damaging. It is within this total complex of issues that the reactions of those who work with victims of rape must be evaluated and systems of support developed.

REFERENCES

Benedek, E. (1984). The silent scream: Countertransference reactions to victims. *American Journal of Social Psychiatry, 4*(3), 49–52.

Best, C., Dansky, B., & Kilpatrick, D. (1992). Medical students' attitudes about female rape victims. *Journal of Interpersonal Violence, 7*(2), 175–188.

Boston Globe. (1992, April 24). 683,000 women raped in 1990, new government study findings. pp. 1, 32.

Brownmiller, S. (1975). *Against our will: Men, women and rape.* New York: Simon & Schuster.

Burt, M. (1980). Cultural myths and supports for rape. *Journal of Personality and Social Psychology, 38,* 215–206.

Burgess, A., & Holmstrom, L. (1974). *Rape: Victims of crisis.* Bowie, MD: Robert J. Brady.

FBI Uniform Crime Report. (1988). *Crime in the United States.* Washington, DC: U.S. Department of Justice.

FBI Uniform Crime Report. (1990). *Crime in the United States.* Washington, DC: U.S. Department of Justice.

Foa, E., & Kozak, M. (1986). Emotional processing of fear: Exposure to corrective information. *Psychological Bulletin, 99,* 20–35.

Giller, E. (Ed.). (1990). *Biological assessment and treatment of posttraumatic stress disorder.* Washington, DC: American Psychiatric Press.

Gold, S., Fultz, J., Burke, C., Priscol, A., & Willett, J. (1992). Vicarious emotional responses of macho college males. *Journal of Interpersonal Violence, 7*(2), 165–174.

Hartman, C., & Burgess, A. (1991). Neurobiology in rape trauma. In A. W. Burgess (Ed.), *Rape and sexual assault* (Vol. III, pp. 1–12). New York: Garland.

Herman, J., Perry, J., & van der Kolk, B. (1989). Childhood trauma in borderline personality disorder. *American Journal of Psychiatry, 146*(4), 490–495.

Howe, A. C., Herzberger, S., & Tennen, H. (1988). The influence of personal history of abuse and gender on clinicians' judgments of child abuse. *Journal of Family Violence, 3*(2), 105–119.

Hunter, M. (1990). *Abused boys: The neglected victims of sexual abuse.* Lexington, MA: Lexington Books.

Jackson, H., & Nuttall, R. (1993). Clinician responses to sexual abuse allegations. *Child Abuse and Neglect, 17,* 127–143.

Kelley, S. J. (1990). Responsibility and management strategies in child sexual abuse: A comparison of child protective workers, nurses, and police officers. *Child Welfare, 69*(1), 43–51.

Kendell-Tackett, K. A., & Watson, M. W. (1991). Factors that influence professionals' perceptions of behavioral indicators of child sexual abuse. *Journal of Interpersonal Violence, 6*(3), 385–395.

Kilpatrick, D., Veronen, K., & Best, C. (1988). Factors predicting psychological distress among rape victims. In F. Ochberg (Ed.), *Post-traumatic therapy and victims of violence* (pp. 113–141). New York: Brunner/Mazel.

Kilpatrick, D., Veronen, L., Amick, A., Villeponteaux, A., & Ruff, G. (1985). Mental health correlates of criminal victimization: A random community survey. *Journal of Consulting and Clinical Psychology, 53,* 866–873.

Nuttall, R., & Jackson, H. (1992). *Personal history of childhood abuse among clinicians.* Manuscript submitted for publication.

Putnam, F. (1989). *Diagnosis and treatment of multiple personality disorder.* New York: Guilford Press.

Scully, D., & Marolla, J. (1984). Convicted rapists' vocabulary of motive: Excuse and justification. *Social Problems, 31,* 530–544.

Teicher, M., Glod, C., Swett, J. C., Surrey, J., & Brasher, C. (1989). Childhood abuse and limbic system dysfunction. *American Psychiatric Association Abstracts,* 142–212.

PART III

Countertransference Reactions in Work with Victims of War Trauma, Civil Violence, and Political Oppression

The four chapters that comprise Part III focus on a different aspects of war trauma or civil violence. Although the victim populations described have all been exposed to the grotesque horrors of violent aggression, they each present different challenges and clinical concerns to the therapists who work with them.

In Chapter 9, J. David Kinzie describes the psychiatric treatment program for Asian refugees at the Oregon Health Sciences University in Portland, Oregon. Begun in 1978, the program has grown steadily, with a current caseload of over 400 patients, including Cambodian victims of the Marxist Pol Pot regime (the Khmer Rouge), Vietnamese refugees, and many others seeking help as a result of having been interned, starved, beaten, tortured, or forced to witness horrible acts of genocide. Over 70% of this population suffer from post-traumatic stress disorder (PTSD) and comorbid states. The staff consists of transcultural psychiatrists who are aided by ethnic mental health counselors. Kinzie details the difficulties of working with trauma victims from a non-American (Anglo Western European) culture and the unique types of countertransference problems that arise in clinical work. These various themes are discussed in the chapter and include (1) sadness and depression; (2) anger, irritability, and hyperarousal; (3) unique shared experience; (4) excessive identification with the patient; and (5) intolerance of other patients. Kinzie goes on to characterize the "broader life effects" on staff members, which can range from vicarious traumatization to a sense of understanding the metaphor of the "Asian wise man."

In Chapter 10, Inger Agger and Søren Buus Jensen describe their work with Chilean therapists who attempt to carry out professional responsibilities in an environment in which state terrorism uses the internment and torture of political dissidents as a commonplace tool of oppression. This oppression, of course, extends to mental health professionals, who work at great risk, in secret, to aid those who have been victimized by the system. Agger and Jensen first discuss the concept of the "wounded healer," a concept originally described by Carl Jung. Next, they describe the field diary technique with which they monitor their own work with traumatized therapists. This fascinating and groundbreaking method—now a "historical document"—chronicles the day-to-day struggles in their research with victimized professionals. As such, the excerpts provide a kind of X-ray of their emotional reactions and profound countertransference processes and captures the *in vivo* essence of their day-to-day work. This rich and innovative work also include an analysis of primary, secondary, and tertiary traumatization within a repressive political state that creates constant terror, fear, and apprehensive mistrust of self and others, and describes the struggle to maintain professional integrity and dedication.

In Chapter 11, Michael J. Maxwell and Cynthia Sturm discuss the clinical treatment of U.S. war veterans, including ex-service personnel from World War II, the Korean and Vietnam Wars, and the more recent Persian Gulf War. Based on their work in the Department of Veterans Affairs hospitals and outpatient programs, as well as in private practice settings, they present critical issues in the management of patient care and countertransference. These themes include but are not limited to the following: (1) countertransference blocks to establishing the therapeutic relationship, (2) gender considerations, (3) uncovering and containing the trauma story, (4) managing suicidal patients, (5) the management of role boundaries, and (6) therapist self-care and personal transformation.

In Chapter 12, Wybrand Op den Velde, G. Frank Koerselman, and Petra G. H. Aarts discuss countertransference with a very unique population of World War II veterans—Nazi resistance fighters living in the Netherlands between 1940 and 1945. The authors note the somewhat surprising fact that after the war, many of the resistance fighters were met with "indifference, hostility, and rejection." Later, as these men sought pension and compensation, their claims for war-related trauma and PTSD were disbelieved, denied, or outright rejected. Op den Velde et al. discuss four factors that contribute to this societal and medical milieu: (1) general reactions toward victims of man-made disasters, (2) rejection and denial of the special position of war, (3) Dutch Calvinistic mentality and morale, and (4) prevailing medical opinions regarding the origin of traumatic neuroses in the post-war years. According to the authors, the psychosocial and medico-legal consequences of these four factors was to create an atmosphere in which it was enormously difficult to determine legitimate service connection for psychiatric impairment due to resistance fighting. This set the stage for two major types of transference–countertransference dynamics, which they have labeled as *paranoid* and *narcissistic*. Of special significance in this chapter is the recognition that historical circumstances and cultural traditions can exert influence on how mental health professionals construe the coping process of those affected by trauma (i.e., resisting Nazi occupation in World War II) and on survivors' attempts to secure psychological help, as well as pension and compensation.

9

Countertransference in the Treatment of Southeast Asian Refugees

J. DAVID KINZIE

Therapists working with Nazi Holocaust victims after World War II found themselves profoundly affected when hearing firsthand accounts of massive human aggression and destruction. As therapists, it was no longer possible, or perhaps even desirable, for them to remain totally objective about individual persecution and torture. Their reactions were described by de Wind (1971) and later by Chodoff (1975), followed by a thorough description by Danieli (1984) of the psychotherapeutic difficulties in treating these victims.

In many ways, Indochinese war victims and refugees had similar experiences to the Nazi survivors. They were involved in years, often decades, of warfare. Many were singled out because of their ethnic, religious, or social class affiliations. Their means of escape from persecution were often extremely dangerous. The greatest similarities, however, were in the concentration camps of the radical Marxist Pol Pot regime where millions lost their lives due to starvation, disease, constant forced labor, or execution. This terrible trauma has been well documented in the popular press (Becker, 1986; Hawk, 1982), in psychiatric literature (Kinzie, 1988; Mollica, 1988), and in a movie, *The Killing Fields*.

Since 1978, the Department of Psychiatry at Oregon Health Sciences University (OHSU) has operated a psychiatric clinic for Southeast Asian refugees. Over this time, the clinic has greatly expanded, and currently (1993) has a caseload of 500. The goal has been to provide treatment in a culturally sensitive manner: The clinical work is performed by experienced transcultural psychiatrists aided by ethnic mental health counselors (Kinzie & Manson, 1983). The clinic identified early post-traumatic stress disorder (PTSD) in Cambodians (Kinzie, Fredrickson, Ben, Fleck, & Karls, 1984), its effects (Boehnlein, Kinzie, Ben, & Fleck, 1985), and its course (Boehnlein, 1987; Kinzie, 1988). The treatment of refugees by individual (Kinzie & Fleck, 1987) and group therapy (Kinzie et al., 1988) has also been reported, as well as some aspects of psychopharmacology (Kinzie & Leung, 1989).

Most recently we reported on a survey of PTSD in the entire clinic population (Kinzie et al., 1990). We were greatly surprised by the amount of trauma previously unreported and by the high prevalence of PTSD (70% of the clinic population). We felt that some of the nonrecognition among even experienced psychiatrists was possibly due to countertransference difficulties, a problem we had begun to recognize earlier (Kinzie & Fleck, 1987).

The goal of this chapter is to further explore the difficulty of therapists and counselors in working with extremely traumatized patients. Clinicians' multiple reactions—social, professional, and intrapsychic—will be discussed, as well as possible adaptive approaches.

THE TRAUMA

The following accounts are typical of those given by Southeast Asian refugees in our clinic during their evaluations.

Patient A., a 45-year-old widowed Cambodian female, was referred for depression. She had multiple symptoms of major depressive disorder, anxiety, and irritability. She also suffered nightly nightmares of the torture she had been subjected to in Cambodia. She was an attractive woman, appearing younger than her age, who spoke some English and was well-mannered, poised, and socially gracious. However, when she began describing the past, she became profoundly sad and cried profusely. She and her husband and six children had been well-to-do before Pol Pot came to power. During this political upheaval, her husband was executed and her parents and she and her children were put into a concentration labor camp. Subsequently, her parents and one child died of starvation. A male child was also beaten and executed. The patient was tied to a stake, beaten, tortured, and told repeatedly that she was going to be killed, before finally being released from the camp. She and her surviving children had no place to stay the first year. They lived under a tree, with very little food, and only survived by bartering small amounts of jewelry. After living for 4 years under Pol Pot, she and her children were able to escape to Thailand when the Vietnamese invaded.

Patient B., a 44-year-old widowed Cambodian female, was originally seen for multiple pains and aches, poor sleep, and depression. She described vivid nightmares occurring nightly: her husband was tied up and forced under water to drown as he called out her name and she was powerless to help him. Other times she saw visions of her children being beaten to death and calling out her name; again she was unable to help them. These thoughts also became increasing intrusive when she was awake. She had married young and had had seven children from this marriage. When Pol Pot came to power she was immediately separated from her family; two children died soon after from disease, and two others, 9 and 12 years old, were executed. She had heard that they called out her name to help them before they were beaten to death. Later a 3-year-old died of starvation. Her husband was executed a year later; she heard that multiple shots severed his head. Although her dreams were of her inability to help her family when they died, she in fact was not with them. She was threatened with death herself, two siblings were executed, and her mother died of starvation. In the interview, she appeared controlled and restricted in affect as she began to tell her story. Then she cried as she talked about the death of family members and became more visibly anguished as details were revealed in the interview.

Patient C., a 39-year-old Vietnamese female, was separated from her husband in Vietnam. She was an attractive, well-mannered, intelligent woman, who knew some English. In a painful interview, she told her story in both anguished and depressed terms, frequently crying, with attempts to hold back her tears. During the more traumatic descriptions, she appeared to lose control.

She and her 2-year-old son escaped by boat from Vietnam. The boat sank after being attacked by pirates who robbed the refugees. Only four people survived. Her son died in her arms from drowning. In the water she swam toward a distant light that turned out to belong to the same Thai pirates who had attacked the boat. She was brutally raped and left on a lonely beach until rescuers found her and took her to a refugee camp, where she stayed for 3 years.

During that time she wrote to her family about the loss of the child (but not about the rape). Learning that her father died soon after he received the letter, she felt that his concern for her contributed to his death. She tried to forget the past but was unable to shake the memories, which had persisted and worsened since coming to the United States.

How should we react to such emotional and tragic presentations? How can therapists remain objective and helpful when exposed weekly to new trauma stories? What are the long-term effects on these therapists? Personal observations and the observations of counselors and psychiatrists within our clinic may shed light on these questions.

METHODS

Recently, to better understand the implications of countertransference as experienced by our clinic counselors and psychiatrists, I devised and administered a short questionnaire with both open-ended questions and a checklist. The questions were about personal and professional changes based on the therapists' reactions during sessions with traumatized clinic patients, and the possible need to limit work with the refugees. The checklist included 15 items on common countertransference themes. Additionally, I asked what these therapists found to be helpful in working through some of the difficulties they experienced.

BACKGROUND: THE THERAPISTS AND MULTIETHNIC ORIENTATION

The counselors in the OHSU program included six from Southeast Asia, four of whom were refugees themselves (three survived difficult experiences in their home country prior to their escape to the West). They served as interpreters for the clinic psychiatrists and as group leaders, case managers, and individual counselors. They had 3 to 11 years' experience in the program, and were well educated. One had a master's degree and two were in MSW programs.

When the counselors serve as interpreters in the clinic, perhaps their most difficult emotional role, they are required to accurately translate the refugees' stories. Such stories are often vivid reminders of the counselors' own lives in the same countries. In essence, they are forced to reexperience some aspects of their own traumatic past.

As counselors, they are practical problem-solvers as well as empathic listeners. They have not been trained, however, in the subtle interpersonal and intrapersonal dynamics of intense psychotherapy.

The four senior psychiatrists in the clinic, including myself, were all board-certified, had worked with the patients from 4 to 13 years, and had broad cross-cultural experience. One was born and raised through his early years in Southeast Asia. The results of the questionnaire, along with conversations with fellow psychiatrists and personal observations of clinic functioning, formed the basis for much of this chapter.

RESULTS

The counselors gave a limited range of responses to the questions. They either responded that there was "no change" or that changes were positive, that they were better able to help refugees. The checklist also showed a limited range of responses. One counselor answered all questions with "never" and one answered all but one with "sometimes." Only one counselor rated one item (sleep disturbance) as "often." Despite the paucity of responses in the written questionnaires, working with the counselors showed them to be dedicated to their work and more articulate about what they did. But irritability, impatience, and frustration were sometimes observed in their sessions with the patients as well as in staff meetings. One counselor commented that a patient could not have PTSD because she only spent 1 year in the Pol Pot camp. Once, in a difficult interview, a new counselor picked up a magazine, started to read it, and ignored the intense history being given. Some counselors felt a frantic need to provide services, overextending themselves to the point of being overwhelmed, while denying the feeling.

Our clinic psychiatrists had a wider range of responses, either writing in detail or meeting with me to discuss complex cases. Use of the questionnaire and our discussions raised many issues for all the psychiatrists, who were intensely aware of the problems involved. On the checklist, all four of the psychiatrists indicated "often" regarding their feelings of sadness and depression, and in answer to other items, "patients bring back painful memories" ($n = 3$), and "feelings of horror and disgust" ($n = 2$). "Sometimes" or "often" were noted by three psychiatrists for the following items: sleep disturbances, being too detached, denial, aggression or irritability, anger and hostility, overwhelmed, and loss of impartiality. Anger toward patients was seen only in two questionnaires ("sometimes"), and none felt relief about missed appointments, or described guilt or shame. A surprising finding was that the refugees' stories affected the psychiatrists' relationships with other patients (see below).

Despite the more overt acknowledgment of stress reactions and countertransference feelings, the behavior of the psychiatrists did not show overt problems. They functioned appropriately and effectively in their work with their patients.

PERSONAL REFLECTIONS

By definition, countertransference feelings are personal, subjective, and private. To be conscious of such feelings in therapy requires a high degree of self-awareness, personal security, and training. Furthermore, by sharing such feelings, which are often negative, with colleagues, one runs the risk that such openness may be misinterpreted as professional incompetence or personal weakness. These factors make it tempting to hide the thoughts on the one hand, or to overcompensate and excessively display them on the other. Additionally, countertransference feelings may be confused with countertransference behavior. Because a therapist feels a specific feeling, it does not follow that specific behavior, for instance, rejection of the patient, results. Indeed, it is probable that the recognition of such feelings prevents most nontherapeutic actions. However, a therapist is never totally confident of his or her behavior in a highly emotional setting.

With this background, I would like to add some personal remarks regarding the effects of working with traumatized refugees. I will give brief, relevant information to help frame my remarks and then add my countertransference reactions.

After a medical internship in a sometimes violent city (Oakland, CA), I was a civilian general medical officer in a provincial hospital in Vietnam. Medically and personally it was a rich, though disturbing, experience. The medical facilities were primitive, the problems were often life-threatening, and death by disease was common. Death, however, was even more common because of the war, and violence became increasingly apparent, as did concern for one's personal safety. After 9 months, I was transferred to Malaysia, where I was a general practitioner for the aborigines living in the jungle areas. After a residency in psychiatry, I taught at the medical school in Malaysia.

My Asian connection was deepened further by living 6 years in Hawaii. The Vietnam War seemed to maintain a tragic hold on my thoughts, and when the refugees started coming to the United States in 1975, I felt a strong need to help. With the aid of a Vietnamese psychiatric resident, himself a refugee, I started an Indochinese refugee clinic in 1978.

Our early interest was straightforward by psychiatric standards: treating psychosis and depression. Only through the process of interviewing and treating a seemingly endless number of refugees, did the many psychic effects of war, the traumas of desperate escape, and the difficulties of refugees in a foreign country become clear. Over time, the patients' needs for psychiatric and medical care grew larger, as did our range of services. We began treating Asian patients in a type of clinic that would have been encountered in Asia. But the arrival of Cambodian survivors from the Pol Pot camps in 1980 changed all that. Evil had made a quantum leap, and the patients—victims and survivors—revealed intense degrees of numbing, anguish, and arousal, which we had not faced before. I began to monitor my professional reactions more frequently and experienced the need for more caution in many areas of life. I felt as if the security of a stable, predictable belief system had slowly dissolved. My reactions to this experience, shared by my colleagues, are summarized below.

Psychotherapeutic Effects

Sadness and Depression

Often psychiatrists describe a general sense of sadness in treating trauma-tized refugees. The sadness not only springs from empathy with the pa-tients, but also from a deeper realization that what happened to the refugees should not have been endured by any human being.

Anger, Irritability, and Hyperarousal

Anger and irritability are often linked with the sadness, which leaves a sense of something awful has happened, that an unpunishable evil has been committed. The result is a heightened sense of arousal with irrita-bility. This is almost never directed at patients but at the perpetrators, usually unknown, who committed such acts. The fact that the anger has no clear focus, no clear enemy, often leaves the feelings vague and in-choate. Typically, such feelings last long after the patient has left, spilling over into other activities and into the therapist's personal life.

The Unique Shared Experience

Although not originally troubling, a profound sense of sharing a unique experience with the suffering, slowly trusting fellow human often de-velops. A personal sense of uniqueness, or even the privilege of hearing such extremely private stories, results. The vulnerability and guardedness revealed during the encounter lead the therapist to be profoundly moved, often developing an awesome sense of responsibility for the patients, the trauma, and the relationship. The ongoing respect is more than confidentiality. Not only can the therapist not ethically tell anyone about the encounter, there is simply no way to adequately describe the ex-perience. This uniqueness is a profound burden affecting other patient relationships and other areas of life.

Excessive Identification with the Patient

The patients' accounts of their traumas, their vulnerability, and their tenuous survivor status can lead to overidentification and overprotective-ness by the therapist. The therapist says, in effect, "With what you have been through, we will protect you, we will take care of you," which leads to excessive caseloads and working late in the evenings to meet patient needs. This can further lead to an obsessive need to anticipate problems—medical, psychiatric, and social—and to develop programs to handle them. The "savior" self-image results in loss of objectivity. This can result in overidentification with the entire program, because "There is no one else who can do it as well as we can," or "don't challenge us, we know how to treat this better than you do," and it may also lead to an intolerance of outsiders and other therapeutic approaches.

Intolerance of Other Patients

A frequent side effect is more difficulty with nontraumatized patients due to an attitude of intolerance of those whose problems seem, by comparison, trivial or minor. Concern about relationships, inability to "find one's self," conflict in the workplace, or somatic complaints pale when contrasted with the huge losses of position, health, family, and culture. This intolerance and impatience is probably most acute when involving patients with disturbing behavior personality disorders. Intellectually, human misery is misery, especially for the suffering individual, but it is hard not to make quantitative judgments that are accompanied by loss of empathy for the usual, mundane human problems.

Broader Life Effects

A friend once reminded me that the role of a physician was to deal with the terrible things in life, the disfiguring wounds, the physically injured, the distorting and painful effects of cancer, the grotesque neonates with congenital defects. The psychiatrist deals with the terrible aspects of the human mind—psychotic distortions, organic cognitive impairment, hopeless depressive ruminations, and the like. There are also the victims of trauma, haunted by terrifying nightmares, repetitive intrusive thoughts, autonomic hyperarousal, and an enduring sense of numbness from which there is often no escape. Other physicians, such as a cynical surgeon or a cold oncologist, sometimes seem "wounded" by their professional contacts. Psychiatrists dealing with trauma can also be "wounded," with major reactions.

An Intolerance of Violence

There develops a strong aversion to violence, with an increased sensitivity to conflict. There can be a total intolerance to war and violent conflicts in movies, television, and even some news reporting. War scenes, especially with multiple killings and torture scenes, are almost all completely avoided by our clinic psychiatric staff. The increase in arousal from murder, rape, and assault news reports has left such discomfort that we avoid hearing the problems whenever possible.

A Personal Sense of Vulnerability

Life is no longer the same. If beatings, starvation, torture, and mass killings can happen to our patients, they can happen to us. There is an increased awareness of the dangers of hatred and brutality that lie behind the mask of civilization we all wear, a sense of being more vulnerable to life's dangers. We do not take 20-century America's security for granted nor, indeed, the family and social relationships we depend on for support. Often I think that if, like my patients, I had lost my parents, family, and friends, what would I have in life? In my more extreme, frightening fantasies or dreams of concentration camps, I am being tortured or seeing family members killed. The catastrophic events have become believable and real.

Reminder of Past Painful Memories

The patients' accounts often bring back suppressed, painful memories of our pasts. Some are merely embarrassing, some involve being humiliated, and some involve being treated in a severe or brutal manner. The most painful of memories, guilt, involves personal actions that were harmful to others. The affects of these memories seem to be reactivated by the affect involved in the patients' stories.

The Psychiatrist Living a Myth

Lindy (1989) described transference reactions of veterans, with the patients taking on the mythical stories of Abraham, Jonah, or Joshua, for example. Psychiatrists, with their unique knowledge and the burdens they encounter in trauma victims, may also take on private, mythical roles. These may be tragic, such as Sisyphus condemned to continually rolling a stone up a hill only to see it fall down again, or Job being tested by God to endure meaningless punishment. They may also be heroic, such as the Seven Samurai of Japanese lore, trying to protect a small group of helpless people against powerful outlaws.

A Sense of Failure of Modern Medicine and Psychiatry

Modern medicine has been optimistic about its ability to understand and control many diseases and disorders. The successes have been spectacular and psychiatry has shared in this, buoyed by advances in the neurosciences and psychopharmacology as well as more sophisticated models, for example, the biopsychosocial model of human pathology. However, nowhere in the medical and psychiatric education did we deal with the factors that would cause humans to inflict massive suffering and death onto others. There were no systematic approaches to helping trauma victims. Much clinical exposure was devoted to treatment of gunshot wounds, and to medical approaches for management of infections and malnutrition, but there was almost total silence about the psychological effects. Even specific nomenclature was absent. Although the first edition of the *Diagnostic and Statistical Manual of Mental Disorders* had a diagnosis of *gross stress reaction,* it was removed from the second edition, because such horror from the Nazis was thought to be a tragic aberration that would not occur again. It was possible to go through 8 years of medical and psychiatric education and to be unprepared for, even surprised by, the serious psychiatric impact of psychological traumas.

When faced with the increasing number of people involved in massive trauma, the psychiatrist with little preparation blames educators and training for the deficiency. This is especially true when it becomes apparent that treatments are often ineffective and the patients' impairments are chronic and severe. Medical optimism subsides and a sense of frustration emerges.

Failure of Western and Human Culture

Nozick (1989), in *The Examined Life,* describes how the Holocaust changed everything for modern man; it radically and dramatically altered humanity. Life did not have the same sense of hope and ever-growing optimism afterwards. Innocence had been lost, and the human species was desanctified. A similar theme was described by Lifton (1979) about the nuclear age and the use of nuclear weapons, with man taking on an "identity of the doomed." The Age of Enlightenment, with its hubris of Western culture confident of its values and its future, ended with these modern tragedies.

However, the tragedies seemed to be suppressed in the '50s and '60s. Through television, the Vietnam War brought home the violence and atrocities of the Asian civil war, along with the violence and atrocities perpetrated by Americans. Once again our culture and society did not seem enlightened nor did our outlook on life seem hopeful, or even civilized. There was something terribly wrong about our understanding of human nature. With the knowledge of Cambodia, especially the graphic descriptions by Pol Pot survivors, it became clearer that our culture and its philosophy had not begun to grapple with the terrible, evil capacities of man. Psychotherapists continually hearing the account of atrocities realized that Western culture and its educational system and values were seriously flawed. The result was a sense of betrayal about the basic assumptions of our modern culture and society. (The ethnic Chinese psychiatrist on our clinic staff has stated that most Asians have always known life was filled with evil—they are not particularly surprised by recent events.)

Countertransference Is Not Necessarily Countertherapeutic

Although most of my comments describe the negative thoughts and feelings the therapist may have in working with traumatized refugees, there are positive therapeutic implications. Clearly, countertransference and, more precisely, awareness of countertransference do not imply therapeutic failure. It seems likely that awareness of such feelings, combined with clinical expertise, promotes the therapy process (Gabbard, 1990; Hamilton, 1985; Kernberg, 1965). It is important to note the successful coping methods used, based on my personal experience and on the comments of my colleagues.

Dealing with Normal Therapeutic Issues

Not all of the therapeutic sessions are filled with descriptions and reactions to traumatic events. After the first session, many problems are related to symptoms, adjustment to American culture, and the universal aspects of life such as raising children, working, and marital life. Therefore, there is not a total, constant pressure of graphic and agonizing descriptions. The normal therapeutic content helps to neutralize the stress on the therapist, with the added advantage of being more familiar territory.

Satisfaction with the Patient's Improvement

Although we probably have never "cured" anyone of the chronic effects of trauma, our efforts have helped most of the patients. The therapist's interest, the consistency of treatment, reduction of stress, socialization experiences, and medicines have had a major impact on intrusive symptoms. Sleep and appetite improves, nightmares and startle reactions diminish, and the patients are visibly grateful. The personal and professional rewards are quite satisfying—sometimes "joyful" is a more accurate word. These successes have a positive effect on both the therapy and the therapist.

Scientific Curiosity

Intellectual detachment is a danger in working with the patients, but in more acceptable terms, studying therapeutic approaches and patients' reactions offers an academic reward. The scientific method of withdrawing to study the phenomena gives a needed detachment but keeps the clinician involved and fulfills another altruistic goal of helping through research and publication. The broad approach often sustains the therapist through the pressures of immediate clinical situations.

Limiting the Number of Patients

All our clinic psychiatrists felt the strong necessity to limit the number of traumatized patients carried in a general psychiatric practice. There was concern that our clinic had reached the limit, which one of us suggested be no more than one-fourth of the patients carried. However, as the clinic load reached capacity, the number of new patients diminished, thus reducing the number of stressful encounters without further limiting.

Personal Growth

Through our clinical association, each of us on the staff has had the opportunity, actually the requirement, to grow personally, to come to terms with the potential for evil in our fellow humans and within ourselves. We have also learned more about suffering and the limitations of available help. Our capacity to take in and contain (Bion, 1957; Hamilton, 1990) the powerful experiences and emotions of our patients has been both taxed and expanded, but there is still a limit to those capacities. Our awareness that we can grow personally through our work has helped (Bion, 1957).

Support from Each Other

A genuine sense of respect combined with our active interest in each other's lives, social and professional, provides a strong supportive network among our therapists. This network helps us through difficult times; the sharing of experiences reduces our feelings of isolation and loneliness.

Probably the most important personal qualities for the therapist are maturity, equanimity, and warmth, which allow us to roll with the vicissitudes of life but still be involved. The mature defenses described by Vaillant (1977)—suppression, altruism, asceticism, and humor—seem to be very evident in my colleagues, psychiatrists and counselors alike, and to be exactly what is needed to work with these difficult and admirable patients.

ACKNOWLEDGMENTS

I am very grateful for the suggestions and critical review by Dr. Paul Leung, Dr. Jim Boehnlein, Dr. Laurie Moore, and Ms. Cris Riley. The helpful considerations about the therapist's growth came from Dr. Greg Hamilton.

REFERENCES

Becker, E. (1986). *When the war was over.* New York: Simon & Schuster.

Boehnlein, J. K. (1987). Culture and society in posttraumatic stress disorder: Implications for psychotherapy. *American Journal of Psychotherapy, 41,* 519–530.

Boehnlein, J. K., Kinzie, J. D., Ben, R., & Fleck, J. (1985). One-year follow-up study of posttraumatic stress disorder among survivors of Cambodian concentration camps. *American Journal of Psychiatry, 142,* 956–959.

Chodoff, P. (1975). Psychiatric aspects of Nazi persecution. In S. Arieti (Ed.), *American handbook of psychiatry* (2nd ed., Vol. VI). New York: Basic Books.

Danieli, Y. (1984). Psychotherapists' participation in the conspiracy of silence about the Holocaust. *Psychoanalytic Psychology, 1,* 23–42.

de Wind, S. (1971). Psychotherapy after traumatization caused by persecution. *International Psychiatric Clinic, 8,* 93–114.

Gabbard, G. O. (1990). *Psychodynamic psychiatry in clinical practice.* Washington DC: American Psychiatric Press.

Hamilton, N. G. (1985). *Self and others: Object relations theory in practice.* Northvale, NJ: Jason Aronson.

Hamilton, N. G. (1990). The containing function and the analyst's projective identification. *International Journal of Psycho-Analysis, 71,* 445–453.

Hawk, D. (1982). The killing of Cambodia. *New Republic, 187,* 17–21.

Kernberg, O. F. (1965). Notes on countertransference. *Journal of the American Psychoanalytic Association, 13,* 38–56.

Kinzie, J. D. (1988). The psychiatric effects of massive trauma on Cambodian refugees. In J. P. Wilson, Z. Harel, & B. Kahana (Eds.), *Human adaptation to extreme stress.* New York: Plenum Press.

Kinzie, J. D., Boehnlein, J. K., Leung, P. K., Moore, L., Riley, C., & Smith, D. (1990). The prevalence of posttraumatic stress disorder and its clinical significance among Southeast Asian refugees. *American Journal of Psychiatry, 147,* 913–917.

Kinzie, J. D., & Fleck, J. (1987). Psychotherapy with severely traumatized refugees. *American Journal of Psychotherapy, 41,* 82–94.

Kinzie, J. D., Fredrickson, R. H., Ben, R., Fleck, J., & Karls, W. (1984). Post-traumatic stress disorder among survivors of Cambodian concentration camps. *American Journal of Psychiatry, 141,* 645–650.

Kinzie, J. D., & Leung, P. (1989). Clonidine in Cambodian patients with post-traumatic stress disorder. *Journal of Nervous and Mental Disease, 177,* 546–550.

Kinzie, J. D., Leung, P., Bui, A., Ben, R., Keopraseuth, K. O., Riley, C., Fleck, J., & Ades, M. (1988). Group therapy with Southeast Asian refugees. *Community Mental Health Journal, 24,* 157–166.

Kinzie, J. D., & Manson, S. M. (1983). Five years' experience with Indochinese refugee patients. *Journal of Operational Psychiatry, 14,* 105–111.

Lifton, R. J. (1979). *The broken connection: On death and the continuity of life.* New York: Simon & Schuster.

Lindy, J. D. (1989). PTSD: Phenomenology, dynamics and transference. *Journal of the American Academy of Psychoanalysis, 17,* 397–413.

Mollica, R. F. (1988). The trauma story: The psychiatric case of refugee survivors of violence and torture. In R. Ochberg (Ed.), *Post-traumatic therapy and victims of violence.* New York: Brunner/Mazel.

Nozick, R. (1989). *The examined life: Philosophical meditations.* New York: Simon & Schuster.

Vaillant, G. E. (1977). *Adaptation to life.* Boston: Little, Brown.

10

Determinant Factors for Countertransference Reactions under State Terrorism

INGER AGGER
SØREN BUUS JENSEN

It is a sad fact that in the world today psychotherapists often have to carry out post-traumatic therapy under severely stressful conditions. Wars and different types of state terrorism are common phenomena in many countries, and psychotherapists will—along with the rest of the population who live in these environments—become traumatized to a greater or lesser degree. This raises a number of important questions about the psychotherapeutic process under these traumatic conditions, namely: Under state terrorism, how are supportive institutional settings developed in which it is possible to carry out psychotherapy for the victims of the regime? To which kinds of trauma are therapists and patients exposed? What are the personal characteristics of the patients? How do the traumatic experiences of the therapists affect their relationships with patients?

We draw on the experiences of a number of Chilean therapists who have had to develop their work under conditions of state terrorism. During our three recent periods of fieldwork in Chile, we interviewed 40 clinicians who worked with survivors of the recent dictatorship's widespread human rights violations.[1] Our experiences from a total of 6 months of fieldwork in Chile are the empirical basis of this discussion.

[1]The fieldwork was carried out as a part of our research project "Human Rights and Mental Health: The Chilean Human Rights Movement as an Exemplary Model for Mental Health Work in Developing Countries." The project is supported by grants from the Danish Research Council for the Humanities and the Danish International Development Assistance (DANIDA), of the Danish Ministry of Foreign Affairs.

We believe that the experiences gained in the Chilean human rights movement are valuable for other therapists who have to work in places where human rights are violated. We also believe that the Chilean experience can highlight some general aspects of the problem of subjective countertransference in post-traumatic therapy—especially in relation to therapists who are on a "survivor's mission" (see, e.g., Catherall & Lane, 1992).

This question relates to the problem of the "wounded healer." Before discussing the Chilean experiences, we will discuss the wounded healer, an issue that becomes relevant under conditions of state terrorism. Moreover, we will describe how we ourselves experienced this problem during our research process in a "traumatized" society that was just at the beginning of democratization. Countertransference reactions (CTRs) are not only felt by therapists; they also develop in researchers who interview traumatized people, be they therapists or other survivors of trauma.

From the stories and writings of the Chilean therapists, we will give an overview of the institutional contexts for psychotherapeutic help to victims that gradually built up in the years just following the military coup. The "underground" quality of these institutions was an important determinant for the CTRs of the therapists. Thereafter, we will describe the various forms of repetitive traumatic events, which became part of daily life in Chile after the military coup, and we will present case examples of trauma to which therapists and patients were exposed. We will then examine some personal characteristics of the patients. These characteristics were especially related to the patients' obvious need to find a therapist whom they could trust from a political point of view. Finally, we will examine some important personal characteristics of the Chilean therapists, especially their view of themselves and their work as it developed during the dictatorship.

THE PROBLEM OF THE WOUNDED HEALER

Using a metaphorical expression, therapists who have themselves survived trauma have been called "wounded healers." We have borrowed this concept from the works of Kleinman (1988), Maeder (1989), Comas-Díaz and Padilla (1990), and Jung (1963/1983). The problem of the wounded healer has been discussed from two different perspectives. On the one hand, wounded healers are expected through their own traumatic experiences to have a greater empathy with the suffering of their patients. They can transform their own wounds into healing power and hope, as seen, for example, in certain types of shamanism (Comas-Díaz & Padilla,

1990). Many Christian saints have also used their own weaknesses and sufferings as a means of become more compassionate and strong (Maeder, 1989). On the other hand, some wounded healers are found to have a compelling *need* to help others (Kleinman, 1988). They are unconsciously attracted to the psychotherapeutic profession in order to gain emotional release through their relationships with their patients. This relationship also becomes a way of avoiding their own trauma, which becomes isolated and encapsulated (Maeder, 1989). From this point of view, it would be difficult for wounded healers to maintain "sustained empathic inquiry" (Chapters 1 and 2, this volume).

However, Carl Jung addresses this issue in *Memories, Dreams, Reflections* (1963/1983), in which he, at over 80 years of age, writes that "only the wounded physician heals" (p. 155). The patient must mean something to the therapist. If the therapist is not affected by the patient's message, he or she will not be able to help the patient. Evidently, Jung finds that the therapist's own wounds are a condition for a genuine empathic stance. From his own experience of a life-long search for self-realization, however, Jung also emphasizes the necessity for the therapist to understand himself or herself, because "the patient's treatment begins with the doctor, so to speak. Only if the doctor knows how to cope with himself and his own problems will he be able to teach the patient to do the same" (p. 154). And Jung continues:

> It often happens that the patient is exactly the right plaster for the doctor's sore spot. Because this is so, difficult situations can arise for the doctor too—or rather, especially for the doctor. Every therapist ought to have a control by some third person, so that he remains open to another point of view. Even the Pope has a confessor. (p. 156)

In essence, the problem of the wounded healer is the problem of how therapists manage their subjective CTRs to patients. This problem is common in all psychotherapeutic contexts, not only under the traumatic conditions of state terrorism.

In the following, however, we will concentrate on the factors that determine the CTRs of the wounded healers who have to carry out their very necessary work in the stressful environment of state terrorism. The urgency of the situation can make this problem seem a bit luxurious. It is, however, still important to be aware of these dynamics because they may, if unrecognized, add to the severity of stressors already present. This was verified by our interviews and discussions with a number of therapists in Chile who had worked under the traumatizing conditions of state terrorism. Likewise, we as researchers had to realize that the same dynamics were reflected in our reactions to the object of our research.

THE RESEARCHERS AND THE RESEARCH PROCESS

The aim of our research project was to study, on the basis of the experiences of people in the Chilean human rights movement, how people develop new ways of resisting power abuse, how they begin to take fate into their own hands, and how they heal the wounds following human rights violations. More specifically, we wanted to understand how concepts of trauma, therapeutic strategies, and therapeutic relationships were developed under state terrorism. From this Chilean case example, we attempted to develop a model that was applicable to other societies in which human rights are also abused (Agger & Jensen, 1993). The scientific value of this model is measured by its explanatory power in local contexts other than Chile.

The object of our research was the community of a human rights movement in a certain societal context. This community is different from and more than the sum of its individual members. Therefore, we could not limit ourselves to interviewing individual members of the community. A human rights movement consists of social relations between people, and it was the *collective consciousness* and the *moral community* of this movement that were our prime targets. It is this collectivity and this moral community that have, we assumed, a certain resisting and healing quality. We see the typical themes of the Chilean human rights movement—the emphasis on the close relationship between the private, the professional, and the political levels, and the linkage of human rights and mental health—as another way of expressing the importance of collectivity and moral community for individual and societal healing and resistance to power abuse.

Research Methodology and Countertransference Processing

To get the "feel" of this community, it was, therefore, important to experience daily life in a traumatized society as well as participate in formal and informal events of the human rights movement. In total, we interviewed 76 people. Of these, 40 were therapists, 23 were representatives of survivors' organizations, and 13 represented other aspects of the human rights movement.

Among the 40 interviewed therapists, 13 (33%) were men and 27 (67%) were women. Some 13 (33%) were psychiatrists and 6 (15%) had other medical specializations; 13 (33%) were psychologists; 4 (10%) were social workers, and 4 (9%) had other educational backgrounds. Of the interviewed therapists, 14 (35%) had been exiled and 11 (28%) had been tortured; 8 (20%) had both been tortured and exiled. Among the 19 interviewed medical doctors, 10 (53%) had been tortured.

During the interview process we ourselves experienced a whole range of CTRs: feelings of being drawn into the interviewees' world with a temporary loss of boundaries, feelings of denial and avoidance in the face of horrible trauma stories, feelings of guilt and anger toward the interviewees. A recurrent theme was a feeling of complicity: were we traumatizing them through our interviews?

We could usually discuss these different types of reactions with each other after the interview, so that in this way we acted as each other's supervisors. The fact that we were two researchers (and therapists) together during the interview was a great help in managing the reactions that emerged in the confrontation with trauma stories of death, severe losses, and torture.

Our debriefing talks were often held immediately after the interview in a nearby café—sometimes accompanied by a greatly needed glass of *pisco* to reduce the level of arousal. Thereafter, one of us (IA) often felt an urgent need to sleep, while the other (SBJ) had a need to order his experiences by writing the field diary. Sometimes, the confrontation with the evil of the trauma story was transmitted into our relationship, probably because of *projective identification*. Although we might be in a good and peaceful mood prior to and throughout the interview, without any external reason we could end up in a quarrel a few minutes after leaving the emotionally charged interview situation. The recognition of these processes made it clear to us that researchers, as well as therapists, who work in the area of extreme, man-made trauma, badly need debriefing talks and/or supervision to stay alert and receptive, and indeed simply to, on the symbolic level, survive.

The Field Diary Technique of Monitoring Reactions

The diary that we wrote during fieldwork was a valuable tool for monitoring these reactions. By analyzing them we learned something about ourselves but also something important about the reality we encountered. In this way, we also became our own informants.

After returning from fieldwork, when we consulted the diary at our desks, we recalled and reexperienced events, thoughts, and emotions. A new perspective had now become part of the process. The temporary encounter between "them and us" was over. A new distance from the experiences had developed, the recorded data in the field diary had been processed, and a new dual vision of what happened became part of reality.

We are both subjects and objects of the research process. We cannot "read" another world from an objective stance but must read it through ourselves as redefined and redefining subjects (Hastrup, 1992). The field diary told us one story, it was our first draft of a map of an unknown territory. We listened to our voices, but we ourselves had changed.

Excerpts and Illustrations of Countertransference from the Field Diary

In the following, we will present excerpts from our field diary followed by our later reflections *(in italics)*.

Excerpts from Field Diary I: Fieldwork March–April 1991

Do they really understand what we want to do? Have we overcome their mistrust and the old, bad experiences of being evaluated by Europeans? Will it give us problems to interview some staff members and not others? Will we be able to establish a contact with the "wounded healers" that enables us to perceive the dynamics of the therapeutic relationships?

It feels as if we are starting a therapeutic process: the first assessment/interview was a success, the "patient" will return, but have we also succeeded in establishing a viable contact and working alliance?

Thousands of questions come up. It is an overwhelming experience to start fieldwork. We are still not quite sure whether we really have a project.

We are received very warmly in the next institution. The director emphasizes that she has complete trust in us. We have made it! We are on the track! We are quite confident now. We have already appointed about 10 interviews for the next week and have been invited to participate in several events. The project will come off!

The relief, the enthusiasm, the engagement—we were on the track, and we were sucked into a whirlpool. We were unable to say no: The impressive leader and our strong wish to get the project going made us schedule too many interviews. We did not realize the risk of exhaustion when we entered the powerful space of the "wounded healers." This over-involvement created the basis of our first research wound.

The testimonial method that we are using in the interviews is unique. This method enables us to use our professional backgrounds in a combination of data collection and establishment of contact. We are really on to something. We get some very moving and insightful stories. This "qualified interview" is a very interesting way of doing research. Maybe we have, however, underestimated the amount of energy that this method requires.

The interview today turns out to be an intense experience and afterwards we discuss ethical questions. How far can we go, when we do not have any contract about therapy and she apparently needs to talk?

Here we were in touch with an important problem of our research method. Our training as therapists and researchers allowed us to create an atmosphere of trust. Our position as "outsiders" who had been invited into this culture offered the interviewees a setting in which they felt safe to tell their stories. However, the strength of the encapsulated traumata, on some occasions, caught all of us (including the interviewees) by surprise, although, as professionals, we all should have anticipated that.

When we started the interview we understood that they have talked about us in the institution and discussed how it is to be interviewed by us. From the way she tells us about it, we also understand that they think that the interviews are all right.

We are evaluated by them, we are placed in certain roles, a transference process is developing between the community of the institution and us. We ourselves are developing CTRs in the balance between overinvolvement and the fear of being rejected by them.

We are exhausted now. It is hard work with too many harsh stories. We must learn to respect our own tiredness. The risk is that we privatize our pain from listening to all these trauma stories—that we direct the anger from this pain against ourselves or each other.

Today, we were on a tough job. Our interviewee, a psychiatrist, was skeptical. We have not met that reaction before. We knew, beforehand, that she had been severely tortured, and she was clearly defending herself, primarily by intellectualization. She did not want to go into her private story. We knew that the director had told her to tell us "everything."

Her anxiety and lack of trust must be seen in the perspective of the request from the director to "tell them everything." This was a request that had been given in solidarity with our work, but at the same time, it created a trauma-symbolizing situation. She felt forced to offer information that she was not ready to share with us. Her taking care of herself was interpreted by us as directed toward us, and we felt narcissistically wounded when she did not readily idealize our aim and work. Our overinvolvement and fear of rejection provoked our CTRs—maybe even a situation of projective identification. Her perception of us as violators and transgressors of her boundaries made us feel—and maybe even act—as transgressors or violators, although we from the "outside" could have been seen as a "neutral," considerate couple doing a very empathic interview. When the tape recorder had been turned off and the trauma-symbolizing situation was over, all three of us were able to develop another contact. We were back into a pro-

fessional exchange situation into which the strong emotions did not interfere. Maybe we could have started the interview all over at this point. Maybe we would have been back in an equivalent situation, if we had tried.

We have both had dreams about how to manage sexuality. We begin wondering about what they do *not* tell us: "the really forbidden"; the secret spaces; some of the strange things happening in the torture houses, for example, in the place nicknamed *la venda sexy* ("the sexy blindfold"). Our fantasies begin pouring out. Something happens during torture that we do not understand—maybe they could avoid other types of torture by agreeing to the sexual part.

We know about sexual torture. Part of our professional background has been to bring this theme to the surface (Agger, 1994; Agger & Jensen, 1993). We nearly "forget" about this theme in Chile. It is too difficult to ask the questions and maybe also to listen to the answers. The sexual undertones are still part of "the conspiracy of silence," part of the unspoken—maybe words can never express it.

We also, however, "forget" about another theme: the process of turning into a collaborator during torture. The theme of "talking" during torture, of giving information, of betraying your comrades and your ideals. "Forgetting" this theme was even more noteworthy, because we retrospectively can see that we struggled indirectly with it throughout our interviews: the problem of how much pressure we could exert on our interviewees to get information.

At home, and at a distance, we begin wondering whether the problem of having "talked" during torture is not the real trauma, the real conspiracy of silence, and that the sexual torture methods, although deeply traumatizing, are somewhat manageable in comparison. Maybe it is an illusion, on the part of the therapist, that you get to the deepest layers of the trauma when the sexual part is disclosed and integrated. Maybe the patients will even disclose this point to avoid telling about that which really damaged their soul.

Now, we have interviewed several clinicians from this institution, and we are beginning to wonder if they maybe are developing aggressive feelings toward us: could we possibly become "scapegoats" for the problems that we sense this institution has? Are we doing any harm to them?

We are struggling with the "problem of complicity": did we ourselves become violators when we asked them to disclose their trauma story? Maybe most of this was in our imagination—or was it real?

Our thoughts at this moment were concentrated on emotional interactions: transference, countertransference, and projective identification. We now interpret that our struggles were part of the reality of therapists who work in this area. The overinvolvement combined with exhaustion. The guilt combined with anxiety. The outbursts of anger toward ourselves and each other. The problem of the wounded healer had become part of our daily life. Our own old wounds came closer to the surface, and we were brought into contact with feelings that contributed to a deeper understanding of ourselves and why we were right there doing that kind of research. The universality of the problem of the wounded healer became clearer. We felt, in our own bodies, that the empathy of the wounded healer deepens the ability to understand the wounded patient. We were, however, also confronted with the continuous dilemma of the wounded healer: either to be sucked into powerlessness without resources to take a step back and go into a process of counteridentification, or to be overcome with the grandiose feelings of being a specially gifted healer—or researcher.

Today, we write a letter of thank-you to the institution. We try to prevent the resistance that we are imagining, "stabs in the back" or whatnot?

We also did an interview that was a bit too short. We could have gotten much more valuable material. We broke the interview off by reminding *them* of the time limit they had given us when we started the interview.

Retrospectively, we realize that this is a pseudoproblem. We were simply exhausted and could not take any more. Our preoccupation with keeping the interviewee's timetable was our own way to secure that the interview ended fairly soon; maybe there are also other mechanisms at work, such as projective identification.

The psychiatrist who was so defensive writes a dedication for us in a copy of her book: "For our colleagues who are dedicated to the same wish for knowledge as we are," she writes. It seems as if we are forgiven, but maybe we never did anything wrong?

We close the field diary. Listening to our own voices from that time, we have become aware that we are no longer the same. The researchers have an impact on the object of research. Likewise, the research process will have an impact on the subjects doing it.

We will now turn our attention toward the reality of our object of research, toward the map that we drew of this territory. It is our narrative about the development of the Chilean mental health network, under state terrorism, based on the interviewees' stories of how it all began (see also our final report, Agger & Jensen, 1993).

INSTITUTIONAL FACTORS UNDER STATE TERRORISM

When a dictatorial regime seizes power, it affects all the institutions in the country, whether governmental or nongovernmental. Therefore, this new situation will also influence the institutions that normally help people with psychological or psychiatric problems. It will become difficult or even impossible to find a supportive institutional context in which victims of the dictatorship can receive treatment. Therapists working in the existing institutions may commit acts of treason if they help people who are defined as enemies of the regime. It therefore becomes necessary to create new institutional settings—sometimes in the form of underground networks—to help victims.

The particular historical circumstances of how such networks or institutions are developed will, of course, vary from country to country. We do, however, find it important to show how a system of therapeutic assistance is gradually born in the midst of chaos. Before therapy can even begin, there must be a setting for it.

Evidently, the context of terror in which this development takes place will affect the internal structure of the insurgent institutions, which will exist in an environment that is directly oppositional to the efforts of the therapists. The possibility of being supportive, flexible, collaborative, and nurturing (see Chapters 1 and 2, this volume) toward each other within the institutional contexts will to a large degree be determined by the life-threatening situation of both patients and therapists.

In the following pages we briefly illustrate the stages of the development of insurgent institutions in Chile in the years just following the coup on September 11, 1973.

The Political Coup of 1973 and Its Consequences for Mental Health Workers

On the day of September 11, many doctors in the hospitals in Chile were on strike. In the months leading up to the coup, the right-wing factions (with the aid of the United States) had tried to destabilize the democratic government of Salvador Allende in various ways, such as calling strikes. The only doctors on duty in the hospitals that day were those people who supported Allende and who, therefore, refused to go on strike.

The coup started in the early morning, and by midday the new regime put the country under martial law and imposed a curfew, which was not lifted until the third day of the coup. This meant that doctors who were in the hospitals when the coup began had to remain there for 3 days. As one female psychiatrist told us[2]:

[2]Almost all interviews were carried out in Spanish and have been translated by the authors.

"A few of us stayed there the whole time. We thought that victims, wounded people would arrive, but nothing happened. Well, of course the military arrived and searched all of the hospital. When they lifted the curfew every one of us went off to find out what had happened to the rest, to our family, to our friends. To find out who needed help, take care of security cases, transfer people. We kept on doing this all the rest of September and October."

Other professionals, such as psychologists and social workers, heard the news of the coup on the radio in the morning, and many stayed at home. When they returned to their workplaces they found out that they had been dismissed. A psychologist who worked at a psychiatric clinic for children told us:

"On this day, the 11th, I went to the hospital to work like every other day in spite of all we had heard, and when I arrived at the hospital, I saw colleagues whom we considered to be our friends arrive in military clothes. The situation was terribly confused. We sat in a group together and heard Allende's last speech on the radio and we did not know what to do. People did not go home, we did not know whether to go home or to stay, or if this situation meant a complete rupture. In reality we were in a state of terrible shock.

It was strange, but at the same time the people at the hospital who were connected with the military also organized themselves, and our clinic—the psychiatric service of the hospital—was accused of having hidden arms and of having a political function. It was a psychiatric clinic for children! We saw children, nothing more. They accused the people who worked there of being terrorists and communists and of being highly dangerous people.

Before the curfew was imposed, we went home without knowing what would happen to us. This we found out when the curfew was lifted again, because on the lattice entrance gates of the hospital there had been put up lists with names of people. There were an A-list, a B-list, and a C-list. The A-list contained names of employees of the hospital who had the confidence of the new regime. The B-list contained the names of the employees toward whom they were doubtful, and the C-list contained the names of the employees who were terrorists and very dangerous. Well, I was on the C-list. . . . The clinic was closed. This meant that I could not work any longer, and the same happened at the university where I had a teaching post. It also happened to my husband. We had to leave our house for security reasons and live elsewhere. We had a feeling of complete defenselessness. After a month we succeeded in getting away to exile in Europe."

Many were arrested in their homes on the day of the coup. Among those were several doctors and other mental health care professionals. In the following days hundreds of people approached the churches to ask for help. Most of the priests had tried to do everything possible, but the task was so great that their efforts were inadequate. Therefore, they decided to collaborate with each other, and during the first weeks of the coup two committees were established: the National Committee for Refugees (Comité Nacional de Refugiados) and the Committee for Peace (Comité por la Paz).

In the beginning, the primary purpose of the National Committee was to save Latin Americans who lived in Chile and who had supported Allende's government. This meant getting them out of the country. The primary purpose of the Committee for Peace was to help Chileans who, as a consequence of the coup, had ended up in difficult economic or personal situations. Soon both committee began giving legal and social assistance to victims in general. The word of the existence of the committees spread quickly, and an increasing number of people began arriving with their burdens of anxiety and uncertainty. They were looking for their relatives: husbands who had been arrested during the night, sons or daughters who had disappeared.

Everyone thought that this situation would only be transitory. Among the people who worked on the committees were priests, lawyers, and social workers, who thought that each day would be their last day of work. They worked as volunteers, and some of their most important practical tasks were to help look for the people who had disappeared, to identify corpses, and to go to funerals. But perhaps their most important job was to listen and to comfort.

The work continued as the requirements grew, and the lawyers on the committees began to take on the defense of prisoners facing the war tribunals. A social worker said that the best she could do was to give people space to pour out their anxiety. But at the same time, she had the feeling that the situation was a complete horror. It was in every way a new experience for the professionals who worked for the committees. They had to build up a practice relying completely on their own resources in an attempt to confront the realities of the dictatorship.

By mid-1974, hundreds of people had disappeared. In actual fact they were murdered by the regime, but the military never recognized these murders (and still does not). Torture had become common practice, and it was now known that the secret police, the DINA, had places for torture at unknown locations.

At this time, family members of the disappeared people began to organize themselves in groups connected to the Committee for Peace. Both committees represented and were protected by the church, an important institution in Chilean society, but this new organization of family members represented another valued social institution, the family (Orellana, 1989).[3] During the following years, other groups of victims also began organizing themselves according to type of trauma. These groups developed nationwide and became a core element in the struggle for justice in the human rights movement. They had medical, social, and juridical support from professionals, and at the same time these groups offered a new network for support on the emotional level. In the groups people could share their pain and receive empathy from other victims of the same kind of traumas.

During the first months after the coup, people who had been tortured began to be released from the prisons, and there were no institutions to give them medical or psychotherapeutic help. So, soon after their creation, the committees needed help from doctors. Trustworthy people were contacted and asked to take care of emergency cases on a voluntary basis. Among such cases were also psychiatric emergencies. As a female psychiatrist told us:

"There was a group of psychiatrists who had a private clinic. They were members of the now illegal Communist Party and all of them except one had sought asylum in foreign embassies. As I had been dismissed from my job at the hospital, he asked me if I would join the work in his clinic. They began to send patients anonymously to this place, without any record but with a letter of identification from which we knew that they were sent by the Committee. In the beginning they sent family members of prisoners, of people who had disappeared, or of people who had been murdered. At the same time, comrades who had been wounded in confrontations with the military began to come, and they needed medical attention. Later on, people who had been imprisoned began to come, a good percentage with panic reactions. I remember the case of an ex-prisoner who had been almost mutilated, and his panic reaction was so enormous that he wanted to shoot at the first soldier he met so that the military would kill him. So what I did was to get him into an embassy—so the treatment, if we can call it that, the therapy, consisted of getting him into an European embassy. We did this with many cases because we were not able to keep them or treat them. We got them into the embassies, and some returned to their normal life in Chile when they felt better, others left the country to go into asylum."

At the end of 1975 the dictator Pinochet ordered the activities of the Committee for Peace to stop, but its work was carried on, almost immediately, by the Catholic Church under the powerful protection and

[3]Other groups of family members organized themselves later on, for example, "Family Members of the Political Prisoners" (1976) and "Family Members of the Executed" (1978).

auspices of the Archbishop of Santiago. This new, nongovernmental organization was called the Vicarage of Solidarity (Vicaría de la Solidaridad).

The Development of Alternative Mental Health Agencies

In 1975, the National Committee had developed into an organization called the Foundation of Christian Churches for Social Assistance (Fundación de Ayuda Social de las Iglesias Cristianas; FASIC). It was an ecumenical organization and some of its social assistance programs were supported by the United Nations. Perhaps for this reason its activities were not stopped.

As part of their work, the Vicarage formed a medical team that mostly gave emergency help to victims. This team could also refer patients to the private practices of psychiatrists and psychologists who were part of the network that had been built up.

In 1977, FASIC created its own mental health team, the medical psychiatric program, but until then it also referred patients to an external network of clinicians. The professionals working on this FASIC team did outstanding work, formulating the first theories about psychotherapeutic assistance to victims of the repression. One of the leading former members of this team, the psychologist Elizabeth Lira, recalls the emotional state of the team in the years of emergency following its creation:

> Our team was directly threatened many times, and we were only able to think of how we could protect patients and the information about them, but we were not aware of our own risk, and thus we were not able to protect ourselves. This threat generated a deep anguish in therapists that invaded life beyond the therapeutical field. (1992, p. 4)

At a meeting in Santiago in 1980 about "Political Crisis and Psychological Damage," therapists from FASIC presented their now famous paper on "The Testimony of Political Experiences as a Therapeutic Instrument" (Cienfuegos & Monelli, 1983).[4] They had observed that giving testimony in a meaningful context seemed to have a beneficial effect on victims of human rights violations. In these early years, testimony was regarded as an important therapeutic technique. "Testimony provided a link between the political and the psychological, between the public and the private" (Lira, 1992, p. 3).

At the Vicarage, several members of the staff went on trial and some

---

[4]The paper was published in Spanish (1983) and in English (1983). For reasons of security it was published under the pseudonyms "Ana Julia Cienfuegos and Cristina Monelli."

were imprisoned. One of the doctors was imprisoned and tortured, and one social worker was murdered. The government put pressure on the church by accusing the whole staff of being communists, but the prestige of the church was so great that it was possible for the organization to subsist.

Later on, psychologists and psychiatrists also became members of the medical team of the Vicarage, but as their primary focus was on emergency help, people who needed more intensive treatment were referred to FASIC's medical psychiatric program and later also to other nongovernmental organizations, which were now in the process of being formed and which had specialized mental health teams.[5]

The explicit political purpose of all these institutions was to fight for human rights, denounce violations of human rights, and investigate the strategies of the repression and its effects on the victims. For the patients, the clear political position of these institutions helped create the trust that was a necessary condition for the start of a therapeutic process.

THE NATURE OF THE STRESSOR

Under state terrorism the nature of the stressor has some characteristics that differ significantly from stressor events usually associated with post-traumatic stress disorder (PTSD). For this reason, many professionals who work with victims of organized political violence question the suitability of this diagnosis in its present form (Becker, 1992; Lansen, 1992; Simpson, 1993; Summerfield, 1992).

CODEPU (1989), one of the human rights and mental health organizations, divides the stressors into the following four categories: direct repression, indirect repression, social marginalization, and individual marginalization. The final objective of all these instruments of terror is to create fear and disorganization (Lira & Castillo, 1991; Orellana, 1989).

Among the most important instruments of *direct repression* we can list the following nine items in ascending order of severity: (1) violent arrests, (2) forced exile, (3) intimidations, (4) arbitrary imprisonments, (5) torture, (6) the "disappearance" of prisoners, (7) executions, (8) the kil-

---

[5]The Foundation for the Protection of Children Damaged by the State of Emergency (PIDEE) was formed in 1979. The Team for the Denouncement, Investigation, and Treatment of the Tortured and His or Her Family (DITT-CODEPU) was formed in 1984. The Center for the Treatment and Investigation of Stress (CINTRAS) was formed in 1986. The Latin American Institute for Mental Health and Human Rights (ILAS) was formed in 1988. The Collective for Mental Health and Family Therapy of CODEPU was formed in 1990.

ling of opponents under false precepts, and (9) death during torture. Where the immediate aim of the first five instruments is to break the opponent psychologically, the aim of the last four is to eliminate her or him physically (Orellana, 1989).

Among the terror instruments of *indirect repression,* we find deprivation of food, housing, and health care; dismissal from work; distortion of facts; and manipulation of information.

Both direct and indirect repression start a process of marginalization on the social and the individual levels. *Social marginalization* describes the process by which people are deprived of their social and political power. *Individual marginalization* describes the process by which people, as a consequence of the other repressive strategies, experience a loss of skills and knowledge, cultural integrity, and self-esteem (CODEPU, 1989).

As noted by Lira and Castillo (1991) in a recent book released by ILAS, another mental health and human rights organization, these strategies of power result in a pervasive fear throughout society, which is felt on all levels of human relationships. As one female social worker told us:

"We lived in that way for 16 or 17 years with a lot of shock, a lot of fear. All that time, I had fantasies about the death of my husband, always. During that period he was involved in one of the socialist parties. For me, therefore, it was a question of living in a continuous state of suspense. At any moment, something could happen to him, and this got even worse in 1989 when they assassinated one of the other leaders of the party. All this terror, all this panic was a permanent state, but we also—and this we were very sure of—would not avoid doing things because of fear. Neither did I demand that my husband stopped his activities nor did I believe that it was my duty to tell him so.

"One obviously transmits all this fright and insecurity to the kids. Our children were extremely frightened by all this. At that time, we had two, and the oldest was aware of everything we went through, because we transmitted it to him. Personally, I think that I transmitted a lot of insecurity to my oldest son. Only recently, he has begun to feel more safe, more relaxed when he sees armed policemen in the streets. Now he no longer automatically thinks that something will happen to him or his father."

Our own observations in Chilean society made us very aware of the necessity to extend our perspective on traumatization. We saw, and experienced ourselves, how efficiently the repressive strategies have been infiltrated into all of the society. We found that we needed to be much more specific in the analysis of the many different ways traumatization can occur on various levels.

Traumatization can, therefore, be described from different perspectives. One perspective describes the *distance* of the stressor from the "object" (a person, a couple, a family, a group, a society). Another dimension describes the *frequency* of the stressor events. A third dimension describes the *context* in which the stressor events take place.

The distance of the stressor from the object describes how close the object is, physically, psychologically, and/or socially, to the stressor event. In *primary traumatization* the object is the direct target of the stressor, for example, the murdered person, the executed, the disappeared, the tortured, the exiled.

In *secondary traumatization* the stressor event is the primary traumatization of another object: The object is traumatized through the traumatization of another. The secondary traumatized object has a close relationship to the primary traumatized emotionally or socially. Examples would be a husband, close friend, colleague, or political comrade (see Milgram, 1990).

In *tertiary traumatization* the stressor event is the primary or secondary traumatization of others. In tertiary traumatization the object is not directly connected by emotional or social ties to the target object, for example, occasional observers, rescuing professionals, therapists, or neighbors.

This classification into primary, secondary, or tertiary traumatization says little about the *degree* or *severity* of traumatization (apart from direct physical elimination of the object). The impact of the stressor must be balanced against the cultural context and the resources of the object, for example, personality structure, social network, political commitment, and the degree of repression in society in general. As noted by Summerfield (1992):

> There is no easy predicting how an individual orders traumatic experience. I have met survivors of torture in London . . . for whom the impact of these experiences was exceeded by others: the ominous disappearance of a younger brother, witnessing the gruesome death of a close friend or the defeat of political ideals. (p. 2)

Under state terrorism, the frequency of the stressor events is characterized by an enduring, repetitive, and chronic impact of stressors, which take place in a context of power where fundamental human rights are violated in a systematic and deliberate way.

For therapists who live and work in this context of continuous stress, the nature of the stressor dimension can, thus, also be described from the following perspectives: Therapists may become the objects of direct and indirect repression, of social and individual marginalization, and of primary, secondary, and tertiary traumatization.

Personal Characteristics of Patients

Under these circumstances, the therapists have many personal factors in common with their patients, with both of them being possible target objects of the repression, and both being the objects of a whole range of other stressors. People who identify themselves as possible target objects (e.g., leaders of political parties and trade unions, members of leftist parties, human rights workers—including therapists) experience a continuous social and political threat, a stressor that generates "the paradox of chronic fear" (Lira, 1992, p. 2). Fear, which is normally an emotion that arises in order to cope with a specific external or internal threat, becomes a permanent component of everyday personal and social life (Becker, Castillo, Gómez, Kovalskys, & Lira, 1990; Lira & Castillo, 1991).

What, then, were the symptoms presented by the patients during the first years of the dictatorship?

> Fear, confusion, general distress, personal threat of death and harassment were some of the subjective consequences presented by the affected people. That was the reason why psychological help was included very early. Those services were mainly conceived of as a relief under emergency conditions. (Lira, 1992, p. 2)

From the beginning, the stressor events were described as "traumatic political experiences" (Cienfuegos & Monelli, 1983). We see the use of this terminology as an important feature in the Chilean human rights and mental health work. The introduction of this discourse implies that the symptoms of the patient are caused by those in power: they can be explained by factors outside of the person. The patients are not ill; rather, they are suffering from the dictatorship, as one therapist told us.

Lira illustrates this perspective in the following description of her first session with an old man who consulted her in 1986:

> THERAPIST: (. . .) Why have you come? . . . What has happened to you?
> PATIENT: Nothing. I had a little problem. I was arrested 12 or 13 days. I resisted well there . . . but now, every night I dream of the jail. I don't feel like doing anything. . . . I was also taken prisoner in 1974. Afterwards things were catastrophic. A lot of searches. In the nightmares, I go back to the chains, to the tortures. . . . I want to get out of this jail . . . of this enormous fall on the scale of human dignity. . . . (1992, p. 3)

In her comments to this dialogue, Lira underlines the following aspects: The patient associates his suffering and symptoms directly with the repressive experience. Also, the repressive experience appears "to be a threatening, repetitive and neverending situation, in spite of his efforts to minimize it" (p. 3). Lastly, his depressive final comment "could be understood as a metaphor either of his personal situation or that of the Chilean society" (p. 3).

It is, thus, clear from the beginning of the human rights and mental health work that the ideology links personal symptoms of patients to the sociopolitical context. By the understanding of symptoms in this framework, the first step in the therapeutic process has already been taken. It is important to note that Lira confirms the experience of the patient: also she links his symptoms to the repression. One of the important elements in the testimony method was also to confirm reality. The dictatorship continuously denied that human right violations had taken place.

Personal Factors of Therapists

The dictatorship defined the possible target objects as "enemies of the fatherland." This threatening situation produced a "great closeness between helpers and victims" (Lira, 1992, p. 2). In a very polarized political situation this implicitly or explicitly suggested the attitude that "we belong to the same side," Lira adds.

Thus, the situation of the patients was not much different from the situation of the therapists. Those therapists who began giving assistance to the victims of the dictatorship were all committed to this work for ethical, social, or political reasons:

> We all had some level of participation in the government of the Popular Unity [the coalition of political parties that was the basis of Salvador Allende's government] either as sympathizers or as active members of one of the parties of that coalition. This produced a significant concern for the destiny of the victims. (Lira, 1992, p. 4)

As noted in Chapters 1 and 2 of this volume, empathy is based on counteridentification, and it is this process that permits empathy to be therapeutically useful. The political and institutional context we have described could seem to be an obstacle to the process of counteridentification, which implies that the therapist can also view the patient's conflict with objectivity. The political consciousness of the therapists and the link to a human rights movement seem, however, to have been an aid in maintaining only partial identification with the conflict of patients: the connection between the personal and the political levels also protected, to a certain degree, against overinvolvement in the patient.

Some of the therapists we interviewed told us that it had been difficult for them to find anyone to help them with their own traumata. As one male psychiatrist told us:

> "I was in a prison in a small cell together with 12 other prisoners. The treatment was rough, bitter, intimidating . . . the comrades from the cell were taken out to be questioned. They returned with marks from torture, and then they came to me because I was a doctor, and because I was also a psychiatrist they asked me for advice about how to ease the anguish, depression, and panic which they had . . . and I also had my own feelings. I am a man with depressive tendencies and at times I was feeling quite bad. Unfortunately, psychiatrists many times do not have anyone to talk to about their pain. We have to carry our pain ourselves, take care of others."

The fact that therapists and patients belonged to the same side created a sense of trust between them. This "bond of commitment" and of "ethical non-neutrality" (Weinstein et al., 1987) was a necessity under the conditions of state terrorism. A so-called "neutral" position was not possible. The bond of solidarity gave patients the necessary confidence to consult and the ethical commitment permitted "the translation of meanings between the different levels of contexts involved in the patient's suffering" (Lira, 1992, p. 4). There is, thus, both an emotional bond between therapist and patient and a common discourse that allows them to interpret or translate the individual symptoms into the language of a human rights ideology.

The bond of commitment also had some difficulties. Mario Vidal (1990) from CINTRAS mentions the risk of mutual idealization and seduction. In the context of threat in which both patient and therapist lived, it became difficult for the patient to express aggressive feelings toward the therapist who risked so much to help him or her. Likewise, it was difficult for the therapist to allow himself or herself to experience anger toward the patient who had suffered so much. This could imply that forbidden reactions on both sides induce a reverse conspiracy of silence.

It also became difficult to express aggression toward each other in the professional team. According to Lira (1992) and other therapists we interviewed, feelings in the team could vacillate between narcissistic omnipotence and impotence. This pattern perhaps implies a regressive reaction toward the external threat. Therapists could feel isolated with their own pain in the team:

> We, as therapists were subjects and objects of the same situation. We were dealing with the aggression and destruction of the patients. We were affected both by the patients' suffering and by the political threat, because we belonged to the same society. We had ambivalent feelings

which ranged from total omnipotence to total impotence which circulated between us without a real holding, in the sense that Winnicott gave to this concept. One of the characteristics of the team functioning was that personal isolation was hidden under very sensitive and vulnerable collective ties. We had great difficulties tolerating differences and facing conflicts. We also had difficulties with aggressive feelings, as if they were the legacy of the dictatorship inside the group. (Lira, 1992, pp. 4–5)

It is only now, after the emergency situation of the dictatorship had ended, that therapists have allowed themselves to consider their own situations. "We were not able to be conscious of those perceptions and feelings or to go beyond them under military rule" (Lira, 1992, p. 5). Only when a hope of liberation from the dictatorship became more realistic, did therapists get the energy to turn their attention toward their own traumatization. Presently, Chile is in a democratic process, and supervision is now an important resource for the "safe holding"[6] of therapists (Lira, 1992, p. 10).

CONCLUSION

Returning to our initial questions, we will summarize the relevant conclusions concerning factors that determine the nature, quality, and dynamics of CTRs under state terrorism.

How Are Supportive Institutional Settings Developed?

Our fieldwork in Chile pointed out the necessity to find a protective shield for the development of therapeutic settings. In Chile, the church, the family, and the international community acted as such shields, because they were respected—also by those in power—as important elements of society. Moreover, the ideology of a human rights movement was an important factor in linking the different institutions and in connecting their work to the international community.

In the insurgent institutions, the common external enemy seemed to create an intense feeling of solidarity among therapists and toward patients: they were on the same side. At the same time, both the institutions and the individual therapists were continuously threatened and harassed by the regime.

The emergency situation and the until then unknown experience of

[6]A concept developed by Winnicott. See Wilson and Lindy (Chapters 1 and 2, this volume).

state terrorism and its effect on victims made it necessary for therapists to develop new types of theory and practice. This added to the stressors, which were already abundant. It was, however, possible in this context to develop new approaches (e.g., the testimony method).

Apparently, the linkage of the insurgent institutions to a human rights movement also helped to create a supportive, flexible, and collaborative environment for the therapists. This particular setting would naturally attract professionals with a prosocial commitment. This could, however, also facilitate CTRs characterized by overidentification with patients (see Chapter 2, this volume). Professionals with a tendency toward avoidance and detachment responses would probably not run the risk of getting involved in this kind of work.

The opportunities for the institutions to meet the therapists' need for safe holding and nurturing seemed, however, to have been limited. In part, this may have been due to the political situation, but in part it may also have been due to lack of knowledge, indifference, or unawareness of the problem (see Lira, 1992). All energy went to the patients. Looking back at those times, therapists now expressed the wish to have had more peer support and supervision. However, they also stated that their most imperative need, a safe–holding environment, could perhaps never have been fulfilled, given the political situation.

To Which Kinds of Trauma Are Therapists and Patients Exposed?

It appeared that therapists were exposed to the same kinds of trauma as their patients. They were exposed to direct and indirect repression, to social and individual marginalization, and to primary, secondary, and tertiary traumatization. Their work, which helped of the enemies of the regime, was fraught with danger and could bring on traumatization by direct actions from the regime. The work could per se be traumatizing without an adequate safe–holding environment. The work could, however, also be experienced as healing for therapists because of the commitment to a higher goal, the struggle for prosocial change and human rights.

What Are the Characteristics of the Patients?

Under state terrorism the strategies of repression are not only directed toward individuals. All human relationships that threaten the regime are possible objects of aggression. Therefore, the "patient" can be individuals, families, groups, and all of society. On all these levels of society, people can be exposed to "traumatic political experiences." The society is permeated with fear, and therapists in Chile have worked on all these levels of human relationships with individual therapy, family therapy, and group therapy. Especially noteworthy was the organization of survivors into groups according to type of trauma. Therapists also acted as counselors to these groups. On the societal level, therapists attempted, through advocacy and denouncement, to repair the traumatized society.

How Do the Traumatic Experiences of the Therapists Affect Their Relationships with Patients?

The development of the concept of the "committed bond" between therapist and patients seems very significant to us. In this way subjectivity was integrated into political discourse, and countertransference could become a medium for social change, for example, through therapists' prosocial commitment to denouncing human rights violations.

This bond implied a therapeutic stance of "ethical nonneutrality" toward the patient. This attitude followed naturally from the organizational setting of therapy, which was offered in institutions that were in opposition to the government and its human rights violations. Without this commitment, basic trust and empathy could never have been established.

In this context, we must also recognize the problem of the wounded healer. Many therapists said that their work helped them overcome their own trauma. It was especially their political commitment and participation in the human rights movement that had helped them manage their subjective CTRs. The experiences from Chile seem, then, to demonstrate that the problem of the wounded healer cannot be discussed only from the perspective of the intrapsychic dynamics of the therapist. In a context of human rights violations, this problem must also be related to the political context. To be on a survivor's mission in Chile was not only a question of one's own survival but also of the survival of democracy and human dignity.

Some therapists did, however, describe difficult subjective CTRs on both the cognitive and emotional levels. On the cognitive level, they mentioned the risk of overidentification with patients and of becoming overly committed to helping. The context seemed to facilitate an excessive belief in personal responsibility for the therapeutic process. An ideological and clinical disillusionment could develop, enhanced by listening to a continuous stream of trauma stories. This disillusionment could swing toward an omnipotent perception of self as a rescuer. As we have explained above, we also felt a number of these reactions during fieldwork in a traumatized society.

The therapists we interviewed also mentioned the difficulty of handling aggression in the therapeutic relationship. Emotional CTRs of anger toward patients had to be repressed or denied. Likewise, aggressive feelings in the team toward other therapists seemed to have been difficult to manage. How to contain their own aggression and that of the patients seems, then, to be a problem that is difficult to solve in the context of state terrorism.

The need expressed by therapists to have a safe–holding environment in the team should, then, also include a forum where such aggressive feelings could be expressed. The safe holding should, however, also include supervision with special focus on the dynamics of empathic enmeshment. How to accomplish such safe holding in a context of terror is a question for further research in this field, which, regrettably, is becoming increasingly vital.

ACKNOWLEDGMENTS

We would like to extend our gratitude to the Chilean therapists who received us with so much warmth and openness. A special thanks to Elizabeth Lira and Hector Faundéz for keeping us updated on the theoretical reflections that have been a continuously important part of the Chilean human rights movement. We would also like to give our thanks to Karen Fuller of the United States for valuable suggestions and help in the editing of this text.

REFERENCES

Agger, I. (1994). *The blue room: Trauma and testimony among refugee women— psycho-social exploration.* London: Zed Books.

Agger, I., & Jensen, S. B. (1993). The psychosexual trauma of torture. In J. P. Wilson & B. Raphael (Eds.), *The international handbook of traumatic stress syndromes* (pp. 685–702). New York: Plenum Press.

Agger, I., & Jensen, S. B. (1993). *Trauma and healing under state terrorism: Human rights and mental health in Chile during military dictatorship—A case example.* Report to the Council for Developmental Research, the Danish Ministry of Foreign Affairs.

Becker, D. (1992, June). *The deficiency of the PTSD-concept when dealing with victims of human rights violations and other forms of organized violence.* Paper presented at the world conference of the International Society for Traumatic Stress Studies, Amsterdam.

Becker, D., Castillo, M., Gómez, E., Kovalskys, J., & Lira, E. (1990). Therapy with victims of political repression: The challenge of social reparation. *Journal of Social Issues, 46*(3), 133–149.

Catherall, D. R., & Lane, C. (1992). Warrior therapist: Vets treating vets. *Journal of Traumatic Stress, 5,* 19–36.

Cienfuegos, A. J., & Monelli, C. (1983). The testimony of political repression as a therapeutic instrument. *American Journal of Orthopsychiatry, 53,* 43–51.

CODEPU. (1989). The effects of torture and political repression in a sample of Chilean families. *Social Science and Medicine, 28,* 735–740.

Comas-Díaz, L., & Padilla, A. M. (1990). Countertransference in working with victims of political repression. *American Journal of Orthopsychiatry, 60,* 125–134.

Hastrup, K. (1992). *Det antropologiske projekt: om forbløffelse [The anthropological project: About astonishment].* Copenhagen: Gyldendal.

Jung, C. G. (1963/1983). *Memories, dreams, reflections.* London: Flamingo.

Kleinman, A. (1988). *The illness narratives: Suffering, healing, and the human condition.* New York: Basic Books.

Lansen, J. (1992). A critical view of the concept: Post-traumatic stress disorder. In *Health situation of refugees and victims of organized violence.* Rijswijk, the Netherlands: Ministry of Welfare, Health, and Cultural Affairs.

Lira, E. K. (1992). *Developing a therapeutic approach with victims of human rights violations in Chile under different political conditions: Discernment of the therapist involvement.* Unpublished manuscript, Latin American Institute of Mental Health and Human Rights (ILAS).

Lira, E. K., & Castillo, M. (1991). *Psicologia de la amenaza política y del miedo [Psychology of political threat and fear].* Santiago, Chile: CESOC.

Maeder, T. (1989, January). Wounded healers. *Atlantic Monthly,* pp. 37–47.

Milgram, N. A. (1990, October). *Secondary victims of traumatic stress: Their plight and public policy.* Paper presented at the annual meeting of the International Society for Traumatic Stress Studies, New Orleans, LA.

Orellana, P. (1989). *Violaciones a los derechos humanos e información: La experiencia chilena [Violations of human rights and information: The Chilean experience].* Santiago, Chile: FASIC.

Simpson, M. (1993). Traumatic stress and bruising of the soul: The effects of torture and coercive interrogation. In J. P. Wilson & B. Raphael (Eds.), *The international handbook of traumatic stress syndromes* (pp. 667–684). New York: Plenum Press.

Summerfield, D. (1992, June). *Charting human response to extreme violence and the limitations of Western psychiatric models: An overview.* Paper presented at the world conference of the International Society for Traumatic Stress Studies, Amsterdam.

Vidal, M. (1990, December). Daño psicológico y represión política: Un modelo de atención integral [Psychological damage and political repression: An intergrative model of treatment]. *Reflexión,* pp. 10–14.

Weinstein, E., Lira, E. K., Rojas, M. E., Becker, D., Castillo, M. I., Maggi, A., Gómez, E., Dominguez, R., Salamovich, S., Pollarolo, F., Neumann, E., & Monreal, A. (1987). *Trauma, duelo y reparación [Trauma, mourning and reparation].* Santiago, Chile: FASIC/Interamericana.

11

Countertransference in the Treatment of War Veterans

MICHAEL J. MAXWELL
CYNTHIA STURM

This chapter discusses countertransference in the treatment of war veterans with post-traumatic stress disorder (PTSD) and the impact of countertransference on technical dilemmas facing the therapist. These reactions grow out of trauma-specific transference themes which become activated in treatment as they were both in war and post-war at homecoming. These transference themes include anticipated betrayal, loss, fear, guilt, affect overload, rage, abusive violence, rejection, hopelessness, despair, and the search for meaning. Each theme, as it is enacted within therapy, may elicit one or more trauma-specific countertransference identifications in the therapist, such as omnipotent buddy, faulty policy-setter, judge, failed protector, commanding officer, murderous aggressor, intimidated or abused victim, rescuer, lover/prostitute or nurturing comforter, neutral or tainted authority figure, or a symbolic enemy.

The technical dilemmas facing the trauma therapist include:

1. Creating a therapeutic space safe enough to allow the veteran to tell his or her story without avoiding, endangering, judging, or rejecting either the veteran or the story;
2. Establishing a working alliance and promoting working through without violating boundaries, encouraging acting out, or losing control of the pace, depth, or affect modulation of treatment; and
3. Facilitating work on the validation, spirituality, and meaning of

the trauma experiences without causing the veteran to feel rejected, intimidated, prematurely reassured, or filled with shame or despair.

Different countertransference reactions (CTRs) arise at different stages in the recovery process (Newberry, 1985). They are influenced by the clinician's setting, such as a hospital inpatient unit, outpatient treatment, a veterans outreach center, or private practice setting, and the clinician's professional responsibilities, such as triage, history taking, leading a group, or individual therapy.

This chapter represents an outgrowth of our collective clinical experience with veterans of World War II, Korea, Vietnam and the Persian Gulf, treated in U.S. Department of Veterans Affairs (VA) Medical Center, Veteran Readjustment Centers (VA Counseling or "Vet" Centers), and private practice settings. As a Vietnam veteran, male therapist and a nonveteran, female therapist we have cofacilitated PTSD groups in the VA and have also conducted individual treatment with male and female veterans in VA and private settings since 1977. As such, the ideas in this chapter reflect a partial understanding of conflicts in war veterans.

McCann and Pearlman (1990) use the term *vicarious traumatization* to describe the potential negative psychological impact on the therapist of prolonged exposure to traumatic client material. If not identified, CTRs may exert a deleterious effect on the therapist and can increase therapist vulnerability to burnout and exhaustion. Constructivist self-development theory (McCann & Pearlman, 1990) assists therapists to identify their own salient psychological needs and cognitive schemas that are vulnerable to disruption by CTRs. McCann and Pearlman's framework is one attempt to normalize the experience of CTRs for the therapist.

The concepts of countertransference and trauma-specific transferences have been discussed in Part I of this book. For us, however, the concept of *projective identification* (Klein, 1946), and how the therapist is affected by it, is a key element in understanding countertransferences (Bion, 1959). According to this concept the patient disallows conscious awareness of intolerable affects, which are powerful reactive affects and often nonverbal. These emotions, in turn, may be projected into the therapist's experience of the therapy. Indeed, among war veterans there may be a subtle pressure on the therapist to identify with the intolerable affects being experienced by the client, such as feeling helpless, or to take action rather than find ways to examine these affects. The therapist must understand the patient's projected conflicts and experience, and must attempt to contain and "detoxify" them in a tolerable manner. A primary objective of post-traumatic therapy is to assist in the process of integrating avoided memories and distressing emotions.

We will begin with some background on the trauma experiences of Vietnam veterans, the largest veteran population studied to date, and then discuss CTRs and technical dilemmas characteristic of each stage in the recovery process.

CHARACTERISTICS OF PTSD IN VETERAN POPULATIONS

War veterans as a clinical population present several unique issues (Wilson, 1988). Veterans displaying the symptoms of PTSD typically manifest periods of extreme anxiety, fear, depression and suicidality, anger and rage, sleep disturbances and nightmares, intrusive imagery, and reliving, all of which alternate with numbing, denial, detachment, and possible dissociative reactions (Catherall, 1986; Haley, 1974).

The traumatic characteristics of the combat experience are multifaceted, unlike those of a single-event trauma. The veteran's ongoing exposure to combat and death and dying, and his or her developmental age at time of service, are some of the key factors in evaluating the degree of impact on adaptive functioning (Harel, Kahana, & Wilson, 1993; Wilson, 1978, 1988, 1989).

Therapists treating veterans with PTSD should expect to encounter overcontrolled emotions, rage, numbing, survivor guilt, and anniversary reactions in their patients. Haley (1978, p. 266) describes the "shame, doubt, guilt, fear of violent impulses and reparation/atonement" that are especially associated with participating in or exposure to atrocities in the theater of war. The circumstances of combat and war create moral dilemmas and spiritual crises that often go unaddressed in traditional therapies.

Areas of interpersonal conflict commonly associated with PTSD stem from central problems with trust and loss, a combination resulting in overall personality constriction and social withdrawal. Unresolved grief and loss issues appear almost uniformly in veterans, often enmeshed with complex issues of moral guilt and survivor guilt. Passivity may also be seen as a defense against issues of aggression and assertion (Haley, 1974). Underlying feelings of helplessness and inadequacy, alienation, and avoidance of affect can generate problems with intimacy, marriage, and child-rearing (Goodwin, 1980; Haley, 1978). Difficulties maintaining close relationships, social isolation and withdrawal, and distrust and resentment of authority are also common interpersonal themes. Pervasive alienation is common among Vietnam veterans (Opp & Samson, 1989) because of their difficulties with reentry into American society after the war (Wilson, 1988).

Chronic ego-defensive patterns in PTSD patients may also have begun to "sculpt" their character. Common problems with social adjustment include divorce, chronic economic stress, unemployment, and legal problems related to aggressive acting out (Wilson & Zigelbaum, 1986). These personal difficulties can further contribute to low self-esteem and the veteran's sense of unworthiness.

Prior to recognition by the mental health community, PTSD was frequently ignored, minimized or simply misdiagnosed in the VA system and other mental health settings. As a result of institutional, cultural, and interpersonal barriers, most Vietnam veterans with post-traumatic adjustment difficulties, for example, did not identify or seek help for these problems until many years or decades post-service. In our experience, it is not unusual for combat veterans to be seen initially by a mental health professional several decades after the original trauma. This delay in seeking treatment often means that psychological problems have become entrenched patterns that have affected most or all domains of the veteran's adult adjustment.

Diagnostic comorbidity is a frequent occurrence in veteran PTSD populations (Wilson, 1988). The therapist may observe PTSD symptomatology along with major depression, anxiety disorders, somatization disorders, and/or substance abuse. Chronic substance abuse problems have been reported in as high as 91% of veterans with PTSD (Boudewyns, Woods, Hyer, & Albrecht, 1991). For these and other reasons, PTSD treatment with combat veterans presents unique challenges for the clinician.

Despite the commonalities to be found among veterans, their therapists must appreciate the unique traumatic experiences of each client. Moreover, although this population is largely male, it is important to acknowledge and actively seek out the female veteran (e.g., Vietnam medical nurses, Red Cross personnel, and Persian Gulf soldiers), who may be even more reticent to seek treatment than their male counterparts, partly because such services were designed primarily for male ex-service personnel.

COUNTERTRANSFERENCE BLOCKS TO TRIAGE WORK

In order to manage the care of veterans with PTSD the clinician must first recognize PTSD as a legitimate entity. Similarly, the veteran must recognize the clinician as sufficiently knowledgeable about trauma to be of help in the trauma recovery. Management issues arise throughout the course of recovery as various triage points are confronted. These involve (1) gaining enough history to make the diagnosis, (2) attending to comorbid diagnoses, (3) referral for limited inpatient care during periods of heightened symptoms, (4) judicious use of medication, and (5) ongoing outpatient work. At moments of triage, a variety of themes may be activated that originate in the veteran's war and homecoming experience, such as fearing orders to a new and dangerous situation and anticipating rejection.

Because of veterans' anxieties about triage decisions, therapists can be pushed into complementary countertransference positions, such as compliant "cogs" in an insensitive military machine, or disbelieving members of the homefront. Succumbing to these CTR roles not only impairs triage and makes sound management decisions more difficult, but risks traumatic reenactment of a negative or invalidating homecoming.

Diagnosing at a Veteran Readjustment Counseling Center

Some therapists do not hear about traumatic events during the initial phase and mistakenly rule out PTSD as a diagnosis. As an example, James, a combat veteran counselor, mistakenly ruled out a PTSD diagnosis in a war veteran client despite his anxiety, numbness, and disturbed sleep. Fred, a client at the Vet Center, reported he performed supply duty while stationed in Vietnam and did not volunteer a history of traumatic events. Later, after one of us (MJM) worked with him for several weeks, his trust grew sufficiently so that he shared numerous traumatic situations: His convoy was attacked; friends were killed; others wounded; his codriver was killed by sniper fire. Moreover, his highly explosive fuel truck had been a favorite target for the enemy. James assumed that "supply" meant relatively safe work in a basecamp. He misunderstood Fred's communication. Because Fred was not ready to talk about his war traumas, James believed that he had none. Seeing Fred as nontraumatized reinforced James's countertransference biases about who was and who was not endangered in combat. A variant to the above case is when the therapist labels the veteran's story as PTSD prematurely, failing to appreciate the unique individuality of the patient's trauma experiences.

Diagnostic Considerations at a Substance Abuse Unit

Clinicians in dual diagnostic settings sometimes deny the meaningful presence of PTSD in an effort to focus on other problems. For example, Jerry, a combat veteran with PTSD and intermittent alcohol abuse, described to us his experience in a drug dependency unit. On the fourth day of the hospitalization at a group meeting, responding to the theme of confronting fears, Jerry remembered with clarity his original trauma, the anniversary of which he had been trying to drown in alcohol. He had been pinned down in crossfire; others in his unit were dead; he realized that truly there would be no escape; then he heard the sound of artillery. For 8 hours he remained fixed in his position, most of it in darkness. It was the actual return of the memory of this darkness, the isolation, and the scene of impending death that had been so terrifying. As he tried to share this memory, however, the group leader interrupted, "The group needs to focus on feelings, but not war stories." A group member added, "We're tired of war stories; they exclude us [the noncombat veterans]." Toward the end of the session the group leader said that Jerry would need to be "clean and sober" for a while longer before they would be ready to deal with his Vietnam experiences. In the meantime he would need to proceed with his 12-step Alcoholics Anonymous recovery program. Following the regimen outlined, Jerry attended to his abstinent behavior and a week later once more engaged staff regarding his PTSD. They then explained that they were not trained to treat PTSD and referred him elsewhere. The staff on this dual diagnosis unit were unwittingly participating in a Type I (denial, minimization) countertransference by isolating PTSD and splitting off its meaning from a potential recovery setting.

When these avoidant responses are manifest, patients may retreat or feel that there really is no place to go for treatment. Therapist avoidance may confirm clients' secret fears that their feelings are uncontainable or unacceptable. If they feel denigrated, veterans may respond with anger and disbelief that the therapist refuses to listen to their trauma experience. They may say, for example, "They told me to talk about my feelings but they wouldn't listen when I talked about Vietnam." We have observed that some therapists recovering from substance abuse themselves have isolated feelings without resolving their own war trauma issues.

Hospitalizing Patients as a Private Practitioner

In a private practice, outpatient setting the therapist is often isolated from a team-based PTSD treatment model. Managing the limits of outpatient treatment, and knowing when to hospitalize the veteran for more intensive PTSD work, how to contain suicidal or homicidal dangers, or when to refer for substance abuse treatment, is critical to providing good outpatient care. Countertransference may play a complicating role. Veterans who are fearful or resistant to treatment in the VA setting or inpatient treatment unit can create a double bind for therapists, insisting that therapists overextend their limits by containing dangerous behavior in less restrictive settings. A powerful countertransference may develop in which the therapist and veteran are surviving together in the bush like war buddies, and isolated from the VA (military establishment) (a Type II

CTR, enmeshment). The therapist caught in this omnipotent and suspicious countertransference could fail to make appropriate referrals for hospitalization. He or she may be tempted to not set sufficient limits around threats of violence to self or others, or to collude with the client to avoid substance abuse treatment.

Disclosing Professional Experience with Trauma to War Veterans

In order for the veteran to comply with a therapeutic management recommendation, he or she must be confident enough in the clinician's trauma credentials. Here the Type I "blank screen" CTR is potentially harmful to the process. The clinician's disclosing information about qualifications may include familiarity with the combat situation and its psychological aftermath. We believe that at this phase, what in another context may be called countertransference disclosure, is the appropriate disclosure of trauma credentials.

Nonveteran therapists, fearing they may be cast in the role of war dissenters, may feel uneasy about being direct by saying that although they did not serve in Vietnam, they have learned much about the war and are familiar with some of its aftermath.

Exclusive preoccupation with trauma on the other hand, may represent a Type II countertransference (see Chapter 2, this volume). We have seen many cases in which the therapist will take a patient and focus on the central trauma issues that the veteran brings up in the first few sessions while ignoring other needs that are reality based in their lives (e.g., homelessness, unemployment)

COUNTERTRANSFERENCE BLOCKS TO ESTABLISHING THE THERAPEUTIC RELATIONSHIP

In the initial phase of psychotherapy, the therapist tries to create a safe–holding environment, an atmosphere of trust, and an encouraging attitude toward disclosing the trauma story. Engaging the veteran in the therapeutic relationship must occur prior to uncovering the traumatic memories. Influenced profoundly by their war experiences, veterans may approach this phase with distrust of government institutions, fears of being betrayed by authority, and fears of being rejected for what they had to do to survive in a tactical war of horror. Therapists, therefore, finding themselves in countertransference roles such as aggressor, rejecting peer, hostile judge and failed protector, may have difficulty establishing the therapeutic relationship.

The development of the therapeutic alliance, which Shapiro (1984) defines as "the relatively non-conflictual rational aspects of the relationship between therapist and patient" (p. 87), pivots on the success or failure of the empathic process (see Chapters 1 and 2, this volume). In her work with Vietnam veterans, Haley (1978) notes that the therapeutic alliance enables the veteran to "tolerate remembering, re-experiencing, understanding and working through stressful experiences" (p. 264). Reactive processes characterized by avoidance and detachment often result in failure to establish an empathic stance and are predictive of premature termination in veteran populations.

In establishing the working alliance, it is important for the therapist to convey a sense of trustworthiness and understanding to the veteran and to adopt an open, interactional style of relating. Therapists who hide behind a silent, unemotional blank screen are actually withdrawing from the veteran's pain in a countertransference caricature of professional rigidity. Intentional ambiguity in the therapist's stance will increase anxiety, suspicion, and fears of disapproval. Combat veterans, in particular, will often see this style of interaction as being judgmental, condescending, shaming, or rejecting: "If the therapist is just sitting there thinking and not saying anything to me, he must be thinking I am crazy or what I did was wrong." At the start of treatment, the client needs education and reassurance that signs and symptoms of PTSD are expectable and that PTSD is a normal reaction to traumatic combat experiences.

One of the many psychological effects of the war is the disruption of the soldier's ability to trust others. Shapiro (1984) has identified some of the common transferential themes in therapy with Vietnam veterans, which include distrust of authority, tendency to withdraw from close relationships, and expectation of rejection in interpersonal situations.

In order for veterans to open up about their trauma, they must feel that they will be safe, trusted, believed, supported, and understood without moral judgments. Moreover, veteran clients are typically hypervigilant to overt physical or emotional reactivity in the therapist (e.g., tension, anxiety, irritability, disgust) as well as changes in the therapist's behavior (e.g., loss of role stance, detachment, hostility).

They will respond sharply to these fears according to their own dynamics and trauma history. Detachment reactions protect the therapist from evoking his or her own trauma anxiety, and they minimize the client's affect. Such coping by avoidance (Type I CTR) may reinforce similar avoidance mechanisms in the veteran, nonverbally confirming that revealing traumatic material, even when ready to do so, is "dangerous" or "intolerable," as the veteran feared.

The VA hospital setting can activate strong *institutional transference reactions* (see Chapter 1, this volume), most likely engendering negative or ambivalent feelings. The veteran may identify the government health care system with the military and feel that the hospital system is responsible for his or her PTSD, lack of adequate prior treatment programs, and poor quality care. In this view, the therapist and the hospital setting become complex authority figures, holding both the power to validate the veteran's experience and heal the wounds of war, and the power to deny or minimize the veteran's compensation status; and therapists can be vulnerable to complementary *institutional countertransference* (Gendel & Reiser, 1981). In some ways, the VA hospital is, in fact, like the military. It is an unwieldy bureaucracy, and its clinicians are cogs in the wheel of its inefficiency. In the transference process, the therapist may be viewed as either an extension of the VA system or an ally of the veteran in opposition to that system.

Community mental health centers and private practice settings also present some CTR issues for the clinician that differ from those arising in the VA setting. Private settings may allow for a more personalized approach to the veteran and may help create the safe environment that is often free from institutional transference reaction and is central to treatment. But it may also foster a form of Type II enmeshment, or over-identification reaction.

GENDER ISSUES IN ESTABLISHING A THERAPEUTIC RELATIONSHIP

The gender of the therapist may play a role in inhibiting the male veteran's disclosure of his trauma story. Overly cautious countertransference behaviors may imply the frightened mother or sister who should be spared grotesque trauma (Type I), while overly involved responses may suggest the lover/prostitute or military nurse who knows only too well the veteran's fear, guilt, and vulnerability (Type II).

In terms of transference–countertransference, we have identified some issues specific to gender. With a female therapist, for example, male veterans may be extremely demanding and judgmental, overly seductive or protective, or unnecessarily apologetic for swearing or using sexual language until they know the therapist well. They may be reluctant to reveal either the "killer" or "victim" self, fearing that the "killer" will frighten or disgust the therapist or that the "victim" will elicit the therapist's pity or disgust. Male veterans may also make stereotyped assumptions about females. Moreover, females in "authority" roles pose an interesting dilemma. Clients may intimidate and devalue the competence of, a female therapist, leading her to experience doubt and uncertainty. When patients do view a female therapist as "human," capable of errors and heroics, sometimes different from and other times the same as a man who is returning from the threat of war, this can lead to dissolving unnecessary boundaries that further isolate the veteran from social support, important relationships (Matsakis, 1988), and from himself.

One particularly critical and often ignored, area of countertransference, is sexual attraction and sexualization of the therapeutic relationship (Pope & Bouhoutsos, 1986). The male veteran may relate to the female therapist in sexualized ways, or seek to have a special relationship with her. Because the female nurse in Vietnam was seen as the embodiment of mother, sister, and lover, the female therapist may encounter a strong transference reaction to her as nurturer—the maternal archetype. The male veteran may resist seeing the female therapist as an expert or one with whom he can develop a strong therapeutic alliance. We believe that it is critical for the female therapist to address both negative and positive aspects of gender-based transference patterns, so that she fully understands her own sexual countertransference feelings and is able to find therapeutic ways to discuss issues of self-esteem with the veteran.

The example of one Filipino nurse who encountered these issues illustrates how they can be used in therapy. This woman had become frustrated at a curious combination of reactions combat veterans were having to her. On the one hand, they defiantly said she could not possibly understand their experiences, yet, on the other, they were both boyish and intimate in their manner. She found herself professionally frustrated while personally drawn to them. The unusual combination of affect was striking. Another response of feeling sexually insulted as an Asian woman was pronounced. Was it a complementary countertransference of a Vietnam-based experience? With the help of supervision, she wondered if these veterans were not having an Asian lover/prostitute transference to her. Using this insight, she now responded to her veteran patients, "I think maybe you remember someone from Vietnam who looked a little like me." In response, their walls of defiance broke down and the veterans shared some enormously poignant and painful memories of moments with Vietnamese women who dared to be close with them when war stress had rendered them frightened or numb.

Both male and female therapists must be sensitive to female veterans who may have lived nontraditional roles upon returning home from the war and may also have concerns that affect the treatment relationship. They may feel they were discounted in military service, intimidated, harassed, or even raped. These female veterans fear their special circumstances will not be appreciated or validated.

Issues of treatment specific to gender may include processing of sexual acting out or of episodes of sexual violence against the enemy. These issues need to be addressed with care regarding gender-based transferential issues. For example, the veteran may be reluctant to reveal abusive, violent, sexual experiences of wartime in front of a female therapist out of a fear of judgment or out of a concern that the therapist would not be able to listen. Contemporary problems with sexuality and relationships must be open topics for psychotherapy, not to be avoided by either male or female therapists.

THE ROLE OF COUNTERTRANSFERENCE IN UNCOVERING VERSUS CONTAINING THE TRAUMA STORY

As the process of disclosure proceeds, the therapist faces numerous dilemmas regarding when to *uncover* further and when to *contain* the veteran's labile affect. These tasks include managing acting out, rage, and suicidal ideas, and setting appropriate/necessary limits within the treatment context.

Again, there are specific war stressors (such as exposure to or participation in abusive violence, grotesque images from war, moments of overwhelming fright and sudden loss) that produced this affect overload originally. Potential countertransference identifications (such as the frightened comrade, the counterphobic lieutenant, the intimidated war victim, the attacking enemy) are aroused in the therapist and make this difficult task even more troublesome and demanding.

Because the PTSD client often oscillates between periods of numbing and periods of being overwhelmed with the intrusive recollections, the therapist needs the capacity to shift position in a flexible way to ensure appropriate pacing for the client. Due to the rapid shifts in intensity of emotional material, it is a therapeutic challenge to balance "staying with" the client and, at the same time, keeping "one step ahead" as a therapeutic guide and modulator.

Horowitz (1986) provides a useful outline of therapist options in the various phases of trauma treatment. From a countertransference perspective, the potential errors at the outset of psychotherapy are the tendencies for the therapist to play out the other side of the client's "shift" by assuming an overcontrolled or undercontrolled stance (i.e., problems of affect modulation). *Unwitting collusion* with the client's avoidance as a form of countertransference can be a powerful nonverbal communication that the material is not tolerable, as the client fears. Conversely, if the therapist adopts a stance that pushes the client too quickly, the client can be retraumatized and feel unable to tolerate affect appropriately, intensifying PTSD and associated symptoms. One may be pulled by the competitive needs of the veteran to speed up treatment, or one may risk evincing shame and self-loathing if the slower pacing appropriate to realistic clinical needs make the veteran feel inadequate, cowardly, or hopeless.

The patient who is undercontrolled in responding to trauma issues and tends to act out against self or others may lead the therapist to adopt a Type I overcontrolled treatment style. If the therapist avoids focusing on traumatic memories that are unsettling out of fear of being unable to contain the patient's affect, treatment may become unnecessarily extended.

Problems in Facilitating Disclosure

In the early stages of treatment, it is common for war veterans to recite traumatic events with "flat" affect. This may reflect their ability to detach or numb their feelings, or it may be a means of testing the therapist's reaction to their trauma story. The therapist who is uncomfortable with unresponsive clients may feel it necessary to "push" the client in order to break through the detachment. Yet what is obvious to the therapist—that detachment masks feelings—may not be within the client's awareness because of the enormity of the painful affect. In fact, telling patients that they feel something that they actively repress may arise out of CTRs. In order to demonstrate the appropriate feeling response, the therapist, for example, may tell a patient he is grieving about witnessing the death of his buddy, but the level of denial and the role it serves in protecting the self must also be assessed clinically. Therapists must recognize that the veteran's unemotional response is not necessarily an unwillingness to deal with pain. It may be that this veteran does not feel safe or that he fears he will be unable to contain or control his feelings. Affective reactions may also mask deeper conflicts about guilt and responsibility.

In the early stages of treatment, the therapist may counterphobically project his or her vulnerability onto veterans by trying to get them to express their emotions before they feel safe or trust the therapist. Furthermore, therapists, fearing their own trauma, may counterphobically intrude or excessively uncover trauma material too early in the treatment process. Because either response impedes adaptive functioning and change, this can overwhelm the client's capacity to cope, impair the development of a sense of interpersonal trust, engender regression, reenact or reinforce the traumatic experience, and risk premature withdrawal from treatment. It is also possible that the therapist's own trauma wound may force him or her to halt a trauma story just as it is unfolding.

For example, Jack, a Vietnam veteran, urgently reported to his therapist that he woke up in the night sweating, with a nightmare: "I see my buddy screaming and the V.C. [Viet Cong] cutting off his head. Isn't there anything you can do?" Feeling overwhelmed and struggling to contain his own war images of grotesquely truncated limbs and genitals, the therapist could barely tolerate his own memories. Pressured to discharge his own unmanageable affect, his therapist said, "I've been through pretty grotesque things there too." In this case, the counselors' discharge of his affective response stopped the client's emerging story just as it was beginning. Two wounded veterans could not at that moment maintain the momentum of the treatment. Both needed time to withdraw.

Problems in Containing Rage

In treating aggressive and angry veterans, a therapist can project onto the veterans feelings of fear, anger, aggression, and rage, leading to a rupture of empathy. Here the therapist's projections are a Type I CTR and are disruptive of treatment, as the following examples illustrate.

A veteran came into a session explosively angry, threatening violence against the VA. The benefits he had been receiving had been declared "a mistake" and the VA was now billing the client for monies he needed for daily living. On the one hand, the therapist realized that mistakes in all bureaucracies do occur. On the other hand, he recognized a tendency to overidentify with his client's sense of betrayal and rage; when mistakes had occurred in Vietnam, they had had devastating results for his client. The question this therapist must ask himself is how devastating this will be for his client in the present.

When dealing with aggressive and angry veterans, there may be a tendency for staff to fall into an intermediate CTR position with a patient whose rage reactions they may not be able to control. For example, Larry, because of prior anger outbursts, was given preferential treatment by staff on the inpatient unit. Larry's outbursts reenacted his holding an advancing enemy squad at bay after his fellow squad members were killed. In the transference projection the staff was like the Vietnamese forces whom he helped stop. But this enmeshed clinical situation kept Larry's progress at a standstill. Larry could not move beyond his trauma until staff could feel less intimidated. In the private practice setting, the therapist must manage fearful CTRs aroused during periods in which anger or reactivity of the veteran are heightened, such as anniversary dates, by planning for the possibility of short-term inpatient treatment.

Problems in Managing Suicidal Ideas

Issues of control in the veteran and the therapist are highlighted when there is a threat of danger to self or others. In severe PTSD, chronic suicidal ideation is not uncommon and requires ongoing assessment. In settings where therapists regularly work with veterans, desensitization may lull the therapists into forms of denial. On the other hand, therapists unfamiliar with chronic suicidality may overreact to the veterans' fears of loss of control.

In our experience, veterans with chronic PTSD will openly discuss suicidal ideation as a means of conveying their frustration with their inability to make changes in their lives. At times, therapists operating from a rescuing countertransference position may have a tendency to protect the patient, or, operating from a despairing, "fellow victim" countertransference, they may feel that they are not able to treat a suicidal patient. It is important for the therapist not to "scare" the client by overreacting (Type II CTRs) to the threat or concern that has been expressed. This is not say that the therapist should take lightly the threat of suicide (Bongar, 1991), but in the case of a client with chronic PTSD the therapist should respond with a degree of caution and explore the lethality of the client's thoughts. The client may be expressing frustration with the situation and using the talk of suicide as a means of freeing himself or herself from the confines of trauma-related psychopathology. In clients with chronic PTSD, the years of avoidance, numbing, and suppression of feelings typically leave them feeling hopeless and helpless. Suicidal ideation may be an expression of undermodulated affect or a wish to join a buddy, or even the enemy, in death.

Combining the problems of uncovering versus containing and managing suicidal ideas, one patient said, "Doc, if you tell me I did those things in my dreams, I'll have no choice but to execute myself." The therapist heard his patient's fear of further uncovering, yet also heard the extraordinary pain of the young man caught in a war filled with horror. The therapist's nonverbal communication did much to contain the affect simply by empathizing with the veteran's pain and efforts to control the idea of suicide. The veteran scrutinized the therapist less for an answer and more to see if he could contain the pain. Carpy (1989) argues that the ability of the client to see the therapist being affected by the client's emotion and adequately containing it validates the reality of the traumatized state of the veteran and assists the integration process of warded-off material.

COUNTERTRANSFERENCE AND THE MANAGEMENT OF ROLE BOUNDARIES

Just as affect is often at the breaking point in these therapies, and requires careful dosing and pacing, so boundaries such as the time and space of the treatment seem insufficient to contain the trauma. Often the therapist must decide what to do when one of the boundaries is being stretched.

Contributing to the picture are, of course, the war traumas themselves, such as extra efforts that saved or might have saved a comrade's life, wishes to see and fears of seeing a comrade after a dangerous mission. The therapist here is sometimes cast in the role of failed protector or wished-for rescuer; the therapist who succumbs to this countertransference pressure loses some of the objectivity needed to keep the treatment from spinning in a phase of enmeshment that interferes with growth and autonomy.

One of the difficult tasks of managing the working alliance is to confront the veteran with the limits or boundaries defining the outpatient therapist's role. In particular, Vietnam veterans, continuing to view life and therapy with the urgency of a combat zone, find themselves in apparently life-endangering situations, expecting "heroic" actions from themselves and the therapist. In wartime, any failure to act could cost a life, and current behavior is still measured against such high standards. For example, veterans in one therapy group decided to meet between group sessions, willingly sacrificing their time for a buddy in trouble, and they put pressure on the therapist to attend this extra group meeting to help one member work through a difficult traumatic memory. They attacked the leader for failing to rescue the veteran, for hiding behind his (officer) role and keeping his hands clean. They evoked guilt and the impulse to overextend. Aware of this tendency, the leader said, "We all have those in Nam we wanted to save. We'll get back to this next time."

Another veteran waited until the end of a meeting to disclose an important trauma story. "I was with 'Sarge' the one I didn't get along with. Well, we were on patrol . . . and he and I were talking about whether or not we should go into the village. Well, this sniper shot him in the head, . . . he was standing right next to me." The therapist feared his ending the session at the designated time would be like the sergeant getting shot. It would leave his client and the group leaderless with tough decisions ahead. Further, there was the veiled threat, through metaphor, that someone (a sniper) would blow his (the sergeant's) head off if he stopped on time. The therapist wanted to hear more and also felt intimidated in the countertransference. The therapist, using his countertransference understanding, responded, "That sounds like an important memory: not liking someone, losing him suddenly and being on your own. I'll be here at our next regular time; let's continue it then." In a situation like this one, it is important both to set the limit, yet assess clinically the client's ability to manage the emotional material during the week. Therapeutic issues around limit setting with war veterans revolve around testing the therapy relationship in regard to the therapist's genuineness, affective availability during working through, and ability to contain and not be overwhelmed by the traumatic material.

COUNTERTRANSFERENCE REAPPRAISAL
AND RECONSTRUCTION

Special dilemmas confront the therapist in the latter stages of trauma therapy. The clinical challenges involve validating the war experience, striving for the remembered rather than the forgotten warrior; the search for personal meaning, including atoning for guilt and shame; and integrating the war experience into a more hopeful future. Among the technical dilemmas in which countertransference feelings play important roles are assessing blame and guilt, assessing the impact and value of compensation, and setting a termination date. Again, countertransference identification as judge, treasurer, or priest distort the therapist's empathy.

Working through war-related trauma recovery frequently requires an examination of issues of accountability, blame, and guilt (Williams, 1988). Opp and Samson (1989) have identified "profound guilt" as a particular concomitant of PTSD in combat veterans, developing a taxonomy of five types of guilt seen in the clinical setting; survivor guilt, demonic guilt, moral/spiritual guilt, betrayal/abandonment guilt, and superman/superwoman guilt.

The countertransference can mirror the guilt of the veteran. Issues for the therapist may relate to his or her own survivor guilt, (e.g., of having survived Vietnam), not being a combat veteran, as well as having presumably been successful in being educated and employed. Feelings of inadequacy and shame on the part of the veteran may engender guilt for the therapist and be associated with thoughts about his or her own sense of deservingness. Opp and Samson (1989) raise the issues that the veteran's internal sense of failure, unworthiness, and fear of success may perpetuate survival guilt. The client's tendency to self-sabotage may pull the therapist to reactions of rescue or detachment.

Self-blame is also seen in relation to specific combat incidents. Scurfield (1985) has discussed the "defensive way" in which blame can be cognitively attributed internally or externally in order to avoid painful affect. One population noted to have a particularly strong internalizing tendency is medical personnel who served in Vietnam. Our clinical observation is that self-blame and remonstration allow the veteran to avoid feelings of helplessness and futility in the face of overwhelming casualties. A common CTR is to attempt to reassure veterans prematurely that they have "done all they can" rather than to tolerate the ambiguity of such situations.

Therapists who are compelled in a countertransference mode of enmeshment, for example, to rescue clients out of their own guilt, risk fostering dependency rather than adaptive personal growth and maturation. For example, Sam, a Vietnam veteran client, was reenacting elements in the disarray of American fall-back positions during the period before the end of the war. Now he moved from place to place in the city in his truck and got into hassles with local residents as he "set up camp." The counselor, trying to save Sam to compensate for having failed to save buddies in his own Vietnam unit, found himself following Sam in his own vehicle to keep him out of scrapes. Increased dependency without insight, change, or growth followed.

Concerns about benefits and disability are often difficult to separate cleanly from the therapy process, especially with Vietnam veterans who failed to receive societal recognition for their sacrifices. Clearly, the delicate balance between genuine validation of affect versus fostering regressive entitlement is also a sensitive issue. This issue is highlighted as the clinician is asked to play a role in the veteran's work life and income status.

A therapist may fail to recognize and validate the importance of advocacy out of fear of engagement and can rationalize this on grounds of neutrality. This can lead to a sense of betrayal and existential despair in the veteran. For example, Mark, a hard-working veteran, feared he would lose his job because he suddenly, out of character, became threatening on the job. If fact, he was unconsciously reenacting an ambush situation from Vietnam. When the doctor refused to write a note to his employer, Mark left therapy in dismay. The doctor had rationalized that the refusal to write the note was consistent with his professional stance of neutrality. But on further reflection, he realized that it was the countertransference of becoming an enemy to Mark and his rage that had led him to withdraw.

MEANING AND SPIRITUALITY

A form of Type I CTR is to *collude in isolating the war experience* of the veteran from the totality of the current functioning. We have found a consistent pressure to assist veterans in "burying" the war, rather than to examine the meaning of this experience for themselves as adults. Scurfield (1985) documents the need for a "whole-life perspective" in PTSD treatment that integrates the veteran's war experience within the context of adult development and creation of meaning and purpose.

At the same time that one is assessing the trauma client, it is helpful, if not essential, for therapists to assess some of their own characteristics that may impact treatment of the veteran. From our perspective it is useful to encourage awareness of objective and subjective countertransference issues, and to understand the motives for working in the field (McCann & Pearlman, 1990). Van Wagoner, Gelso, Hayes, and Diemer (1991) refer to this component as "self-insight." This preparation may also involve methods of "self-checking" to determine the therapist's CTR reaction, as well as consultation with colleagues familiar with the population and treatment (Kernberg, 1965). Therapist characteristics include such things as attitudes about Vietnam and other wars; the use of violence; the effects of war on young men; and the political dimensions of war that activate potential countertransference "nodes" in the therapist. Further, with veteran populations, familiarity with slang and military terms, and the geography and idiosyncracies of the country in which they fought, are all integral to developing therapeutic empathy. Knowledge about comorbid conditions and how to deal with acting out, flashback/dissociative episodes, and potential violence to self or others is essential for the therapist. Familiarity with adult developmental theories (e.g., Erikson, 1968) can help the therapist to understand the impact of the trauma, current developmental challenges facing the veteran, and the likely interaction of these issues (Wilson, 1988).

THERAPIST SELF-CARE AND PERSONAL TRANSFORMATION

Self-care for the provider may represent one of the most effective methods to reduce counterproductive reactions, therapeutic errors, and vicarious traumatization (McCann & Pearlman, 1990). Making countertransference more conscious through initial and periodic self-checking confronts the denial of therapist vulnerability.

Guilt and overresponsibility (Type II CTRs) can interfere with responsible self-care, especially if the therapist places the needs of the client over his or her own. A multifaceted model of self-care addresses these issues. First, having avenues for debriefing of traumatic material is important for "detoxifying" therapeutic experiences, strengthening the healthy boundary between professional and personal life, and reducing vicarious traumatization. In both institutional and private practice settings, we have found this need for debriefing to be acknowledged, but infrequently implemented. Second, the isolation of private practice and the pressures of institutional schedules may prohibit sharing between therapists. Team approaches may best address the needs of therapists treating PTSD and, as well, provide a supportive community that can acknowledge countertransference issues. Third, structured peer supervision fulfills several key needs for the therapist. The supervision dyad or group can assist the therapist to contain feelings and reactions and support the conceptual working through of difficult clinical interventions. In addition, we have found such groups to be helpful in normalizing therapist CTRs, developing realistic expectations for the work, and serving the therapists as an observer of their successes and stress level. Individual needs of the therapist may impact his or her work (McCann & Pearlman, 1990) and necessitate clarification and working through in peer supervision or individual therapy. This model can help to balance the transferential pulls of the veteran PTSD population, as well as assist the therapist in dealing with his or her own institutional transference—for example, in a private setting, knowing when to refer, separation of compensation issues, dangerousness, loss of perspective, and disillusionment.

REFERENCES

Bion, W. R. (1959). Attacks on linking. *International Journal of Psycho-Analysis, 40,* 93–109.

Bongar, B. (1991). *The suicidal patient: Clinical and legal standards of care.* Washington, DC: American Psychological Association.

Boudewyns, P. A., Woods, M. G., Hyer, L., & Albrecht, J. W. (1991) Chronic combat-related PTSD and concurrent substance abuse: Implications for treatment of this "dual diagnosis." *Journal of Traumatic Stress, 4,* 549–560.

Carpy, D. V. (1989). Tolerating the countertransference: A mutative process. *International Journal of Psycho-Analysis, 70,* 287–294.

Catherall, D. R. (1986). The support system and amelioration of PTSD in Vietnam veterans. *Psychotherapy, 23*(3), 472–482.

Erikson, E. H. (1968). *Identiy, youth and crisis.* New York: W. W. Norton.

Gendel, M. H., & Reiser, D. E. (1981). Institutional countertransference. *American Journal of Psychiatry, 138*(4), 508–511.

Goodwin, J. (1980). The etiology of combat-related post-traumatic stress disorders. In T. Williams (Ed.), *Post-traumatic stress disorders of the Vietnam veteran: Observations and recommendations for the psychological treatment of the veteran and his family* (pp. 1–18) Cincinnati, OH: Disabled American Veterans.

Haley, S. A. (1974). When the patient reports atrocities. *Archives of General Psychiatry, 30,* 191–196.

Haley, S. A. (1978). Treatment implications of post-combat stress response syndromes for mental health professions. In C. R. Figley (Ed.), *Stress disorders among Vietnam veterans.* New York: Brunner/Mazel.

Harel, Z., Kahana, B., & Wilson, J. P. (1993). War and remembrance: The legacy of Pearl Harbor. In J. P. Wilson & B. Raphael (Eds.), *The international handbook of traumatic stress syndromes* (pp. 263–275). New York: Plenum Press.

Horowitz, M. (1986). *Stress response syndromes.* Northvale, NJ: Jason Aronson.

Kernberg, O. F. (1965). Notes on countertransference. *Journal of the American Psychoanalytic Association, 13,* 38–56.

Klein, M. (1946). Notes on some schizoid mechanisms. *International Journal of Psycho-Analysis, 27,* 99–110.

Matsakis, A. (1988). *Vietnam wives.* Kensington, MD: Woodbine House.

McCann, I. L., & Pearlman, L. (1990). *Psychological trauma and the adult survivor: Theory, therapy and transformation.* New York: Brunner/Mazel.

Newberry, T. B. (1985). Levels of countertransference toward Vietnam veterans with posttraumatic stress disorder. *Bulletin of the Menninger Clinic, 49*(2), 151–160.

Opp, R. E., & Samson, A. Y. (1989). Taxonomy of guilt for combat veterans. *Professional Psychology: Research and Practice, 20,* 159–165.

Pope, K. S., & Bouhoutsos, J. C. (1986). *Sexual intimacy between therapists and patients.* New York: Praeger.

Scurfield, R. M. (1985). Post-trauma assessment and treatment: Overview and formulations. In C. R. Figley (Ed.), *Trauma and its wake: The study and treatment of post-traumatic stress disorder* (pp. 219–256). New York: Brunner/Mazel.

Shapiro, R. B. (1984). Transference, countertransference, and the Vietnam veteran. In H. J. Schwartz (Ed.), *Psychotherapy of the combat veteran* (pp. 85–101). New York: Spectrum.

Van Wagoner, S. L., Gelso, C. J., Hayes, J. A., & Diemer, R. A. (1991). Countertransference and the reputedly excellent therapist. *Psychotherapy, 28,* 411–421.

Williams, T. (1988) Diagnosis and treatment of survivor guilt: The bad penny syndrome. In J. P. Wilson, Z. Harel, & B. Kahana (Eds.), *Human adaptation to extreme stress: From the Holocaust to Vietnam* (pp. 319–336). New York: Plenum Press.

Wilson, J. P. (1978). *Identity, ideology and crisis: The Vietnam vet in transition* (Vols. 1 & 2). Cincinnati: Disabled American Veterans.

Wilson, J. P. (1988). Understanding the Vietnam veteran. In F. Ochberg (Ed.), *Post-traumatic therapy and victims of violence* (pp. 227–254). New York: Brunner/Mazel.

Wilson, J. P. (1989). *Trauma, transformation, and healing. An integrative approach to theory, research, and post-traumatic therapy.* New York: Brunner/Mazel.

Wilson, J. P., & Zigelbaum, S. (1986). Post-traumatic stress disorder and the disposition to criminal behavior. In C. R. Figley (Ed.), *Trauma and its wake: Theory, research, and intervention* (Vol. II, pp. 102–147). New York: Brunner/Mazel.

12

Countertransference and World War II Resistance Fighters: Issues in Diagnosis and Assessment

WYBRAND OP DEN VELDE
G. FRANK KOERSELMAN
PETRA G. H. AARTS

In this chapter we will discuss the phenomena of countertransference in those who are professionally responsible for the treatment, psychotherapy, and medico-legal examination of survivors of Nazi persecution during World War II in the Netherlands. Massively traumatized people may invoke intense emotions in medical and mental health experts, sometimes leading to unfavorable effects within the relationship of the mental health professional and the survivor. These reactions are by no means unique and are described in other chapters in this book (see Chapter 1, this volume). However, in the Netherlands particular socially and culturally determined factors cause additional problems in relation to countertransference issues. We will discuss special forms of countertransference, which include paranoid and narcissistic reactions in the mental health professional, and explain their relationship to historical events and societal attitudes toward those who fought against Nazi oppression: the Resistance fighters.

THE CONCEPT OF COUNTERTRANSFERENCE

Freud (1910) introduced the terms *transference* and *countertransference,* describing the processes of interaction between the patient and the doctor within the therapeutic setting. Transference became an important and central tool for the psychoanalyst. By means of interpretation, the analyst utilized the reactions, emotions, and attitudes of the patient toward him or her in order to help reveal and work through the patient's underlying intrapsychic needs and conflicts. Countertransference—the analyst's intense feelings toward the patient—was understood as the result of unresolved neurotic conflicts in the analyst, and it was usually considered an obstacle to adequate therapeutic empathy. In the early days of psychoanalysis, countertransference was thought to be triggered solely by the patient's transference reactions. Today, however, the interaction between therapist and patient is understood to be much more complex. The therapeutic work with war victims reveals that strong countertransference reactions (CTRs), regardless of the individual therapist's and patient's pathology, are evoked during the working through of traumatic memories. These CTRs may be divided into two general patterns—avoidance (Type I) or overidentification (Type II)—that are equally applicable to the Dutch situation (see Chapter 1, this volume).

With regard to countertransference, Kernberg (in Sandler, 1988) once said:

> Twenty years ago there were bitter fights around the traditional concept that countertransference should be defined as the unconscious reaction of the analyst to the transference of the patient, but now we see countertransference reactions as part of a broader concept that also includes realistic reactions to the transference and to other aspects of the patient's life as well as the analyst's. Countertransference is a broad spectrum of reactions. (p. 195)

Following Kernberg, we do not restrict countertransference to the narrow definition (i.e., the therapist's responses to the patient's transference). Instead we include other aspects such as cultural and heuristic influences on the therapist's mental reactions to psychic trauma in general and to traumatized patients in particular. As a result of these specific factors in the Netherlands, a development of the avoidance type of response into a paranoid collusion countertransference, and a development of the overidentification type of response into a narcissistic collusion countertransference could take place. We will discuss these forms of countertransference more fully later in the chapter.

WAR VICTIMS AND COUNTERTRANSFERENCE

A striking example of countertransference manifestations toward war victims is given by W. G. Niederland (1980). Since 1953, the West German government provided restitution for disabled German victims of Nazi persecution, German Jews included. Medical experts were appointed to assess the degree of disability and the degree of relatedness of this disability to the actual experiences during persecution. Since many Jews of German origin left or never returned to Germany after the war, a number of physicians outside of Germany were requested to report on applicants for restitution under the German indemnification law. In his capacity as a psychiatrist in the United States, Niederland examined a Jewish man in his late 50s who had emigrated from Germany to the United State a few years after the war. After a relatively long symptom-free interval, the man suffered several breakdowns and was finally hospitalized in a renowned psychiatric clinic, where he was not the only survivor patient. A 12-page file on the man's history and condition was sent to Niederland along with this patient. Apart from the various diagnoses and a report about his medication and treatment, the biography comprised the main part of the file. Pages were filled with his personal and family background; his childhood moods and fantasies, his achievements at school, the frequency of masturbation, and his relationships with the opposite sex were described extensively. However, about the man's experiences during the war there were no more than seven words: "X was in Auschwitz for three years." That "X" also was the sole survivor of a previously extended family was a fact Niederland only learned from the man himself.

It is most unlikely that ignoring the causes of this man's serious condition stems from maliciousness, simple indifference, or lack of empathy. Instead, Niederland's description is an example, as Wilson, Lindy, and Raphael (Chapter 2, this volume) have pointed out, of the empathic withdrawal in therapists when confronted with severely traumatized patients: withdrawal through avoidance, denial, and a focus on pre-morbidity. Indeed, it is illustrative of intense anxiety and affective distress that a confrontation with the extremes of human vulnerability and malice can evoke in each of us.

GENERAL REACTIONS TOWARD WAR VICTIMS

The encounter with trauma victims may elicit strong emotional reactions in family members, relatives, significant others, professional helpers, and even strangers. These reactions range from disbelief to pity and over-involvement and go hand in hand with distress, anxiety, and denial, often leading to the tendency to avoid confrontation with the experiences of the traumatized individual (Danieli, 1980). These reactions place victims in an isolated position, and deprive them of the possibility to exchange and discuss their experiences in an empathic climate. A complicating factor in the case of war survivors lies in the very fact that they have fallen victim to a catastrophe that was caused by fellow humans. Traumatic experiences such as systematic persecution, torture, captivity, malnutrition, battering, and so forth, were deliberate actions of one group of people toward another group. This may enhance the tendency of others to avoid confrontation. The general reactions toward victims of traumatic stress are discussed in Chapter 2.

THE POSITION OF WAR VICTIMS IN DUTCH SOCIETY

After 5 years of suffering during the occupation by Nazi Germany (1940–1945), Holland was liberated. Most people experienced the liberation as a victory of good over evil. Those who had actively fought against the Nazi occupiers, in particular the civilian Resistance fighters, had reason to be proud of their personal contributions to the victory and might have expected to be treated and appreciated as heroes. However, they often experienced exactly the opposite, being treated with indifference, or even hostility and rejection. Today, many of them express bitterness, disappointment, and a sense of isolation. For them the fourth phase of the trauma recovery process, giving meaning to the traumatic experience, was hindered by this unusual general reaction pattern of Dutch society. They were deprived of understanding, appreciation, and the necessary care for their physical and mental sufferings. Four dimensions of this phenomenon will be discussed as they pertain to countertransference processes.

1. General reactions toward victims of man-made disasters.
2. Rejection and denial of the special position of war victims in the Dutch society.
3. The peculiar Dutch Calvinistic mentality and morale.
4. The prevailing medical opinions regarding the origin of "traumatic neurosis" in the post-war years.

These factors add an important social dimension to coping with war trauma. In several aspects these four factors are closely interrelated. In the Netherlands, this gave rise to additional types of transference in victims of man-made disaster, a dimension in which therapists and medical doctors are not well trained. As will be explored further, this social dimension is responsible for particular patterns of countertransference in medical doctors and psychotherapists, which are different from those usually encountered in the treatment of trauma survivors.

Rejection and Denial of a Special Position
of War Victims in Dutch Society

To most people in Holland, the German invasion in 1940 came as a surprise. At the beginning of the military occupation, life went on as usual for most people. The special regulations and restrictions of the German occupiers were experienced as a nuisance. However, during the year 1940 the suppression and persecution of the sizeable Jewish community began to be implemented. A part of the population reacted with aversion. These events stimulated the development of active resistance to the Nazi occupation (Warmbrunn, 1963). Numerous Jews, Resistance participants, and opponents of the Nazis were arrested, often after betrayal. They were sometimes cruelly interrogated, tortured, and subsequently executed or put into concentration camps, where many of them perished. Others had to live in hiding for years.

Although the great majority strongly disapproved of the acts of the Nazi occupiers, only a minority (3%) of the population was actively involved in the Resistance. In the margin the silent majority played its own, but no less important, role in this constellation of perpetrators and persecuted. The fact that they were, or at least seemed, indifferent, that they feigned ignorance and did not protest actively seemed to legitimate the cruel and criminal acts of the perpetrators.

After the liberation by the Allied armies in 1945, the Dutch hardly found time to reflect on the war era or to deal directly with their emotions. The disorganized and plundered country immediately claimed all their energy for reconstruction. In a way every citizen considered himself or herself a victim of war. Many concentration camp survivors suffered from severe malnutrition, infectious diseases, and exhaustion. Medical treatment was based on the principle of rest and good food. Mental problems of war victims were seen as temporary burdens that would disappear spontaneously.

The earliest encounters of Dutch medical professionals with war victims fell outside the scope of psychotherapy. With regard to indemnification laws for disabled war victims, applicants for such pensions had to undergo medical examinations to determine the relationship of their disability to their war experiences. Often, lengthy procedures accompanied by multiple medical examinations were part of the application for a war pension. This led to additional forms of disruption of understanding and empathy.

Collectively as well as individually the people tried to forget the 5 frightening years of Nazi occupation. The vast majority of the Dutch population had strongly disapproved of the behavior of the Nazis, yet only a few expressed their opinion, or offered active resistance. Most people simply lacked the courage to risk their lives for ideals like freedom and a just society. And the silent majority did not appreciate being reminded of their own lack of courage and the resulting guilt feelings. Thus, the social appreciation of war victims as well as war heroes became beset with ambivalence. The result was that the war victims were largely ignored as a special group of people in need of support and care. As a consequence, many war victims learned to stifle their emotions, enhancing their feelings of neglect and rejection by society in general. This isolation was further strengthened by the feelings of guilt and shame characteristic of many war victims. A kind of societal conspiracy of silence emerged.

This particular situation created a considerable burden on the process of working through war traumas. In this respect a study of Dutch-Jewish war orphans is of particular interest (Keilson, 1992). A remarkable result of this study is the fact that the conditions following the traumatization, being either supportive or deficient, could predict the incidence and severity of later symptomatology in these young survivors of war. Keilson introduced the term *third traumatic sequence,* as opposed to the first traumatic sequence, the anticipation of the traumatic event, and the second, the actual period of persecution. This study demonstrates the importance of social support in coming to terms with war trauma, a finding repeated in more recent studies of U.S. war veterans (Wilson, 1989).

However, instead of receiving social support, most war victims became trapped in the conspiracy of silence. Only recently, there is a growing acceptance of the sad fact that people can have long-lasting and severe breakdowns as a result of their psychic traumatization during World War II. Until this time, however, survivors lacked the necessary support and acknowledgment of their sufferings during and after the war. In this sense, Keilson's third traumatic sequence was indeed an additional trauma for many Dutch war victims.

The Significance of Calvinism in Dutch CTRs

The Low Countries, well known for their never-ending but overall victorious struggle against the devouring powers of the water, show another distinguishing, cultural characteristic, which is less commonly known but is crucial to understanding the peculiar mentality and attitude of the Dutch. Like many other Northern European countries, Holland was strongly influenced by the anti-Catholic Reformation of the 16th century. In Holland, it was especially the ideas of Calvin that hit the core of the culture. Since the posthumous publication of Max Weber's major study, *Die Protestantische Ethik und der Geist des Kapitalismus* (Protestant ethics

and the spirit of capitalism), the Dutch successes in international com-
merce and the resultant accumulation of wealth are commonly explained
as the result of the prevailing standards of productivity and thrift to
previously unknown heights and put an end to the old-fashioned Catholic
aversion against financial profits. It marked the waning of the Middle Ages
and the birth of modern times.

However, the lack of aristocratic traditions in the Dutch Republic
explains the persistent success of Calvinism and much of the Dutch mentality up to the current era. In contrast to all the other European nation-
states, the Dutch Republic in the 17th century developed as a bourgeois
society. There was a general and strong aversion against any overt display
of power and wealth, as was habitual in those countries where the aristocracy was a ruling class. Spending money solely for joy and pleasure was
disdained. Life in the Low Countries was a "duty" for all classes, the rich
and the poor, that had to be endured without complaining and even in
humble gratitude. Gratification, happiness, and the pleasures of leisure
belonged to the realm of the divine hereafter, if one was lucky enough to
get there. For a life led in soberness and abstinence, and in dedication to
labor in the here "below" and to the spirit of God, was no guarantee
whatsoever of a secure place in heaven. This injustice within Calvinist
creed was to be accepted without questioning, as were the hardships of
life. The influence of this mentality on the present Dutch population
should not be underestimated. For centuries the material and therefore
mental world of the Dutch, from the lower to the upper middle classes,
was determined by standards of industriousness, soberness, and introver-
sion. Even the nonreligious and the Roman Catholics in the Netherlands
are more Calvinistic in their attitudes and convictions than they would
probably care to know. Over the ages, wealthy but (at least seemingly)
pious burghers, instead of an exuberant aristocracy, have been models of
envious identification.

For centuries heroism (other than the stoic kind), fervent national-
ism, or any strong worldly conviction or dedication have been strongly
disparaged by the Dutch. A typical Dutch proverb demonstrates this mentality, though nowadays it is also said with sarcasm or irony. Translated
into English it would probably read like this: "Act normally! That is
already mad enough." The aversion against the display of strong emotions, whether of joy or of criticism and lament, is still prevalent in the
Netherlands. But it is not expressed in the phlegmatic, humorous way the
British are thought to deal with or ward off their affects, but, on the
contrary, as a rigid and humorless repression of emotions. The expression
of feelings—in particular, pride—is denounced and considered to be a
weakness of character and pathos. Suffering is appreciated as a burden
that must be endured in silence. It is this particular Calvinistic mentality

that illuminates the CTRs of the Dutch authorities and health professionals toward victims of World War II.

Although the Dutch Government openly expressed a "debt of honor" toward all war victims, the redemption of this debt took the form of a payment. War pension laws for disabled veterans of the Resistance and persecuted people passed the Chambers. Those war victims who were obviously crippled or disabled could ask for financial compensation for subsequent loss of income, but compensation was only granted when a causal relation of the disability and war experiences was proved beyond reasonable doubt. The measure of disability, and the evidence of its relation to deprivations during the war, were based exclusively on medical and historical verification. Although this procedure of application satisfied many urgent material needs in the immediate post-war years, over the years the award of a war disability pension became the only means for survivors to receive formal recognition of their emotional isolation and suffering. Yet, many of these war victims were treated as ordinary disability benefit applicants. They often experienced the procedures and medical examinations as humiliating and insulting, and the resulting financial compensation, if any, as an insufficient gratuity. When turned down, they frequently sought an outlet in lengthy legal procedures against the government's Endowment Funds.

The relationship between applicants on one side, and the officials and medical experts of the Endowment Funds on the other side, is beset with aversive CTRs. The war victims, now mostly elderly people, have the obvious need to speak about their traumatic experiences, but for a long time, the officials, doctors, judges, and legal counselors were only interested in medical facts and historically verified data. As a result, a complete rupture of empathy between victims and their official caregivers occurred. Many war victims experienced the application procedure as "a continuation of the war," or an "affirmation of hostility and rejection." On the other hand, medical and legal experts involved in the assessment of applicants may have strong feelings of resentment and anger toward these "troublesome, thwarting, and always discontented" war victims, partly caused by the animosity of the applicants. They further feel that these war victims are unreliable, and that they exaggerate the importance of their role in the Dutch Resistance or of their sufferings during and after the war.

PSYCHOLOGICAL TRAUMA IN PSYCHIATRIC TEXTBOOKS

From the early ages on, many works of literature and art have revealed the sometimes devastating impact that shocking events can have on human integrity. However, until recently, mental health experts have generally ignored this common awareness. Especially in the second half of the 19th century, when psychology and psychiatry were academically institutionalized, a physiological approach to mental disorders was prevalent in Europe. At that time psychiatry in the Netherlands was dominated by German Kraepelinian nosology. Within this organic–biological frame of thought, the often disrupting effects of psychic trauma were indeed inexplicable.

A study of the literature on survivors of persecution of World War II reveals the general lack of understanding, empathy, and support, including the inadequacy of treatment in the first few decades after the war, to be the result of the prevailing, obsolete psychiatric nosology (Grubrich-Simitis, 1981; Hoppe, 1971; Luchterhand, 1970). The most important factor was the prevalence of physiological interpretations of the so-called traumatic neurosis. Only organic damage, such as cerebral dysfunctions as a consequence of head injuries or dystrophia caused by prolonged malnutrition, was held responsible for lasting psychiatric disorders in these patients. In the absence of evidence of such organic brain damage, any direct connection of the symptomatology to the traumatic experiences of persecution was denied. A short reaction after the exposure to a shocking event was expected, but so was an immediate recovery to the former physical and mental equilibrium. No generally accepted textbook of that time described psychic trauma as a possible cause of decompensation in otherwise healthy patients. Only since the second half of this century, has there been a gradual shift toward a more psychodynamic focus on human development and existence.

However, even in the immediate post-war years, some mental health experts—most of them prompted by their personal experiences during the war—have shown deep insight into the pathogenesis and dynamics of symptomatology in victims of Nazi persecution. They often quite effectively utilized psychoanalytic concepts and theories to understand and clarify the behavior and symptomatology of survivor patients. Psychoanalysis could offer the necessary frames of reference. Concepts such as the deterioration of ego functions, breakdown of the stimulus barrier, regression toward archaic superego functioning, different patterns of identification, and various mechanisms of defense, supported the maturing understanding in the underlying etiology and psychodynamics.

But the varying diagnostic classifications of the symptomatology, such as concentration camp syndrome, identity diffusion, chronic reactive depression, psychosis, and reactive change of personality, may well have sounded too scary for many of their mental health colleagues. The very idea of humankind being so vulnerable that serious and even permanent psychic damage could develop as a consequence of distressing events is not only a frightening idea, but also a narcissistic blow. Furthermore, the confrontation with the atrocities of World War II and its survivors deeply challenged the belief and trust in the linear progress of Western civilization. These narcissistic injuries and fears, combined with the normal tendency to deny our own physical and psychic vulnerability, can still be additional motives for the ongoing, general negation of psychic trauma as a cause for various psychiatric disorders other than PTSD to date (Aarts, 1990).

Based on the works of philosophers of science such as Popper, Lakatos, and Kuhn, it is apparent that other factors than scientific variables have a certain influence on the sciences. The questions we ask and the answers we seek, indeed, what we perceive and do not perceive, are to a certain extent determined by factors that are beyond the objects and theories of our research. These nonscientific factors can be of a political, cultural, or religious nature, but in addition rivalry among scientists and *jalousie de métier* can, more often than we wish to admit, cause scientific growth or stagnation. Therefore, we should consider psychiatric textbooks on psychic trauma not only as a product of objective scientific progress, but also as the result of subjective human thought and affect. The textbook, is in fact, a coproduct of medical expertise and nonscientific CTRs. As such, psychiatric curricula also lend support to rationalizations and intellectualizations as a result of CTRs in the leading mental health experts. An example of such CTRs, emanating from theoretical convictions and beliefs, is described by Stein (1991). As Wilson, Lindy, and Raphael have pointed out (see Chapter 2, this volume), empathic failures, as a consequence of affective countertransference within the therapeutic setting, also involve cognitive defenses. Intellectualization and rationalization may serve as cognitive tools to deny either the severity of the patient's symptomatology and traumatization, or the relatedness of the symptoms to the preceding traumatic event. Psychiatric textbooks could indeed for a long period of time serve as cognitive tools in such CTRs.

Even psychoanalysis, with its emphasis on the psychodynamics of the human psyche, only temporarily and reluctantly accepted external traumatic events to cause lasting disturbances in the human mind. After dismissing the "seduction theory" at the turn of the century, Freud (1919) only acknowledged the potential pathogenicity of external shocking experiences when confronted with soldiers suffering from traumatic neurosis—so-called shell-shock—during World War I. However, this acknowledgment did not lead to the integration of adult psychic trauma into psychoanalytic theory on pathogenesis. The works of his forerunners, such as Charcot and especially Janet, written more than a century ago, were covered with dust, until their insights into the traumatic genesis of hysteria were recently rediscovered, undusted, and appreciated (van der Kolk & van der Hart, 1989).

For decades the focus of psychoanalysis remained as near as it could to drive theory and the defenses against the conflicts that drives generate in every human being. Only the minds of children were thought to be sufficiently vulnerable for external disrupting stimuli to cause long-lasting or permanent psychic damage. Indeed, the possible disintegrating effect of external stimuli on the adult personality cannot easily be integrated in drive and structure theory, where only internal conflict was at the core of neurotic pathology. Even years after World War II, the psychoanalyst Edith Jacobson (in Ulman & Brothers, 1988) argued, with respect to the condition of female inmates in Nazi prison, that "the women prisoners were not directly traumatized by their shattering experiences in prison, but rather were traumatized by identifying themselves with sexually aggressive fantasy images unconsciously organized around repressed memories of the primal scene" (p. 54). Zetzel (1970) stated that "external events, no matter how overwhelming, precipitate a neurosis only when they touch on specific unconscious conflicts" (p. 64). Indeed, for the purpose of adequate psychotherapy with trauma survivors the intertwining of preexisting internal conflict and the subsequent subjective meaning of a traumatic event cannot, and should not, be denied. But we should beware of a reversal of cause and effect, which might serve as a new legitimation of defensive CTRs in mental health experts.

In effect, it was not official psychoanalytic theory that helped establish a general acceptance of adult psychic trauma; it was the direct confrontation of mental health professionals with survivors of the many wars and atrocities of this century. As the philosopher of science Feyerabend (1988) states, "Where arguments *do* seem to have an effect, this is more often due to their *physical repetition* than to their semantic content" (p. 15). On the other hand, it must be said, that psychoanalysis was the only school that, since Freud, at least tried to establish a comprehensive theory of trauma. But the theory dismissed the possibility that a mature personality could fall prone to the disintegrating effects of overwhelming external stimuli. The theory on psychic trauma was primarily focused on the effects of traumata during the formative years of childhood (see Furst, 1967).

For a long time, cognitive defenses in medical and mental health professionals were supported by the general denial of psychic trauma in psychiatric textbooks. Only since the introduction of post-traumatic stress disorder (PTSD) in 1980 in the third edition of the *Diagnostic and Statistical Manual of Mental Disorders,* has acute, chronic, and delayed post-traumatic symptomatology found general recognition.

According to textbooks in the immediate post-war years, post-traumatic psychic and somatic symptomatology either were understood as manifestations of organic brain damage, or, based on the prevailing psychoanalytic theories, the problems of victims of persecution were primarily seen as the result of a reactivation of neurotic conflicts originating in childhood. As a consequence, in the practice of examination and treatment, a genetic predisposition for mental disease (i.e., *Anlage*) in the survivor was thought to be the primary cause of the symptomatology. In other cases, patients who complained about disabling aches were believed to be exaggerating and even simulating their symptoms when an organic substrate could not be found. The so-called *compensation neurosis,* which manifests itself in the wish to be freed from further efforts and responsibility for one's own material and immaterial well-being after a shocking event, was one post-traumatic sequela that was generally recognized, including in the pre-war textbooks. As a result, many victims of war were deprived of proper understanding and treatment of their post-traumatic symptoms and were often denied the award of a special pension.

Case Example

A 62-year-old man, living abroad, was referred for a psychiatric report by a Foundation of Resistance Veterans. His application for a Special War Veterans Pension has been dismissed twice.

According to his file, he was 20 years old at the beginning of the German occupation of the Netherlands in 1940. At that time he was a second-year university student in mathematics. His impartially verified war history revealed that in 1942 friends asked him to help with the printing and distribution of an illegal newsletter. Later on he became involved in the aid to members of the Allied Air Forces, who had crashed over occupied territory. On several occasions he accompanied these people to safe hiding places. One day he was unable to escort a group of British pilots because he was ill, and his best friend took over his task. This friend and the pilots were caught by a German patrol and arrested. For a long time he was unaware of their fate. He had to go in hiding because his friend might confess his name during interrogation or under torture. Nevertheless, he continued his Resistance work. During subsequent escorts of groups of air crewman he felt very anxious, particularly if the men were careless and spoke English in public.

After the liberation in 1945 he was told that his friend had been executed and the British flyers incarcerated in a German prisoner-of-war camp. He then was restless and tense, and he suffered from insomnia and concentration difficulties. He could not continue his study and took a job in an insurance company. He married and had two children. Because of problems with his superior, he started his own private insurance agency. He worked day and night and was at first rather successful. Around 1970 this changed. He made some financial miscalculations, started to quarrel with clients, and got into financial troubles. He complained of extreme fatigue, stomach problems, and vomiting. However, medical examination revealed no abnormalities, and he was advised "to take some rest." He continued his work and his financial situation grew worse. In 1978 he applied for a Special War Veterans Pension. The medical consultant of the War Pension Endowment Office asked his family physician for information. The family physician reported the complaints, the negative results of medical examination, and that he never had heard anything about stressful war experiences. On the basis of this information a Special War Pension was rejected. Five years later, after intensification of his complaints, he was forced to quit his work entirely, and he applied again for a Veterans Pension. He was examined by the medical consultant of the War Pension Endowment Office, a nonspecialist. The rather brief report read: "The applicant speaks matter of factly about his war experiences, and shows no emotions." The Resistance work was described as being of minor importance and not contributing to his complaints. The disability was understood as a manifestation of a neurosis originating in his childhood. His personality was described as obsessive–compulsive, aggressive, uncooperative, stubborn, and hostile, with a tendency to malingering. For the second time his request for a Veterans Pension was turned down.

A tall man, dressed in a rather old, but originally expensive, suit that was now too large for him, entered my consultation room. His attitude was formal and somewhat suspicious. He gave brief answers to my introductory questions, and I began to feel uneasy. He suddenly shouted, "Why are you asking all these questions? Everything is in my file!" My feeling was, "He is entirely right. What I am doing must be a nuisance to this man." In a certain way I wanted to receive his sympathy, not his anger. He started telling about his previous experiences concerning the official verification of his Resistance work, where he met with disbelief and hostility and had to provide proof for acts done in secrecy. He had lost any faith in his family physician, who did not support his claims. The previous medical examination was "worthless, lasting only ten minutes." I invited him to tell more about this. He got rather tense and angry, and he described how he felt neglected and humiliated. He emphasized the stupidity of his family doctor and the examining officials. The doctor of the Endowment Office gave him the impression that he tried to lure him into a trap, because he asked many questions about his childhood and his work, but not about the war time. After the rejection of his pension claim his anger never disappeared, and conflicts with his wife and children increased. He had never had much contact with them, and now he started to see himself an outsider in his own family. He felt increasingly inadequate and worthless. The discussion of these feelings took a lot of time.

I made an appointment 1 week later. After he left, I felt very tired and angry about the insincere way he had been treated. I understood his feeling of not being taken seriously and his loneliness. I experienced a strong need to gain his respect, perhaps even friendship. In the second and third session his complaints, life history, and war experiences were the focus of attention. He was raised by rather wealthy, but cold and demanding parents, who gave all their attention to their grocery shop. The care of their only child was left to ever-changing female servants.

He was able to express his anxiety and guilt about his executed friend, who had taken his place during a dangerous mission. I asked him why he continued the resistance work after the arrest of his friend. He mentioned a feeling of loyalty, a desire not to abandon people in difficulty, hate toward the Nazis, and shame about his fears, and that he was afraid to fall into "a kind of emptiness, in which life had lost any meaning." He needed the intense comradeship and commitment of his fellow Resistance participants.

After the war, he experienced his work as a challenge: "I had to win the game." He never felt like the same person he was before. He never talked about the painful events, because "I do not like to bother people with my misery." He loved his family but was unable to show or share emotions. He stated that he suffered from insomnia and almost every night he had repetitive nightmares, mainly one about pursuit by German patrols, or another in which his executed friend tried to hand over a present. He was always irritable and fatigued, and he described his vomiting "as a way to get rid of my disgust."

I was pleased when he told me how he appreciated "complete understanding." I felt reluctant to write my expertise report and postponed it. I was afraid of losing this case and of being seen as a traitor. Somehow I had lured him into confidential confessions about his innermost feelings, regarding his far from happy childhood but also about positive appraisal of the commitment with his fellow Resistance comrades, an intensity of contact he had always missed since then. I observed in him a tendency to exaggerate his complaints, to blame all of his difficulties on the war, to minimize his early life experiences, and in fact, I doubted if I was at all competent to write this report, notwithstanding my considerable experience. I referred this man for treatment to a colleague, whom I knew as an adequate and empathic psychotherapist.

Furthermore, this case was discussed at a group meeting of psychiatrists, who had much experience with the treatment and medical examination of war victims. All agreed that this man suffered from a delayed PTSD. Despite his life full of conflict, there was no evidence of traumatic events other than his Resistance participation that could be responsible for his disability. The reaction of the previous examining doctor was an example of paranoid countertransference, and my reactions were considered to be an example of narcissistic countertransference.

Based on my report his case was reopened, and he was granted a Special War Veterans Pension.

CTR PATTERNS

In general, Dutch war victims have been exposed to existential threat. They experienced extreme measures of fear, sometimes once and acutely, but often repeatedly and for extended periods. They used several psychological mechanisms of defense to ward off these unbearable feelings. Most of them continued to use these coping patterns after the war, thus saving themselves from nightmares, flashbacks, and other manifestations of persistent anxiety. However, later on in their lives, occasionally even after some 50 years, their psychological resistance becomes vulnerable, and thus they are caught by the memories of their former fears. PTSD then develops in its full power.

Yet, PTSD is not the only way in which post-traumatic maladjustment may reveal itself. Mechanisms of defense may be very successful concerning their primary goal: protecting the subject from unbearable fear. Biologically they represent a function comparable to retracting a limb in reaction to pain. But when pain goes on, the retraction gets useless and continued muscle contraction will produce pain itself and prove to be harmful. The same holds true for psychological defense against anxiety. Anxiety as a biological signal stimulates the subject to avoid danger, to react with fight or flight. But when anxiety belongs to past events, when it is the product of a former period of one's life, it no longer serves an objective goal. Nevertheless, subjects do experience the anxiety and arousal as real, and in reaction will be prepared to fight or to avoid some imminent threat, which in fact belongs to their past. And the more helpless they are as a consequence, the more they will at last become depressed. Interpretation of the real world as though it were the world of one's former nightmares is, in fact, neurotic behavior. Anxiety and depression are then neurotic reactions, neurotic feelings. For those who were existentially traumatized in an earlier period of their life, this, as a general rule, is one other possible outcome besides PTSD. Depression and generalized anxiety (accompanied by psychosomatic and somatoform reactions) with these patients result form their neurotic interpretation of their actual world by the standards of their never-extinguished former traumas. Their post-traumatic neurotic *modus vivendi* can be characterized by two features: (1) the nature of the once real threat, and (2) the nature of their once adequate but now maladaptive responses.

Dutch war victims generally experienced a continuous threat of, or even real confrontation with, extreme humiliation and/or annihilation. They responded to the threat of death with conscious alertness. To humiliation they responded with special consciousness of their task and position, of the values they were fighting for, or of anything that might support their threatened self-esteem. This, of course, is not only characteristic of Dutch people in World War II; it also fits the case of any prisoner of war, of any hostage. Characteristic of Dutch war victims is the way in which these two types of defensive reactions, with respect to these two forms of real threat, resulted in later neurotic patterns of adjustment within modern Dutch society. As we explained above, Dutch war victims were compelled to seek "justice" within the medical system, with the help of medical legislation. They were confronted with medical authorities, whom they found in the position to grant or to refuse the commemorative financial endowment. These doctors were perceived often as powerful and godlike. Hopefully they would be on the "good" side; possibly, however, they could be on the wrong side, trying to humiliate or annihilate the victims again. Transference-splitting into all-good and all-bad is a common defense against overwhelming threat. It is typical of the idiosyncratic Dutch situation that doctors should become the object of these war victims' transference reactions, which because of the intensity and duration cannot fail to awaken the doctors' counter-transference.

Countertransference is not only a reaction to a patient's or claimant's behavior; it is also the expression of one's interpretation of that behavior against the background of very personal emotions. In the Netherlands, doctors are part of the social system in which the recognition of one's behavior during war has been made dependent upon a medical diagnosis. Some 50 years after World War II, the population as a whole seems deeply concerned with the moral issues of that time. This applies not only to the generation that was adult during the war, but also to young people as more and more of them want to attend ceremonial commemorations of a war they only heard about from their parents. All this tends to create an environment in which it is almost impossible to stay neutral. The impact of this trend on the average doctor must therefore be almost irresistible, when he or she is confronted with the claim for a medical diagnosis that essentially constitutes a recognition of bravery. Consider how much more difficult it will be for a doctor who was involved personally in the questions of right or wrong during World War II, or who had similar traumatic experiences?

In the last decade we have seen some specific, related transference–countertransference combinations. One might even speak of the complementary neuroses of war victims and doctors. These complementary traumatic neuroses may be seen as particular forms of the avoidance and overidentification types of countertransference, shaped under the influence of existential threat and loss of honor in a Calvinistic context. The Swiss psychiatrist Jürg Willi (1975) coined the term "collusion" in addressing the phenomenon of the complementary neurosis. In matrimony and other close relationships the neurotic needs of one partner may be satisfied by neurotic solutions of the other. But in the same way, one could also regard some complementary combinations of transference and countertransference neurosis as collusions. In these cases, countertransference represents a doctor's personal, neurotic problem that is specifically enhanced by the patient's transference claims.

In the Netherlands two types of transference–countertransference collusion between victims of World War II and their doctors have been discerned. The political and cultural situation that we described above offered the ground upon which such collusions could develop. We give a description of these two types below.

Paranoid Collusion

In this type of collusion former war victims expect humiliation from anybody who possesses some kind of power. They live in constant fear that the other may even deny their right to exist. For them life becomes a continuous struggle against authorities. At the same time, however, they intensely long for recognition of their bravery, of their contribution to the nation.

But official recognition depends almost entirely upon a doctor's declaration that they are medically ill and that this illness is caused by suffering experienced during the war in Resistance efforts or in a concentration camp. Thus, that doctor is bestowed with immense power.

Caught within the trap of unbearable dependency, patients try to ward off range and fear by anticipating rejection. So they accentuate their complaints, exaggerate their physical disabilities themselves and treat the doctor with suspicious arrogance. They try to prove their bravery by proving themselves to be ill.

By chance this patient may meet a doctor who personally adheres to high standards of strength and bravery. Such a doctor will find the claim of illness to be incompatible with a claim of courage and therefore will distrust the patient. The doctor may also perceive any tendencies of his or her own to give in as a personal weakness, as a personal defeat. The stronger the war victim's claim, the stronger the doctor's resistance will be. He or she may even declare it impossible, as a general rule, that a war trauma can cause illness or PTSD after a delay of several years. Sometimes the doctor himself or herself suffered during the war. In that case the doctor may experience the patient's behavior as a form of treason and consequently treat him or her with thinly disguised contempt.

It is obvious that both the doctor and the patient/war victim will become entangled in a mutual neurotic struggle. The paranoid preoccupation of the one will provoke the same reaction in the other. Transference and countertransference determine each other, maintaining the vicious circle of their paranoid collusion.

Narcissistic Collusion

Neurosis can be characterized by the neurotic *theme* and the neurotic *solution.* In narcissistic collusion the theme is the same as that of paranoid collusion: fear of annihilation and humiliation. However, in this situation the solution is different. The claim of illness (as required in the Netherlands) is no longer perceived as humiliating but rather as a distinguishing mark. The patient not only claims to be ill; he or she claims to have a very special illness. His or her war-related complaints cannot be understood by ordinary doctors. The doctor has to be a person of outstanding and very rarely met capacities, nearly a genius. To this patient, it is not the doctor but the outside world that represents the enemy. The grandeur of the patient's war-caused disability and his or her paranoid contempt of the "normal" (medical and political) world represent a neurotic solution to the problem of how to live with constant fear of humiliation or annihilation.

By chance this patient may meet a doctor who has a personal need for grandiosity and for being singled out from the anonymous mass of his or her ordinary colleagues. Such a doctor may even claim that he or she is the only one able to treat war victims, that only he or she recognizes the real impact of their suffering (which in the Netherlands is equivalent to recognition of bravery) and heroism. These doctors may declare it impossible to share their specific knowledge with any colleague. Those who are skeptical or doubt their claims will be suspected of conscious obstruction.

It is obvious that both World War II victims and their doctors have a common interest in maintaining that war-caused illness is a unique condition. In doing so they help each other to ward off the threat of humiliation and annihilation that they (perhaps for different reasons) cannot bear. Transference and countertransference get connected in an interdependent narcissistic collusion.

CONCLUSION

This chapter has been concerned with the vicissitudes of countertransference that in our opinion developed in the particular Dutch sociocultural climate after World War II. We do not know in how many cases these particular collusions played a role. But we have observed that these collusions have been responsible for intense conflict on the individual as well as the societal level. They have been the cause of useless individual suffering and financial damage. Special courts of appeal have treated hundreds of cases in which not a legal but a transference–countertransference problem was the central issue.

The fourth phase of the trauma recovery process is the reappraisal of the traumatic history and the reconstruction of the imagery and emotions into a new, more appropriate structure of meaning and understanding. Rendering meaning to the traumatic experiences and their effects, facilitates the final phase of the trauma recovery process, where a certain acceptance of one's fate and a sense of continuity in life is (re)established. For Dutch war victims, the crucial fourth phase of trauma recovery was seriously hindered by the strong societal ambivalence, the Calvinistic morals, and the then prevailing medical opinions, as described above. As a consequence of the empathic break with authorities and caregivers, the fifth phase of the war victims' trauma recovery process, that of trauma integration, could hardly be reached.

REFERENCES

Aarts, P. G. H. (1990). De kunst van het verwerken [The art of mastering]. In D. H. Schram & C. Geljon (Eds.), *Overal sporen: De verwerking van de Tweede Wereldoorlog in literatuur en kunst* (pp. 296–323). Amsterdam: VU Uitgeverij.

Danieli, Y. (1980). Countertransference in the treatment and study of Nazi Holocaust survivors and their children. *Victimology: An International Journal, 5,* 355–367.

Feyerabend, P. (1988). *Against method* (Rev. ed.). London and New York. Verso.

Freud, S. (1910). *Über Psychoanalyse.* Wein: Gesammelte Werke 8.

Freud, S. (1919). *Einleitung zu 'Zur Psychoanalyse der Kriegsneurosen.'* Leipzig and Wien: Gesammelte Werke 12.

Furst, S. S. (Ed.) (1967). *Psychic trauma.* New York: Basic Books.

Grubrich-Simitis, I. (1981). Extreme traumatization as cumulative trauma. *Psychoanalytic Study of the Child 36,* 415–450.

Hoppe, K. D. (1971). The aftermath of Nazi-persecution reflected in recent psychiatric literature. In H. Krystal & W. G. Niederland (Eds.), *Psychic traumatization,* (pp. 169–205). Boston: Little, Brown.

Keilson, H. (1992). *Sequential traumatization in children.* Jerusalem: Magness Press.

Luchterhand, E. (1970). Early and late effects of imprisonment in Nazi concentration camps. Conflicting interpretations in survivor research. *Social Psychiatry, 5,* 102–110.

Niederland, W. G. (1980). *Folgen der Verfolgung: Das überlebenden-syndrom [Consequences of persecution: The survivor syndrome].* Frankfurt: Suhrkamp.

Sandler, J. (Ed.). (1988). *Projection, identification, projective identification.* London: Karnack Books.

Stein, S. (1991). The influence of theory on the psychoanalyst's countertransference. *International Journal of Psycho-Analysis, 72,* 325–334.

Ulman, R. B., & Brothers, D. (1988). *The shattered self: A psychoanalytic study of trauma.* Hillsdale, NJ: Analytic Press.

van der Kolk, B. A., van der Hart, O. (1989). Pierre Janet and the breakdown of adaptation in psychological trauma. *American Journal of Psychiatry, 146,* 1530–1540.

Warmbrunn, W. (1963). *The Dutch under German occupation, 1940–1945.* Stanford, CA: Stanford University Press.

Weber, M. (1965). *Die protestantische Ethik und der Geist des Kapitalismus* (2 Teilen). München: Siebenstern Verlag.

Willi, J. (1975). *Die Zweierbeziehung.* Reinbek: Rowohlt Verlag.

Wilson, J. P. (1989). *Trauma, transformation and healing.* New York: Brunner/Mazel.

Zetzel, E. R. (1970). *The capacity for emotional growth.* New York: International Universities Press.

PART IV

Countertransference in "At-Risk" Professionals: Rescue Workers, Mental Health Providers, and Persons at the Workplace

The fourth section of this volume focuses on "at-risk" professionals and countertransference that occurs in the line of duty. In contrast to being victims of traumatic experiences, people who are disaster workers, emergency medical personnel, mental health providers, firefighters, police, and employees at the industrial workplace are frequently exposed to or witness traumatic events that happen to others, which involve physical injury, burns, accidents, and death. Duty- or work-related exposure also place such persons at risk to develop post-traumatic stress disorder (PTSD) and associated conditions. Thus, those who are in contact with these "eye-witness," traumatized individuals are prone to countertransference reactions (CTRs) as well. In this regard, it is necessary to broaden the concept of countertransference beyond the setting of psychotherapy to include other venues in which empathic strain and CTRs may occur.

In Chapter 13, Beverley Raphael and John P. Wilson discuss nine dynamic themes common to rescue work. These themes include (1) force and destruction, (2) confrontation with death, (3) helplessness, (4) anger, (5) loss, (6) attachments, (7) elation, (8) survivor guilt, and (9) voyeurism. Disaster and rescue workers are not immune from developing psychiatric disorders, and the authors cite empirical studies that show that between 20 to over 80% of rescue workers show symptoms of prolonged stress response. The recognition of this problem has implications for job performance as well as for the nature of clinical interventions necessary to provide care and an opportunity to work through the emotionally troublesome aspects of rescue work. The authors note that at present there are few controlled studies of such interventions as critical incident stress debriefing (CISD) and similar techniques designed to facilitate stabilization after disaster work.

In Chapter 14, Christine Dunning discusses trauma and countertransference in the workplace. When traumatic exposure occurs, it frequently has a "ripple effect" that draws fellow employees, supervisors, and administrative personnel into its wake. For this reason, social support, counseling, employee assistance programs, and so forth, may be necessary to facilitate recovery of the employee who witnessed a trauma in the workplace. To illustrate just how complicated the effects of trauma in the workplace can become, six case studies are presented to explain the relationship between workplace trauma and various forms of transference and countertransference among coworkers and, especially, supervisors. The chapter concludes with a discussion of how organizations can more effectively manage trauma and countertransference processes within organizations.

In Chapter 15, Yael Danieli presents a training model for mental health professionals who work with PTSD. This informative chapter contains step-by-step instructions on how to identify and manage CTRs. A pioneer in the field, Danieli clearly indicates that therapist training in trauma work must begin with an understanding of the complexity of CTRs.

In Chapter 16, we review and summarize the seminal contributions and insights developed through the collaboration of the authors of this book. Moreover, despite the inevitable differences in the contributions' theoretical or clinical orientation, what has emerged in the process of analyzing the phenomena of countertransference in work with PTSD, dissociative disorders, and comorbid states is the identification of areas of commonality and agreement, as well as areas in which we lack knowledge or empirical foundations in terms of the effects of countertransference in the recovery process.

In moving beyond empathy in our work with trauma victims, new directions for future research are evident. First, the programs on countertransference processes are necessary for education, training, supervisory responsibilities, and medical curriculum. Second, scientifically controlled studies of Type I and Type II CTRs are needed to address many research questions pertaining to psychotherapy outcome, the personality styles of the therapist, various types of interaction effects (e.g., client–therapist, gender, age, race, cultural differences, etc.), and much more.

Third, the presence of countertransference in clinical work and research needs to be both "normalized" and made "normative" because these human tendencies are ubiquitous, indigenous, and unavoidable, much in the same ways as are PTSD symptoms following trauma. In this regard, countertransference to traumatized persons is part a complementary process that may hinder or facilitate the integration of the experience for the client. Finally, new directions for the future are discussed as an outgrowth of this project and the findings it has uncovered.

13

When Disaster Strikes: Managing Emotional Reactions in Rescue Workers

BEVERLEY RAPHAEL
JOHN P. WILSON

The occurrence of violent and traumatic incidents may create powerful affective responses in those who rescue, care for, and counsel the individuals directly affected. These helpers are likely to respond both with their own feelings about the event and to the feelings and experience of those who have been direct victims. Some of these feelings will be dominated by realities, some by social and cultural perceptions about behavior, and some by internalized templates reflecting the helper's own past experience and psychodynamics.

Massive community catastrophes and disasters have a further dimension. They are, by definition, overwhelming to the community's resources and response capacity, at least temporarily. They may reflect the awesome, unpredictable, or uncontrollable forces of nature, or the farthest extremes of human negligence or maleficence. Individuals will respond not only with their own personal perceptions and reactions, but with those determined by the cultural and social context of the affect community (Raphael, 1986).

As a society, we delegate the various trauma-specific roles such as warning, protecting, reassuring, and comforting to individuals or groups located on or called to the disaster scene. Sometimes these persons are carefully trained and professional rewarded for their roles (fireman, policeman, emergency medical squads), sometimes they are volunteers; and sometimes these roles are taken on spontaneously by others on the trauma scene.

Regardless of category, these persons are stepping into intense, trauma-specific roles that place them in contact and interaction both the disaster itself and with disaster victims. Interactions at the disaster scene are intense and may be critical for survival. They are complex, requiring instant decisions of a life-saving or life-endangering nature, leading to powerful and long-lasting affective reactions in the rescue worker. For purposes of this chapter we use the term *rescue worker* in its more generic sense to include all on-site, disaster-specific helping roles: those who warn (such as seismologists and air traffic controllers), those who protect (such as firemen, policemen, engineers, city planners), those who rescue (such as firemen, policemen, emergency medics, life squads), and those who comfort (Red Cross, clergy, mental health professionals). Each of these roles in a given disaster may be carried out by professionals, by community volunteers, or may be spontaneously carried out by others on the disaster scene (including survivors).

Seen in this light, almost all survivors at some point take on or wish to take on rescue roles as part of their own trauma experience. They want to warn and protect others less fortunate than themselves, they want to save or rescue those who may perish, and they want to comfort those in pain and those whose loss is clear. As they later process their own survivor experiences these roles and their performance of them comes under closer scrutiny. In fact, one problem in empathy for therapists of survivors in general is to understand that even enormous personal loss may feel less important at times than the survivor's own sense of failure to rescue someone else.

NINE DYNAMIC THEMES COMMON
TO RESCUE WORK

In this chapter we examine several dimensions or dynamic themes in the disaster experience that affect those who take on the rescue worker role: force and destruction, confrontation with death, helplessness, anger, loss, attachments, elation, and guilt. Each of these is an emotional component of the disaster experience itself; and each evokes strong affective reactions in the rescue worker who attempts to contain the affect by disaster-specific defenses. The resultant strain may tax rescue workers beyond their limits, leading temporarily to actions and behaviors outside the bounds of their rescue (helping) roles and/or producing symptoms that interfere with function and relationships in the months that follow the disaster. These out-of-role behaviors and helper-role-induced symptoms meet the central criteria for what we are calling *countertransference* in the trauma context, although of course, the rescue worker is (under most circumstances) not a mental health professional, and the rescue worker–victim relationship is not a psychotherapeutic one.

For those who educate disaster workers, knowledge of these powerful disaster-specific affective reactions and likely countertransference responses (CTRs) to them is indispensable.

Force and Destruction

The massive nature of community disasters, and the *force and destruction* involved—the disruption of the solidity of the earth in earthquakes, the ripping apart of mountains in volcanic eruptions, the torrential forces of floods, the force of wind of tornados—is likely to create feelings of "primeval" terror. Workers, as well as those directly affected, speak of how they have been overawed by the massiveness of physical destruction after earthquakes, forest fires, hurricanes, and volcanic eruptions, to name a few. Both rescuers and direct victims are awestruck by the spectacle of cities, forests, or farms laid to waste. Infantile fantasies of omnipotent destructiveness may also lurk close to the surface, leading to defensive avoidance, denial, or excessive and driven attempts at restitution or renewal for the affected community (Wolfenstein, 1957).

Confrontation with Death

Disasters also mean *confrontation with death* and, in many instances, with massive, gruesome, and mutilating deaths. The senseless, untimely deaths of children, the young, even the old, often occur in the absence of human dignity, of opportunity for goodbyes, finalization, and culturally defined rites for the dead. "Mass" deaths take meaning in numbers—many persons are killed—but the "number" of dead may seem to diminish the significance of the death of the individual. *Immersion in death* or *death overload* are terms that can be used to describe the way in which victims and rescuers may be overwhelmed by such extensive death (Lifton, 1967; Pine, 1974). The degree to which bodies are mutilated, gruesome, unrecognizable, charred, or incinerated may add further to the stress experienced by rescuers, even those formally trained to deal with body parts, such as disaster victim identification teams (Taylor & Frazer, 1982). Regardless of training, or hardening, or "blooding" to prepare workers to deal with this level of exposure to death, the extent of deaths, the involvement of children or those known to the workers, and the destruction of the humanity of those who were living but are now dead are all too real. Numerous workers also speak of the enormity of "row after row of grey bodies" in morgues after disaster, and even the ordering and cleaning of the dead is not protective (Titchener & Lindy, 1980). Where time has elapsed and putrefaction has occurred—for instance, at Jonestown—the impact of the smell and decaying human flesh will be overwhelming and leave the rescuers not only with a sense of futility, but with readily triggered memories of smells and sights they would rather not have experienced (Jones, 1985). The disaster literature abounds with descriptions of the impact of such exposure on workers and the possible longer-term effects for some in the development of both traumatic stress reactions and disorder.

Clearly such confrontation with death must not only bring distressing affects and the need to process the experience cognitively and affectively, but it is also a confrontation with the worker's own mortality, the mortality of his loved ones, and of human society. Outcomes vary with individual dynamics and sanctioned social response. For example, "black" humor is a frequent mechanism to deal with the horror, as is dehumanizing the bodies, treating them as "meat" when there is no humanity left in the remains. On the other hand, there are also efforts to preserve human dignity. Recent measures with the recovery of bodies after a North Sea oil rig disaster highlighted how positive it was for those working with the bodies to have their own body/person (the deceased) as a focus for a caring reconstitution of human remains (Alexander & Wells, 1991). Thus, the prosocial act of caring for dead coworkers gave some sense of meaning to the tragedy.

Following disasters, some rescuers describe the way in which confrontation with death has not only reminded them of their own vulnerability, but of the value and importance of life and relationships. They have reevaluated their own lives and reinvested their emotional commitment in family relationships and in the achievement of worthwhile goals. Such responses have been identified even after such traumatic events as a major rail disaster (Raphael, Singh, & Bradbury, 1980), a football stadium fire (Shapiro & Kunkler, 1990), a number of natural catastrophes, and the recent Gulf War (Easton & Turner, 1991).

The rescuers' own fears, death overload, or traumatization by images of death may lead to numbing, denial, or avoidance of everything to do with death or, alternately, a driven preoccupation with death, reflecting failing attempts to master this fear. Themes of intense terror, or confrontation with death, may also reverberate with an anxious vulnerability related to childhood experiences of trauma, deprivation of attachments, and difficulties with affect modulation and control.

Helplessness

Feelings of *helplessness* are also prominent for all those who deal with catastrophe. Just as there may be primitive terror in reaction to the overwhelming forces and destruction, so also there may be a recognition of the helplessness of humanity or the self to counter these forces. Such helplessness is further reinforced by the encounter with death. And the rescuers are frequently confronted with inability to carry out the rescue procedures for which they are prepared because of the nature of the disaster, or the relative or actual inadequacy of equipment and techniques (Hodgkinson & Stewart, 1991). Workers frequently report one of the most stressful factors in their experience is their "frustration" that they cannot achieve more. This sense of helplessness may be particularly difficult to come to terms with for those whose personality and training gear them to be action oriented, because much of their self-esteem may depend on successful achievement of their professional tasks. Mitchell and Bray (1990) and other researchers suggest this is a significant pattern for emergency service workers. A further issue is that the shock and trauma of this event may paralyze effective coping so that workers do not fulfill roles for which they are technically competent, and they may suffer substantial guilt afterwards, thereby reinforcing the likelihood of developing morbidity (Hodgkinson & Stewart, 1991). They also may feel that they did not do all they could, and that their actions were inappropriate. While this is sometimes the case, cognitive distortions, including the perception of time, that often occur in such situations may lead people to wrongly believe there were more opportunities than actually existed.

Themes of power and helplessness are likely to reverberate with other social roles defined by the disaster, such as rescue/helpers being powerful and victims being helpless. Workers need to be educated to avoid reinforcing destructive stereotypes of this kind and the feelings of personal inadequacy and grandiose omnipotence that may be associated with them.

During a devastating tornado, members of a hospital emergency room were looking after scores of residents who had been struck by debris, trapped in falling buildings, and witnessed other terrifying experiences that had resulted in death to others. Meanwhile, no electronic communication outside the hospital was possible, and emergency workers had to suppress their fears for their families who were in the path of the storm in order to tend to others. They said nothing to each other about their own fears. Afterwards, symptoms related to anxiety, especially around separations, persisted. None of the workers had connected the symptoms to their experience of helplessness during the tornado until a mental health intervention months later.

Anger

Another common affect is *anger.* This may relate to confrontation with loss of the sense of personal invulnerability. The reality of disasters, even when one is trained, brings a recognition that the individual and his or her loved ones can be affected. There is often both realistic anger and also anger related to projections that more was not done to warn, prevent, stop, or mitigate the effect of the catastrophe—"they" should have handled it differently. In the post-impact phase, this anger often seeks a focus, therefore, scapegoating of workers, systems, authorities, and individuals may occur, which satisfies the intrapsychic demands for control (Raphael, 1986). Rescue workers in a small town in Iowa who had traveled from a nearby city were greeted with hostility by families whose homes and stores had been destroyed by a killer tornado. Residents were cordoned off from their own homes, and they believed that the out-of-town rescuers were lighting matches near exposed and leaking gas lines. They thought that these outsiders were going to blow up their already decimated town.

Anger in rescuers may follow the same course it does in those who are directly affected, particularly in regards to blaming "them"; "they" did not prevent it, and so forth. The rescuer may be drawn into empathic rage toward authorities, those to blame, or those scapegoated, rather than face the reality that the disaster could not be prevented and cannot be undone. Anger may be displaced onto equipment, and/or technical failure as well. The rescuer may fear being overwhelmed by his anger, or he or she may withdraw into bland or technical detail and deny the directly affected person's need to release emotion in a nondistorted way.

Loss

Most disasters bring significant *loss,* including personal, property, community, and symbolic losses. *Grief* is thus a prominent affect, although the initial shock and numbness and the mobilization for rescue, recovery, and survival may block its appearance. Rescuers may be intimately involved with the affected community and may thus suffer personal loss from the disaster. They may find or attempt to rescue friends and even family members, or see the destruction of personal or community property. Such grief is direct and easy to understand. Workers may have to set it aside because of the demands of their tasks and may have difficulty in releasing it subsequently. Grief may also occur over the loss of one of their group as a result of the disaster-related activities. Such line-of-duty deaths are especially poignant, reflecting as they do the loss of a friend and workmate, but they also symbolically pose a potential threat to the self and the group.

The losses of the disaster may reawaken old grief for the worker, with the corresponding need to work it through. Generally, however, workers experience an *identificatory empathy*, grieving for the human condition for other human beings devastated by this event, and for themselves within this context. Although workers can bear this, there are sometimes deep burdens of suffering, especially if they have dealt with many such events. A "macho" approach is often expected in terms of workplace ethos; therefore, these feelings may be difficult to acknowledge. Instead, they are defended against by black humor or defensive denial and avoidance of feeling-related issues.

Loss often evokes distancing, because of the recognition of the possibilities of losing one's own loved ones, or it elicits a numbing affect and an incapacity to recognize or respond to the grief of the survivors. Jerry, a hardened, loyal member of a firemen's unit had the task of removing two bodies after a nightclub fire. They were a couple in their 70s (who had come to celebrate an anniversary). The couple had recognized that escape was impossible so they fell prone on the floor, to avoid asphyxiation as long as possible, then clenched their hands together waiting for death. To remove their bodies, Jerry had to saw their hands apart. As Jerry carried out his task he thought sadly of his own parents who had recently died and his pending divorce with his wife, which left him shattered. But soon a numbing wall fell over him; he avoided debriefing efforts. He later entered psychotherapy, which is described in more detail in Chapter 3.

Loss may also produce an overinvolvement with the bereaved and enmeshment in their grief, or reawakened grief and loss related to the rescuer's own life. A common problem is the excessive preoccupation with material loss and replacement, leading to denial, by both rescuer and rescued, of the need to deal with grief.

Attachments

One of the areas that is as yet insufficiently recognized in the literature yet that powerfully affects rescuers is that of *attachments* and *relationships*. Strong bonds bind rescue teams together, even more so when they face threat, deal with highly distressing tasks, or achieve major goals together. As evidenced in the post-disaster, "therapeutic community" effect, normal society barriers may vanish, so that special closeness develops for those who have "been through" this together (Raphael, 1986; Wilson & Raphael, 1993). Special bonds may also develop between rescuer and rescuee, especially if there has been prolonged, difficult contact during the rescue process. These "special" relationships may simply be that, but if their relationship to the emotional experience of the catastrophe is not understood, those involved may carry this specialness with them subsequently in ways that are threatening to intimate and family relationships or even other workplace ties. This effect may be heightened if there has been dislocation from home and family to a foreign place where emotional reactions to the disaster and to the alien culture may push workers to form close bonds. It is not difficult to understand that ordinary, everyday relationships may pale in comparison. Again debriefing models may be useful to assist people to talk of their experiences and their closeness and to let go of some of this for reengagement with their families and everyday lives. Some debriefing programs also provide for stress faced by spouses, who often feel excluded both because of these bonds and the fact that they were not there and cannot know what it was really like, especially if their loved ones are unable to share the experience with them. This is why it is most important that communication with families is provided so that workplace relationships with workmates do not supersede primary family ties.

Elation

Elation and triumph are emotions that are not usually associated with the trauma, loss, and death of a disaster. Nevertheless they frequently occur and need to be understood. A volunteer pastor had been working with families as they tried to identify next of kin at a large temporary morgue. He had worked for 20 hours without break. Speaking to no one in particular he began moving his legs in the air as if climbing. Looking skyward he said he could do the Lord's work forever, never again would he need rest.

Survival in the face of massive destruction evokes feelings of elation that it was not oneself who died, even if such feelings are only transitory, and almost immediately replaced by shock, guilt, anger, shame, or grief. This elation may be more prolonged where there is a sense of achievement about tasks well done, lives saved, death defeated. It may merge into a euphoria and celebration of life—even to the extent of joyous release and sexual behavior, for a small proportion of people, usually the young.

Shortly after personally walking through aisles and warning nearly 2,000 patrons in a supper club that they must act quickly to evacuate their building, a bus boy received intense media attention for his heroism. Within days he was being praised by the President of the United States. His hypomanic state lasted for months, resulting in severe difficulties in relationships and at work. At a deeper level, the elation, or even feelings of triumph, may relate not only to survival in the face of the deaths of others but a sense of vicarious indulgence of omnipotent destructive fantasies (Wolfenstein, 1957).

Survivor Guilt

Where elation or triumph have been experienced a common reaction, countertransference or otherwise, is *survivor guilt*. This leads to depressive, self-blaming, despairing, or counterresponsive reparative behaviors that are excessive and do little to resolve the emotional reaction underlying them.

Tim, an air traffic controller, was praised as hero after half of the passengers in a commercial jet aircraft crash were saved. In the aftermath, Tim dwelled on those of his actions during the disaster that he felt were less than perfect; the more he was praised, the more guilty he felt for the deaths. He became depressed and alienated from his wife, and he changed career paths, grimly seeking to help families suddenly bereaved. He did all this without relief from his attempts at atonement. None of these reactions made sense until he sought psychotherapy over a year later.

Survivor guilt arises secondarily from a number of different themes discussed. Rescue workers feel helpless that they cannot do more to save victims and are prone to guilt. Rescue workers enjoy the euphoria of intense, close, and successful work in the life and death situation, but later they feel guilt about such feelings in the presence of awesome death and destruction. Rescue workers feel guilty when their own decisions, actions, or omissions unintentionally increased the death toll. And finally, some rescue workers feel a more existential guilt when they realize that they are alive and their comrades are dead.

Voyeurism

Certain themes are not easily accepted, but are also part of the reality of the human psyche. Those who flock to the scene of disaster are often called "ghouls" by the media. They too may be attempting to master their fears of death and their own destructiveness, yet may be condemned because they reflect an aspect of the human condition that we cannot readily accept in ourselves. (see Chapter 1).

Special dynamics are likely to be evoked when the disaster is a consequence of human maleficence. Fear of human destructiveness, when confronted by its outcome as in the case of those who released survivors from the concentration camps, may be overwhelming. It may lead to disgust, anger, denial, wishes for revenge, attempts at restitution, and even hatred of the self as a representative of humanity. The needs for vengeance and justice may override logic and can lead to further cycles of destructiveness unless these issues are recognized, dealt with openly, and, as far is possible, worked through, or unless some constructive and adaptive processes are sought. There is clear evidence from a range of disaster studies that psychological morbidity is likely to be greater after such events, probably because of these and other factors (Raphael, 1986).

MENTAL HEALTH INTERVENTION WITH THE RESCUE WORKER

The above dynamic themes are likely to be differentially present, depending on the nature of the catastrophe and the particular elements of destruction, death, loss, and human intervention. Recognizing their significance both potentially and realistically is essential for those who wish to manage or to assist with the emotional reactions of rescue workers.

Significant social movements have evolved supporting the value of a preventive approach to assist with such reactions and to prevent negative outcomes. Raphael (1977) described a program of psychological debriefing for rescue workers affected by a rail disaster. Mitchell (1983) developed the concept of *critical incident stress debriefing* (CISD), which has become widely utilized in the United States and many other countries. This work proposed a formal, specific mental health intervention to assist workers in dealing with their reactions to critical incidents or disasters. Dunning (1988) has reviewed the various models of "debriefing," which propose interventions to support rescue workers in dealing with their psychological reactions to disasters. These models all operate on the hypothesis that workers are distressed and at risk of psychological morbidity as a consequence of stress experienced in their work, in terms of the traumatic stress reactions.

Morbidity in Rescue Workers

Studies in the United States, Australia, the United Kingdom, and Scandinavia all substantiate the significant impact of disaster stressors on workers. Studies of workers after a rail disaster (Raphael, Singh, Bradbury, & Lambert, 1983–1984) showed that 81% experienced the work as stressful, with 70% showing some strain (symptoms like PTSD). Jones (1985) showed that 32% of the Air Force workers involved in body recovery from Jonestown developed dysphoric reactions. After the Hyatt Regency skywalk collapse, Wilkinson (1983) found that intrusive phenomena, sleep disturbance, and impaired function occurred in more than 40% of rescuers and victims. Large-scale studies of voluntary fire fighters after Australian forest fires showed high levels of disorder even 4 years later, with up to 20% being affected by PTSD. Numerous other studies (e.g., Ersland, Weisaeth, & Sund, 1980; Hytten & Hasle, 1989) also report significant levels of stress reaction in rescue workers. Clearly these levels of morbidity require management both on humane and health care grounds.

Nature of Interventions Utilized

Debriefing intervention systems propose a brief, time-limited focus as the central postulate for psychosocial interventions. These interventions propose a range of phases typified by opening, review, affective working through, and closing. The debriefings are usually carried out in groups comprised of those who have been through the same experience and involve varying levels of educational, directive, psychological/psychotherapeutic, and nondirective methods. Clearly, and as demanded by their proponents, mental health expertise is required by those who carry out such debriefing and need to include knowledge of trauma responses. Models, specifically Mitchell and Bray's (1990), also proposed the involvement of peer support persons.

The earlier models, which utilized a brief intervention focused on the immediate post-disaster period (24–48–72 hours), have been replaced by a broader approach. These earlier methods relied very heavily on military psychiatry models of proximity, immediacy, and expectancy. Although these methods are still used, it is widely recognized that these brief, focused interventions may not be adequate for many people and that delayed or highly personal responses, as well as prolonged effects, call for a more broadly based program. Thus most groups providing intervention now acknowledge and promote the possible need for repeat debriefings over time, plus individualized counseling or referral to specialized care, as well as pre-disaster education and training (Alexander & Wells, 1991; Raphael, 1991; Shapiro & Kunkler, 1990).

As experience has grown, formats have been altered to meet individual needs. The concept of a "safety net" of support and working-through programs, including organizational management, pre-disaster education and training, and post-disaster debriefing and counseling, now appears to be the norm. It is supported by the finding of more positive outcomes for such an approach (e.g., Alexander & Wells, 1991).

These "preventive" interventions are aimed at education, in that most provide information about normal reactions to traumatic events. They also promote review to assist cognitive processing, and they frequently encourage emotional catharsis, although the degree to which this occurs may vary significantly. Effectiveness and goals are discussed below.

Other interventions are also provided to rescue and other disaster workers who may be suffering from their emotional reactions or the development of psychiatric complications. These range from brief counseling programs, usually in crisis intervention models that concentrate on current problems, positive coping, and working through of feelings, to complex psychotherapeutic and behavioral programs for treating developed disorders such as PTSD (e.g., trauma psychotherapy and trauma desensitization by Kleber & Brom, 1987). Rapid eye movement reprocessing (Wolpe & Abrams, 1991) is a behavioral technique described as being successful for some people with established PTSD, but, like most other treatments in this field, it requires further controlled trials.

Effectiveness of Intervention

Sadly, despite widespread utilization of the above methods there has been little systematic examination of their effectiveness. Recent reviews show that, although those evaluations that have taken place suggest that interventions are generally perceived as helpful, this is not so in many instances, and in some cases they are perceived negatively (Raphael, 1991). Thus follow-up of the Hillsborough disaster debriefing programs found that many did not attend, although those who did found them helpful. The more distressed seemed more likely to attend, but their attendance did not necessarily lessen their distress and they were still often prone to long-term distress and related problems (Shapiro & Kunkler, 1990). These findings are similar to those of Hytten and Hasle (1989), who found that when several members of a group who had debriefing were compared with a similar group who had not, there was little difference in distress and intrusive phenomena as measured by the Impact of Events Scale at 6-month follow-up. There are, however, many general reports of the helpfulness of these programs, both in the opportunity they provide for talking through what has happened and sharing it with others who have been through the same thing and the lessening of preoccupation and distress that many report. The provision of debriefing programs also symbolizes the care and concern of the organization and may have value simply in that light.

Reviews of recent work (Raphael, 1991) indicate the degree to which organizational and preparatory measures are important. Duration of shifts, tasks and their value, debriefing on a regular basis, and adequate preparation and training all seem to make a difference to outcome and should be incorporated into programs. This means a sensitive and knowledgeable appraisal by mental health professionals with relevant trauma, organizational, disaster,and dynamic understandings is critical for planning and management of programs for rescue workers and others likely to be affected post-disaster.

Goals and Interventions

Goals and interventions are often poorly defined. They need to address the fact that the event will not be forgotten and will often be a reference point in the individual's life. People and organizations need to gain a sense of mastery, even in retrospect, to integrate their experience into their lives, and to become able to move on from it with appropriate emotional learning and maturation. As indicated earlier, this is often not easy to do. Disaster work may produce a "high," a sense of being the only worthwhile work one has done, and a sense of highly meaningful, personal involvement with intense attachments different from the normal, daily relationships of life. It is often difficult for rescue workers to "hand over" to be affected community, or to other workers, the responsibility for recovery. Interventions need to be sensitive to and deal with not only the need for mastery but also integration of the experience into the significant past. It is often quite difficult for workers to relinquish what has been for them, despite the trauma, so involving and rewarding. Interventions and activities, including social rituals, need to promote recognition of what has been achieved, while at the same time moving rescuers and others towards some sense of completion about the disaster.

Rescue workers, together with other survivors, play an important role in designing and participating in special group level ceremonies honoring the dead in a given disaster. Rescue workers at Sioux Falls, Iowa, arranged with survivors of a plane crash to return to the site a year later for memorial activities. Employees of a supper club fire joined with rescue workers and the community at large to sponsor a concert benefiting children orphaned by the fire; rescue workers supported families who honored those dead in a Honduran Bronx social club arson by a special mother's day ceremony.

Other Factors

Rescue fantasies are significant motivating dynamics for many in the helping professions and in rescue work. These may relate to a wish to rescue
others whom the rescuer as a child could not help (e.g., a sick, abused
parent) or to rescue wounded parts of the self, which the worker identifies
as those he or she assists. Thus when rescue is frustrated, problems may
arise, and awaken anxiety, and anger, and/or withdrawal related to these
earlier themes. Similarly overinvolvement may reflect inner desperation
concerned with undoing the past as well as the realities of the current
challenge.

Those specifically involved with *counseling* may face difficulties at
several levels. The person being helped may be of the same social class and
background as the counselor. Sick and noncoping persons such as those
who traditionally present to care systems for counseling are less likely to
be encountered. Thus these "protective" influences, which reinforce social distance and social role between "sick" and helper, may be diminished. Also there is a lessening of social boundary and role definition in the
post-disaster period. The massiveness of the loss/death/destruction occurring to people with whom the counselor identifies may add greatly to the
personal experience of empathy, and to the likelihood of being overwhelmed by feelings of identification with the victims.

Helping roles and their purpose may be poorly defined. For all these
reasons helpers may be overwhelmed by threatening empathic identifications, and they may lack their usual professional roles in regular counseling settings, which more clearly define how to respond. They may struggle
to deny their human response, seeing it as nonprofessional, but feel their
professional response to be totally inadequate to the magnitude of what
has occurred. Thus, in these settings, some helpers may run the risk of
CTRs dominated by enmeshment and overinvolvement or, alternatively,
withdrawal, avoidance, and denial of the victim's need. In a situation of
acute trauma, the modulation of human and compassionate response with
a caring, supportive, and dynamically aware interaction with those affected requires high levels of personal maturity, professional competence,
and safety and security in one's own inner psychic world (see Chapters 1
and 2, this volume).

Rescuers/helpers at all levels need not only special educational preparation for their roles that takes full account of the issues outlined above,
but also administrative back-up that provides support structures. These
latter must provide for limited tours of duty, debriefing at the end of each
tour, opportunities for case review and referral, periods of relief and
release, and for finalization of the work by rescuer. Report writing, research, and recommendations about appropriate future responses should

be gleaned from workers, as these are not only helpful for future disaster management, but also allow the workers the value of testifying about, documenting, and learning from their own experience.

COUNTERTRANSFERENCE IN THOSE HELPING THE HELPERS

The countertransference issues confronting those who help the helpers, for instance, in providing debriefing, have not been discussed. Nevertheless, they warrant consideration. The same dynamics of destruction, death, helplessness, loss, anger, triumph, and guilt may confront, secondhand, the debriefer or counselor helping rescue workers. The horror of shared images may evoke post-traumatic phenomena in those who hear them secondhand, so it is not surprising that countertransference issues occur. The structure of traditional debriefing may provide some protection, but it also holds the danger of feeling omnipotent and denying any effects of others' distressing experience on the self. Group process understanding is important, as otherwise countertransference issues may interfere with leadership and appropriate group and individual outcomes. Overload of particular debriefings or numbers of debriefings may also occur. Specific understanding of the dynamics of trauma response, transference, and countertransference surrounding the "telling" of the trauma story, of victim–helper dynamics, and survivorship are important. Empowerment and mastery are also critical issues, as well as the value of activities vis-à-vis fantasy and the relevance of each to therapeutic outcomes. Clearly working with rescue workers, not themselves identified patients or clients in many instances, is complex and challenging. Thus education, case review, debriefing of the debriefers need also to be available as has in fact, occurred in many recent disaster responses.

SOME PSYCHOLOGICAL DISASTER SYNDROMES

The *disaster syndrome* is familiar to workers in the field. Although not prevalent in all disasters, this syndrome needs to be understood, as it affects direct victims and may also affect rescue and other workers. In this syndrome, individuals are stunned and may wander the scene of devastation, apparently nonresponsive to stimuli and unaware of personal danger. This state of numbness may last minutes, hours, or days, and it may seriously interfere with functioning and decision making. The person may need to be protected and cared for. Reports of this type of response or related patterns of psychological withdrawal have been described when workers are overwhelmed by the destruction and devastation. Such responses may be more likely for those suffering "culture shock" or a sense of depersonalization in the face of strange places, the loss of familiar cues, helplessness, and inability to communicate in relevant languages. For instance, after a South American earthquake, volunteers from the United States arriving to help with rescue operations were overwhelmed, withdrew into their own accommodations, and had to be looked after by locals. Similar reactions have been described in other such settings.

The *counterdisaster syndrome* is an intense and continuing overinvolvement with disaster roles. It seems particularly likely to occur in disaster managers. It is reflected in a failure to give responsibility to others and a sense that one is indispensable, that the disaster cannot be managed if one steps down, and that nobody else can replace one's understanding or expertise. Frequently the person will demonstrate excessive activity, will be unwilling to sleep or hand over responsibility at the end of a duty roster, and will wish to control even the smallest detail. This may be associated with the "high" that is present in all disaster workers, but which in this case seems to continue as a supercharge until ultimately the person's efficiency is diminished and judgments are impaired; further research could explore this issue. Some workers need to be relieved of duty sensitively, or angry confrontations may arise, leaving the person, who felt they were contributing so much, hurt and offended. Again, training, administration and strict handover, debriefing, delegation, and review can help prevent this. Conversely, studying the reaction of rescue workers is enormously useful to psychotherapists of trauma survivors of all types. Therapists are unconsciously cast into one or more of these trauma-specific roles during the course of therapy (warning, protecting, rescuing, comforting). Trauma-specific transferences take the shape of these helping relationships and countertransferences portray powerful responses evoked in the helper at the time.

CONCLUSIONS

Disasters are always "special" for those who are involved and will always leave an impression and be something of a reference point. If rescuers and other workers are educated in the issues outlined above and organizational and administrative systems provide structure, support, recognition, and care for workers, it will be more likely that this powerful psychological experience will be meaningfully integrated into the worker's life—without undue pain but with appropriate compassion for the human suffering that was involved.

REFERENCES

Alexander, D. A., & Wells, A. (1991). Reactions of police officers to body handling after a major disaster: A before and after comparison. *British Journal of Psychiatry, 159,* 547–555.

Dunning, C. (1988). Intervention strategies for emergency workers. In M. Lystad (Ed.), *Mental health response to mass emergencies.* New York: Brunner/Mazel.

Easton, J. A., & Turner, S. W. (1991). Detention of British citizens as hostages in the Gulf—Health, psychological and family consequences. *British Medical Journal, 303,* 1231–1234.

Ersland, S., Weisaeth, L., & Sund, A. (1980). The stress upon rescuers involved in an oil rig disaster: "Alexander L. Kielland." *Acta Psychiatrica Scandinavica Supplementum, 355,* 38–49.

Hodgkinson, P. E., & Stewart, M. (1991). *Coping with catastrophes: A handbook of disaster management.* London: Routledge.

Hytten, K., & Hasle, A. (1989). Firefighters: A study of stress and coping. *Acta Psychiatrica Scandinavica, 80,* 50–55.

Jones, D. R. (1985). Secondary disaster victims: The emotional effects of recovering and identifying human remains. *American Journal of Psychiatry, 142,* 303–307.

Kleber, R. J., & Brom, D. (1987). Psychotherapy and pathological grief: Controlled outcome study. *Israeli Journal of Psychiatry and Related Sciences, 24,* 99–109.

Lifton, R. J. (1967). *Death in life: Survivors of Hiroshima.* New York: Random House.

Mitchell, J., & Bray, G. (1990). *Emergency services stress: A Brady book.* Englewood Cliffs, NJ: Prentice-Hall.

Mitchell, J. (1983). When disaster strikes: The critical incident stress debriefing process. *Journal of Emergency Medical Services, 8*(1), 36–39.

Pine, V. R. (1974). Grief work and dirty work: The aftermath of an aircrash. *Omega, 5,* 281–286.

Taylor, A. J. W., & Frazer, A. G. (1982). The stress of post-disaster body handling and victim identification work. *Journal of Human Stress, 8*(December), 4–12.

Raphael, B. (1991). Psychological problems of rescuers and other disaster emergency personnel [Editorial]. *British Medical Journal, 159,* 555–560.

Raphael, B. (1986). *When disaster strikes.* New York: Basic Books.

Raphael, B. (1977). The Granville train disaster: Psychological needs and their management. *Medical Journal of Australia, 1,* 303–305.

Raphael, B., Singh, B., & Bradbury, L. (1980). Disaster: The helper's perspective. *Medical Journal of Australia, 2,* 445–447.

Raphael, B., Singh, B., Bradbury, L., & Lambert, F. (1983–1984). Who helps the helpers? The effects of a disaster on the rescue workers. *Omega, 14*(1), 9–20.

Shapiro, D., & Kunkler, J. (1990). *Psychological support for hospital staff initiated by clinical psychologists in the aftermath of the Hillsborough disaster.* Sheffield, England: Clinical Psychology, Northern General Hospital.

Titchener, J. L., & Lindy, J. D. (1980). *Affect defense and insight: Psychoanalytic observations of bereaved families and clinicians at a major disaster.* Unpublished manuscript, University of Cincinnati.

Wilkinson, C. B. (1983). Aftermath of a disaster: The collapse of the Hyatt Regency Hotel skywalk. *American Journal of Psychiatry, 140,* 1134–1139.

Wilson, J., & Raphael, B. (Eds.). (1993). *The international handbook of traumatic stress syndromes.* New York: Plenum Press.

Wolfenstein, M. (1957). *Disaster: A psychological essay.* Glencoe, IL: Free Press.

Wolpe, J., & Abrams, J. (1991). Post-traumatic stress disorder overcome by eye-movement desensitization: A case report. *Journal of Behavior Therapy and Experimental Psychiatry, 22,* 39–43.

14

Trauma and Countertransference in the Workplace

CHRISTINE DUNNING

In this chapter we examine trauma in the workplace. We emphasize the emotional reactions of fellow workers, supervisors, and others whose roles are to document the traumatic event and assist the worker's recovery. In this regard, the nature of countertransference processes will be cast in a new light and expanded to include a new area of research in the field of traumatic stress studies.

The context of trauma recovery is a broad one. In managing PTSD, as in other areas of community mental health, those who first discover and evaluate persons temporarily impaired by emotional stress are often not formally trained mental health professionals. For example, they may be teachers, police, or other "gatekeepers" to the mental health system. In the workplace, such roles are taken by supervisors, coworkers, and investigators. For a traumatized person, these reactions, either supportive or newly traumatizing, have enormous impact on the future course of recovery.

As in the case of disaster rescue workers (see Chapter 13, this volume), we are considering countertransference broadly to include emotional reactions evoked in those directly or indirectly (vicariously) exposed to the trauma, especially those whose regular and expected tasks in the workplace could facilitate or hamper the recovery process.

It is the purpose of this chapter to examine how trauma that occurs in the context of the workplace affects the employee, his or her colleagues, and the organization as a whole. We contend that organizations and their representatives in supervisory roles often manifest strong rational and irrational reactions. Some of these reactions, such as contempt, minimizing, and blame, impair recovery. As such, some reactions may be considered forms of countertransference to the traumatized colleague, who may have been injured or killed at the worksite or elsewhere.

Workplaces vary in the degree to which exposure to hazardous conditions may place the individual at risk for experiencing or witnessing life-threatening or bodily mutilating events. Thus, office work in an urban setting might be low on the scale; manufacturing jobs that use large equipment might be higher, work with known toxic substances higher still; while police, firefighters, and members of the military accept hazardous duty as an expectable part of the job description. Emergency medical technicians and workers in hospital intensive care, trauma, and burn units, although not directly endangered (except by such risks as HIV infection), are especially prone to witnessing trauma, death, and disfigurement in a context so intimate that dealing with vicarious traumatization may be an expectable part of the job description.

Later in this chapter we illustrate strong emotional reactions to work-related trauma in each of these progressively high-risk settings. Case examples show that what is traditionally considered countertransference is not limited to the context of psychotherapy.

Formal access to the mental health care system for those exposed to traumatizing experiences will tend to vary given the nature of the work and the sophistication of the mental health model employed. Low-risk settings may have employee assistance programs not specially attuned to trauma; high-risk settings may have trauma specialists such as mental health consultants who are part of the ongoing management team so that education, briefing, and debriefing are ongoing activities. But in many work settings such consultation and other resources may be totally absent.

With or without formal mental health support, it is coworkers and supervisors who play critical front-line roles in assessing and supporting the trauma survivor and in facilitating recovery.

THE WORKPLACE: AN UNTAPPED RESOURCE IN TRAUMA RECOVERY

Only limited research or literature examines the context of the work situation of the traumatized person as a source of counseling and treatment for post-traumatic sequelae. Most of the literature on post-traumatic therapy has focused on individual and group approaches to trauma resolution, with emphasis on the therapeutic alliance. The inclusion of the family as being central to the treatment of trauma in relation to social support has also been discussed (Figley, 1989). Rarely, however, has the literature examined the impact of work itself—the work environment, colleagues, or superiors—as being central to the perception of trauma, severity of reaction, and likelihood of recovery. This lacuna is surprising because most of us spend the majority of our waking hours in activities associated with work. Indeed, apart from family, no other group provides the individual with a sense of self-worth as do associates at work. The job and those with whom the survivor works are central, not peripheral, to the system in which the trauma victim resolves a traumatic event.

Traumatized workers frequently suffer their greatest debilitation at work. Just as family relationships are affected by post-traumatic reaction, so too are the relationships that one has with those with whom the majority of waking hours are spent, namely, work colleagues. The problems associated with post-traumatic reactions, including difficulty concentrating, short-term memory impairment, hypervigilance, and inability to make decisions, are as problematic at work as at home.

The importance of social support at work as a mitigator of stress has long been recognized in industrial psychology. The human relations school of administration (Likert, 1961, 1967; Mayo, 1933); has contended that supportive behavior by work supervisors can reduce organizational stress dramatically. Kahn and Katz (1960) conducted some of the earliest studies that found that supportive supervision and organizational support from coworkers have considerable stress-reducing effect. In a classic study, Seashore (1954) found that as group cohesiveness increased, anxiety over work-related matters lessened. House (1981) asserts that where efforts at coping and defense fail, social support by supervisor or coworker(s) may alleviate the stress impact on short-term physiological, and behavioral outcomes. Clearly, workers look to those within the work environment to facilitate efforts at defending and coping with stress. This is particularly true when the traumatic event occurs in relation to the job. Whether the traumatic event occurs when traveling to or from employment or as a result of performing within the scope of duty of the job, work trauma is resolved differently than that experienced privately and personally as an outside-work event. The context of work, that is, virtually all aspects of the organization, acts to change and intensify the character of the traumatic experience, as well as providing the venue in which the survivor seeks to understand and resolve the trauma event. Stated somewhat metaphorically, the trauma that occurs at the workplace creates a ripple effect and its wave possesses the power to generate countertransference reactions (CTRs) in fellow workers.

Unique Stressor Qualities in the Workplace

When trauma takes place at work, the event is frequently revisited, especially in the United States, with its high incidence of litigation. The survivors and witnesses to the incident are often subjected to repeated questioning by supervisors, investigators, and health, safety, and insurance reviewers. Beyond these inquiries are depositions as part of lawsuits. Consequently, the circle of vicariously traumatized individuals widens to include others who were not necessarily direct witnesses to the event. The target "patient" might be the physically injured or threatened party; eyewitnesses to the event, such as coworkers or customers; people who may have witnessed a colleague inflicting injuries on others (such as police officers who shoot a criminal); or a common group victimized by violent crime, vehicular accident, or technological disaster.

Traumatic Exposure: High-Risk Jobs

In professions such as police, firefighting, emergency medical response, corrections, or the military, personnel are especially vulnerable to the likelihood of experiencing or witnessing trauma. Jobs in heavy manufacturing, vehicular transport, or chemical handling also are at risk due to increased incidence of accident. Work settings involve the manufacture and use of dangerous chemicals, risk of fire or explosion, or physical work conditions such as deep tunnel worksites, operation of dangerous equipment, or high-altitude construction are also potentially traumatic. The worker is at risk for on-the-job trauma as well as for all the other types of traumatic events that may occur during personal hours outside work, such as violent crime, disaster, and accidents. There is likely to be increased exposure to trauma in workplaces in which there is high transportation use, increased public contact, and increased dependence on safe work procedures, for example, in industries such as nuclear waste management and airline maintenance.

Little is known about the prevalence of psychological damage sustained as a consequence of employment. Although some information could be gleaned from claims filed for disability, Social Security, unemployment, or workers' compensation, no systematic research has documented the existence and prevalence of traumatic, work-related mental disorders. Data potentially indicative of post-trauma behavior, such as increased use of alcohol, tardiness, work absence, hyperaggressivity, and social withdrawal, and of post-trauma symptoms such as chronic pain, sleep disorders, and hypersensitivity to environmental cues have not been systematically examined in relation to a traumatic context. What little documentation exists is generally to be found in sources such as:

1. Court records of those countries that require civil litigation to recover expenses and damages;
2. Crime or medical insurance records that keep track of time, place, and circumstances of the traumatic event if significant to its resolution;
3. Records of employers who choose to document such incidents; and
4. Claims against employment benefits such as workers' compensation or disability or retirement benefits.

Although the number of claims has dramatically increased in the last few years, for the purposes of research, these data are limited in their usefulness because of confidentiality and privacy rights of the individual and the organization, whose interests in exposing or protecting such information may be at odds. As a result, unless a worker who is mentally injured in a work-related setting chooses to pursue action (such as treatment, recovery of lost wages, retraining, redress) or documents injurious situations, it is difficult to discern the full impact of traumatic events on the working population.

In addition to the need for the worker to initiate action to document the work-relatedness of the mental injury, which would then identify the realm of work-induced trauma, research is further hampered by constraints of law regarding the worker's right to pursue such claims. For example, in Florida and Georgia, no rights exists for recovery for mental injuries emanating from accidents (physical threat, witnessing someone being injured or killed) but only for a physical occurrence of a sudden nature (assault, tornado-related building collapse).

Laws covering workers preclude recovery in the majority of cases in which we know traumatic stress reactions are likely to occur. This is especially true when the traumatic sequelae involve behavioral manifestations that are antisocial or disruptive. Hyperaggressivity expressed in verbal confrontations; poor work habits such as tardiness or excessive use of sick leave; alcohol/drug use on the job; and social withdrawal that hampers communication are frequently cited as reasons for discipline and even termination. Yet these same reactions are commonly found to be related to trauma.

Traumatic Exposure and Employee Performance Level

Although issues of performance including employee demeanor, attitude, and behavior may be severely affected by trauma experience, this history is rarely considered in disciplinary and termination proceedings. The trauma experience and its attendant manifestations are not presented as a defense by the employee and are rarely accepted as a defense by an employer in resolving administrative actions addressing work performance. The trauma experience may also be ignored when considering the productivity of the employee. Yet difficulties in concentration and decision making, poor memory, and distractibility are traumatic sequelae that may well affect work performance.

Contrary to what seems to be good managerial sense, the typical response to work trauma (or personal trauma that affects work performance) seems to be left up to supervisors and work colleagues. If the supervisor is responsible and concerned, he or she may pursue such issues as:

1. Installing safety programs that incorporate mental safety and physical safety through training (stress inoculation) and education (informational brochures/posters); these activities instill and restore a *sense of control and safety* in the worker, two issues of importance in resolving trauma litigation (Janoff-Bulman, 1985, 1992); and
2. Instilling social support in the context of work, by developing group cohesiveness, providing employee assistance programs, and conducting formal group support activities.

Special Problems of the Supervisor's Post-Trauma Role

The supervisor's role in trauma recovery is caught in the crosswinds of multiple human, hierarchical, and organizational objectives. Supervisors are likely to be the repositories of powerful trauma-based feelings, especially criticism, guilt, and blame, some of which are also clear manifestations of transference–countertransference reactions. Such CTRs may undercut the potential positive power of social support in the workplace and instead present new hurdles to the recovery process. Supervisors are frequently cast as central to the personal, as well as professional, lives of coworkers. They are thus confronted with both work performance demands and with implementing a more humanitarian way for dealing with employees experiencing psychological problems.

House (1981) found that a good supervisor provides emotional, informational, instrumental, and appraisal support for workers. He further suggests that, like a good therapist, a good supervisor should be warm and empathic. Empathic listening and understanding, as well as a real concern for the worker's welfare, are seen to be important components of effective supervisory support. The likelihood that the supervisor can assume this role depends not only on natural ability but also on the supervisor's life and work experiences, personal values and agendas, and the larger organizational context of the work setting. Whether a supervisor assumes the stance of empathic supporter depends in large part on what management sees as an appropriate role, especially in relation to the organizational responsibilities perceived by administration.

THE ROLE OF EMPATHY AND SOCIAL SUPPORT IN THE WORKPLACE

Individual and group relationships. among coworkers provide the same type of emotional support as families. Indeed, some individuals are more likely to identify coworkers as their closest sources of advice and support than family members. Even without close personal relationships, the work group's attitude can have a major impact on perceptions of competence, self-esteem, and ability. In situations associated with work, the individual is much more likely to look to the work group, work colleagues, or work friends to clarify perceptions of interpretation of events, analysis of responsibility, and review of performance and reaction. Because the family, the therapist, and other sources of support lack information and insight into work norms, values, conditions, and expectations, the worker will turn to his or her colleagues and coworkers for support and integration of the traumatic event. In some instances, coworkers, like supervisors, assume therapeutic functions for the recovering traumatized worker. The healing effect of this alliance is as strong as the worker's perception of need to receive feedback from coworkers and of the coworkers' willingness to perform that role.

THE TRAUMA STORY: DISCLOSURE IN THE WORKPLACE

Others in the work organization have formal responsibility to respond to and assist the traumatized worker; they can also develop an empathic relationship with the worker. A central feature to the development of this relationship is that these individuals expect the worker to tell the *trauma story,* thereby enabling them to fulfill their formal responsibility to respond and/or assist the worker. These positions include persons acting on behalf of the organization or agencies responding with formal responsibility in relation to the trauma. Depending on the extent of contact, the degree of assistance sought, or formal action required, these individuals might be insurance adjusters, human resource personnel, employee assistance program counselors, union representatives, emergency response employees, safety and risk management examiners, and safety/accident investigators. If the traumatized worker is met with blame, disbelief, moral judgments, skepticism, negative evaluations, curiosity, or rejection by any of these participants in the event aftermath, secondary impacts can aggravate the trauma (McCann & Pearlman, 1990a, 1990b). Often these same workers are so affected by the story that they fail to perform their appropriate duties, seeking instead to "save" the traumatized worker, or are so repelled as to inadequately complete tasks related to that worker.

COUNTERTRANSFERENCE IN SUPERVISORY AND INVESTIGATIVE RELATIONSHIPS

The dynamics of the supervisory role suggest that the interactions between supervisor and worker in a work trauma are analogous to those of therapist–patient interactions. Because the trauma, as the focal point of interaction subsequent to the event, is the context of supervisory–subordinate contact, the scene for the potential development of countertransference has been set. Thus, the demand for interactive processes in the supervisory mission makes countertransference almost inevitable. The organization employing the traumatized worker delegates the supervisor to act in different roles such as "diagnostician," "investigator," or counselor. Given the strong relationship between work and the individual (McLean, 1979), it is not surprising that the reaction of the supervisor to the worker is important to the worker and provides a context for confirmation of the meaning of the event for the worker. Clearly, reactions of a positive or negative nature emanating from the supervisor can potentially facilitate or interfere with the process of recovery.

The case illustrations that follow examine trauma in workplaces of increasingly high risk: they involve a warehouse worker, a water treatment plant technician, a forklift operator, police deputies, and staff in surgical and emergency units. In each case the traumatic event reverberated, affecting coworkers, witnesses, helpers, supervisors, and investigators. In these vignettes we focus on the experiences of those people who were secondarily impacted by the trauma, who may have been vicariously traumatized themselves by the event, and who therefore found it difficult because of CTRs to continue to function competently and empathically in their roles. As a result, the traumatized workers' recovery was impaired and the organization became conflicted and less functional.

Case Example One: They Think I'm to Blame

For some time, Mr. A., a conscientious and ambitious warehouse manager/supervisor had been preoccupied with protecting his unit from the impact of higher management policy. He now spent less time orienting new workers than he had previously. After years of an excellent safety record, he had delegated safety orientation to others. At 4:00 A.M., he was awakened at home by a telephone call explaining that Jim, a young man working for Mr. A., was found by the next crew in a refrigerated area, pinned between a forklift and a pallet of ice cream. He was crushed, frozen, and dead. Mr. A. suffered severe guilt after the accidental death. Even though he broke no policies, Mr. A. felt responsible for Jim's death. For 2–3 weeks after the death, he reported paranoid feelings, especially involving what workers and administration were saying about him in relation to the event. Thereafter, when he saw groups of workers talking, he thought they (and the crew who found Jim's body) were talking about him and saying, "There goes Jim's supervisor, it's his fault." In order to avoid these paranoid feelings, he confined himself to his office and avoided the work group. He also discouraged the work group from congregating and talking about the incident among themselves, thus removing both himself and coworkers as a source of support for resolving Jim's traumatic death, a Type I avoidance reaction. Meanwhile, he awoke nightly, reliving the experience of receiving the telephone call at 4:00 A.M. Mr. A. experienced himself as the failed protector regarding Jim's death. He projected his own harsh judgment, that the accident occurred because of his failure, onto others and grew to fear them, and thus isolated himself. In this self-accusatory state, he became unavailable to assist his employees in the psychological task of surviving the trauma. He was not only unable to empathize with their distress; in this Type I CTR, he saw their cohesiveness as dangerous to himself.

Supervisors determine organizational culture and act as facilitators, giving strength and confidence to workers, reinforcing workers' desires to act and do well, to grow through accomplishment, and to become productive and skillful in completing the mission of the organization even after calamity. In withdrawing from the work group subsequent to the traumatic event, Mr. A. ceased to perform those functions, thus impeding an important group process that might otherwise have resolved the trauma. In fact, by interfering in the natural work-group support system, the supervisor's CTRs can thus obstruct the use of the work cohort for social support.

TRAUMATIC CONTAGION WITHIN AN ORGANIZATION

In addition to the primary trauma victim, work trauma often affects others in the workplace. It first draws in the immediate supervisor as the person responsible for both gathering information and determining culpability. Over the course of the investigation, the supervisor is expected to elicit the trauma story in relation to the facts of the incident and to determine the identity of all those involved, not only at the time of the incident but also in the past and future. He or she is then required to assess the situation in relation to the subsequent need for intervention (disciplinary action, training, or revision of equipment or procedures) and to assist in any investigations that might ensue. Both roles, that of empathic listener and determiner of fault, can be influenced by countertransferential feelings of anger because this event happened "on my shift, at my worksite, or because of my workers, thus reflecting on me as a supervisor." Additional influences are frequently stated as contempt for the traumatized worker such as "I've lived through this type of thing before when I worked the 'line' and it didn't bother me, so I reject your whining complaint" (Type I CTR, minimization; see Chapter 2, this volume). But by far the most damaging reaction has to do with the conflict between the neutral stance required of the supervisor and the worker's need to have the supervisor be an empathic listener. This conflict is frequently expressed by the trauma survivor as "employee betrayal" (Lawson, 1987).

Dealing with administrative issues surrounding the traumatic event, such as workers' compensation claims, safety investigations, and insurance benefits, may provoke Type I CTRs, such as denial, avoidance, or counterphobic reactions, in the supervisor, administrator, or others who have an organizational responsibility to hear the trauma story. These CTRs take the form of limiting contact with the worker to verifying facts, completing forms, or participating in administrative, judicial, or safety reviews. Rather than assisting the employee to resolve issues related to the trauma and work, resolution is blocked. Traumatized workers frequently express a sense of being betrayed by the supervisor, administrator, or organization as a whole. When management is uninterested in the condition of the worker or, worse yet, when blame is leveled at the employee for the occurrence of the event or for his or her emotional reaction, the anger associated with the trauma is exacerbated. The assessment of the workplace, of colleagues, and of management as callous or indifferent to the employees' trauma also produces mistrust, anger, resentment, and demoralization.

Case Example Two: Don't Hold Us Accountable for Your Distress

Mr. B. was manager/supervisor of maintenance workers at a water treatment plant. He assigned a team to work on the potentially hazardous task of repairing a leak in a pipeline that carried chlorine gas. In attempting the repair, the workers were exposed to a toxic cloud of chlorine gas but managed to clear the area before the lack of oxygen caused by the leak could overcome them. Despite the lack of physical injuries, one worker, Mike, evidenced post-traumatic stress disorder (PTSD) associated with the event. Plagued with nightmares of being chased and overcome by a gas cloud, Mike became phobic about working in the area of the plant that was traversed by pipelines. Mr. B. listened carefully to Mike's trauma story and his plea that he needed psychological help with his panic attacks. Mr. B. felt torn. On the one hand, he wanted to be supportive of Mike and his need for help; on the other, he needed to protect management from culpability. Other workers, using denial, were minimizing their own symptoms; why couldn't Mike? Further, legal advice to the company cautioned against letting word of the leak get out to local residents who might become alarmed and begin class action proceedings. Mike pressed Mr. B. to have the company pay for his treatment. Mr. B., driven by his wishes to minimize and his allegiance to the higher directives, convinced himself that the request was unjustified and turned it down. Mike felt disillusioned; on top of his post-traumatic stress symptoms, he now had to endure what he considered betrayal from his own, previously trusted, supervisor.

In this case, management maintained a distancing role because of the possible liability the plant could incur as the result of the chemical leak to those in the residential area surrounding the facility. Anger was displaced onto the worker(s) for allowing the event to occur or for increasing management workload.

VICARIOUS TRAUMATIZATION AND COUNTERTRANSFERENCE IN THE INVESTIGATOR

The roles of investigator and analyst in the resolution of a work-related traumatic event also carry risk for indirect traumatization and CTRs, although they would not refer to these reactions with clinical terms usually confined to psychotherapy.

Case Example Three:
How Can I Help When I Must Judge?

An Occupational Safety and Health Administration (OSHA) investigator, Mr. C., was called to evaluate an industrial accident in which a factory worker, Bill, was killed by being impaled by the prong of a forklift. The witnesses to the event as well as the forklift driver were severely traumatized by the accident. All felt responsible for the event, some for failure to shout warnings or to push the victim aside, the driver for not avoiding the victim. As the industry was mandated to participate in an occupational safety investigation, all involved parties were extensively interviewed by the OSHA investigator. Many sought reassurance as to their actions and responsibility in this situation. Mr. C. had arrived on the scene shortly after the accident, had reviewed photographs of the scene, and listened to numerous eyewitness and participant accounts. Despite the need to maintain investigatory objectivity, the OSHA examiner felt considerable pressure to console, comfort, and support the grieving workers. Like them, he reexperienced the impalement in flashbacks. He worked hard to separate his findings from past occurrences, as well as from the anger he felt toward the industry for allowing such a common accident to occur. Mr. C. was thrust by his role into a judging perspective and found himself identifying with other eyewitnesses, and he was temporarily drawn away from his task by this countertransference response.

Common CTRs reported by investigators include being influenced by the empathic need to absolve workers for their part in the traumatic event (Type II CTR, overidentification), a breach of investigatory responsibility, or, at the other extreme, being so angry at workers for allowing the event to happen that a concerted effort is made to exact severe punishment of them for their part (Type I CTR, counterphobic). In effect, the anger causes the investigator to take on the harsh role of accuser, thereby exacerbating the guilt felt by the worker. This reaction is especially likely to occur if the investigator, who has seen many similar types of accidents, is emotionally inured to any explanation of action offered by the worker. The trauma of one or more previous investigatory events may color the analysis of the current incident and influence the manner in which the investigator interacts with the worker. Accusations, statements of blame, refusal to listen to the emotional messages being given by the worker, a facade of indifference, or impressions of anger all act to undermine the social support the worker seeks from the investigator, as well as the willingness of the worker to cooperate with the investigator.

ORGANIZATIONAL COUNTERTRANSFERENCE TO TRAUMATIZED WORKERS

The need to understand what happened, in the context of how others behaved before, during, and after the event, is the traumatized worker's primary motivation to seek clarification and support from coworkers. If the coworkers feel guilt, they may strive to compensate for their part in the trauma by either being extremely available to the traumatized worker or by directing anger at the identified victim to offset their own personal responsibility. This generally places distance between the workers as the coworkers, not wishing to be identified with the event, justify their own actions. The coworkers avoid discussing the event and displace blame onto improper training or equipment, or blame the traumatized worker.

Case Example Four: They Should Suffer in Silence

Sheriff D. found himself confronting the following situation. Two of his deputies, Mark and Bob, were to transport a convicted felon from one presumably secure facility to another. The felon had been slipped a weapon, which he used to shoot Mark and Bob, and then he escaped. The deputies suffered serious physical wounds and developed symptoms of PTSD from their near-death experiences. Initially, both supervisors and coworkers had been understanding and supportive of the mental injuries suffered by the deputies. In telling the trauma story, Mark and Bob sought reassurance from coworkers, who were seen as a safe but authoritative source of analysis of what happened and how they performed. The emerging understanding that the trauma story would have serious implications of liability for the organization and might result in disciplinary action for others altered the exchange. At the point at which the deputies filed for compensation for their injuries, the coworkers and Sheriff D. reversed their positions. Now Sheriff D. criticized the deputies for their performance. Filing for benefits was seen as betrayal of the department and of the police occupation, because these physical and mental injuries should have been borne in silence, in keeping with the unwritten code of the occupation. Sheriff D. withdrew emotional support when he learned of the filing and his anger intensified during the civil process, culminating in overt denouncement upon award of damages. Mark and Bob later explained that the worst injury they suffered from this traumatic event was that Sheriff D. and their coworkers turned against them as their court case progressed.

The reactions of Sheriff D. and the coworkers were in part the result of their "police culture" beliefs: that the appropriate response of a police officer to a physical injury incurred on the job, is to suffer in silence, to bear injury as a "red badge of courage." Officers who had been in similar situations but had not resolved their trauma, especially their feelings concerning the level of support given them by coworkers and administration, were particularly critical of Mark and Bob. The civil process required an investigation to determine the source of the felon's weapon (a prison guard). Some coworkers had known of the personal relationship between that prison guard and the felon prior to the escape. Therefore, many coworkers felt guilty and felt accused of wrongdoing by Mark and Bob. Consequently, the level of anger at the injured deputies increased. Initial emotional support from coworkers turned to outright hostility. Others felt that the pursuit of monetary damages was inappropriate, and they expressed disagreement through withdrawal of support.

These reactions are common as the traumatic event and its subsequent organizational resolution slowly churn through the required administrative and civil processes. Coworkers or unions may initially rally around an affected worker, then withdraw, actively oppose, or blame him or her, given the circumstances. In this case, supporters of traumatized workers abandoned their colleagues at the moment it appeared as if some formal body might assign responsibility or liability to aid the injured parties' claims.

MOBILIZING HELP: FORMAL AND INFORMAL ORGANIZATIONAL CHANGE

One way in which countertransferential issues can be resolved is for coworkers to seek a formal role in providing emotional support for traumatized workers. It is not uncommon for such individuals to become members of formal peer support team programs, to train with employee assistance programs, or to pursue the provision of mental health services for trauma victims through unions or in collective bargaining agreements. Frequently, it is formerly traumatized workers and those who felt their impotence at previous work traumas who are most active in demanding some sort of formal organizational response to workplace trauma situations.

Certain types of workplaces deal with the effects of trauma routinely, such as emergency medical workers and surgical and trauma units in hospital settings. Workers who routinely confront wounds, disease, and imminent death develop their own protective culture, with necessary defenses (intellectual, distancing, protocol, isolation, black humor, and unit *esprit de corps*) that mitigate against the worker being overwhelmed by such exposure. The supervisor, assuming that vicarious traumatization is part of the job, may not remain alert to the impact of especially poignant moments of vicarious traumatization.

Case Example Five: Seeing Them Go Up in Flames

Ms. F., a nurse on surgical unit, was treating a pilot who had survived a plane crash. While she cared for his wounds, the pilot described in graphic detail how, after crashing, he turned around to check the passengers and saw them "go up in flames." The nurse treated the pilot's wounds daily while he cried with pain and poured forth his story. When Ms. F. worked nights, she heard the pilot wake up screaming and saw him sit bolt upright in bed and relive his watching helplessly as the passengers burned. The pilot's account of the crash was so vivid that Ms. F began to feel as if she herself had been there when it happened. Ms. F. was drawn in to the pilot's story as though she were his flight assistant at the moment of the crash. She too would have been helpless to change the passengers' fate. Ms. F. began having traumatic dreams in which she could not prevent fatal accidents. The childhood memory of watching helplessly when her own mother died in an auto accident was revived.

Ms. F. began to miss work; she developed bronchitis and headaches. Coworkers sealed off Ms. F's stress response as they did the troublesome cries of the pilot. Her supervisor had been informed of a deteriorating level of performance. Neither she nor Ms. F. brought up the case of the pilot and the presence of vicarious traumatization. The supervisor did not understand that Ms. F's vague questions about the stress of managing burn patients had such a vivid focus. Ms. F., without an opportunity to process the pilot's crash and its impact on her, left the nursing profession, an extreme example of Type I countertransference (withdrawal).

Case Example Six: A Bundle Wrapped in Blankets

Ms. E. was providing emergency nursing care for David, a young survivor of an urban fire. As she was tending to his wounds, a big, burly police officer walked into the emergency admitting area holding a bundle wrapped in blankets. The officer did not speak or move once he entered the room. He merely stood, eyes fixed in a deathly stare, holding the bundle tightly. Ms. E. approached the officer, unwrapped the blanket and saw a dead, 3-month-old infant, with no sign of physical injury. The baby had apparently died of smoke inhalation. Ms. E., only after prolonged efforts, convinced the officer to let her take the child. At this point, two workers were vicariously traumatized, the officer and the nurse. At a police debriefing, the officer reviewed his actions of finding the child in a smoke-filled room. He became aware of his thoughts during the rescue operation, namely, that one of his own children was approximately the same age and he felt it was his urgent responsibility to get the child to safety. He could not believe the child was dead and stated that he believed that by letting go of the child, he acknowledged its death and abrogated his responsibility. The frozen moment when the policeman refused to let go of the dead baby moved Ms. E. intensely. She felt that he was holding on to the dead child because he did not want to show the mother that he had failed. Ms. E. not only understood the mother's grief, but recognized the traumatizing impact on the face of the policeman, the image of the failed protector.

Both coworkers and supervisors took time to help Ms. E. process the event. They were supportive during a period of reduced functioning at work and nightmares that followed, and they assisted her in getting counseling. Ms. E. came to understand that her vicarious traumatization had several layers of meaning, including her reaction to learning recently that she would be unable to have children of her own. Thus, her frozen moment was also the moment of acknowledging her own "dead baby." Ultimately, Ms. E. found creative expression for her tumult that night, taking additional courses in psychiatric nursing and becoming head of a workplace intervention team within an employee assistance program.

CONCLUSION

Work occupies a unique place in life, and what work means to the worker has significant impact on the worker's ability to resolve the emotional sequelae of trauma. Whether the traumatic event occurs outside of or during work, work issues come into play. Work colleagues and the work group not only are a potential source of support for the traumatized worker, but also frequently act to serve as the mirror in which issues surrounding the trauma are examined and evaluated. Most importantly, the reaction of the organization plays an important role in the ability to resolve trauma.

Because work trauma is a new field of inquiry in management as well as in mental health, it is not surprising that very little consideration has been given to the dynamics of countertransference and its impact on both trauma survivors and work participants. What is increasingly understood is that a ripple effect seems to occur after a traumatic workplace event as the consequences reach far beyond those central to the experience. All those who come into contact with the trauma survivor, who hear the trauma story, and who have formal responsibility (or assume an informal role) not only are potential trauma survivors as well, but add to the traumatic event as their CTRs determine the perception of what has happened, is happening, and will happen as trauma resolution is sought.

REFERENCES

Figley, C. (1989). *Helping traumatized families.* San Francisco: Jossey-Bass.

House, J. (1981). *Work stress and social support.* Reading, MA: Addison-Wesley.

Janoff-Bulman, R. (1985). The aftermath of victimization: Rebuilding shattered assumptions. In C. Figley (Ed.), *Trauma and its wake: The study and treatment of post-traumatic stress disorder.* New York: Brunner/Mazel.

Janoff-Bulman, R. (1992). *Shattered assumptions.* New York: Free Press.

Kahn, R., & Katz, D. (1960). Leadership practices in relation to productivity and morale. In D. Cartwright & A. Zander (Eds.), *Group dynamics: Research and theory* (2nd ed.). Evanston, IL: Ross, Peterson.

Lawson, B. (1987). Work-related post-traumatic stress reactions: The hidden dimension. *Health and Social Work, 12,* 250–258.

Likert, R. (1961). *New patterns of management.* New York: McGraw-Hill.

Likert, R. (1967). *The human organization: Its management and values.* New York: McGraw-Hill.

Mayo, E. (1933). *The problems of an industrial civilization.* New York: Macmillan.

McCann, I. L., & Pearlman, L. (1990a). Vicarious traumatization: A framework for understanding the psychological effects of working with victims. *Journal of Traumatic Stress, 3*(1), 131–149.

McCann, I. L., & Pearlman, L. (1990b). *Psychological trauma and the adult survivor: Theory, therapy, and transformation.* New York: Brunner/Mazel.

McLean, A. (1979). *Work stress.* Reading, MA: Addison-Wesley.

Seashore, S. (1954). *Group cohesiveness in the industrial work group.* Ann Arbor, MI: Survey Research Center, University of Michigan.

15

Countertransference, Trauma, and Training

YAEL DANIELI

Speculating about the nature of shame, one of the 49 countertransference themes abstracted from in-depth interviews with 61 psychotherapists and researchers working with Nazi Holocaust survivors and their children that I conducted during the 1970s (Danieli, 1980, 1982a), I proposed:

> Perhaps the deepest aspect of shame is what I have called the *fourth narcissistic blow*. Freud (1917) speculated about the reasons people rejected and avoided psychoanalysis, stating that Copernicus gave the first (cosmological) blow to humanity's naive self-love or narcissism, when humankind learned that it was not the center of the universe. Darwin gave the second (biological) blow, when he said that humanity's separation from and superiority to the animal kingdom is questionable. Freud claimed that he gave the third (psychological) blow, by showing that "the ego is not even master in its own house" and that, indeed, we have limits to our consciousness. I believe that Nazi Germany gave humanity the fourth *(ethical)* blow, by shattering our naive belief that the world we live in is a just place in which human life is of value, to be protected and respected.
>
> A country that was considered the most civilized and cultured in the western World committed the greatest evils that humans have inflicted on humans and thereby challenged the structure of morality, dignity, and human rights, as well as the values that define civilization . . . all of us, in various degrees of awareness, share this sense of shame. Indeed, this fourth narcissistic blow may have caused many in society to avoid confronting the Holocaust by refusing to listen to survivors and their offspring, [those] who bear witness to the experience and its consequences.

Although all four "blows" forced confrontation with essential truths about human existence, the ethical blow distinguishes itself by massively and mercilessly exposing the potential boundlessness of human evil and ugliness. . . . (Danieli, 1984, p. 31)

I believe that psychotherapists who work with other victims and trauma survivors, particularly of man-made disasters, share this profoundly existential sense of shame, which constitutes, with the other countertransference reactions found in my study, an aspect of the larger *conspiracy of silence* that has existed between survivors, their offspring, and society.[1] Elsewhere, I have reviewed in detail the literature on the conspiracy of silence (Danieli, 1982a), and described its harmful long-term impact on the survivors (Danieli, 1981, 1989a), their families (Danieli, 1981a, 1981b, 1985), and their psychotherapies (Danieli, 1984, 1993).

In order of frequency, some of the major categories of countertransference phenomena systematically examined in my study were:

1. *Various modes of defense* against listening to Holocaust experiences and against therapists' inability to contain their intense emotional reactions (e.g., numbing, denial, avoidance, distancing, clinging to professional role, reduction to method and/or theory);
2. *Affective reactions* such as bystander's guilt; rage, with its variety of objects; dread and horror; shame and related emotions (e.g., disgust and loathing); grief and mourning; "me too"; sense of bond; privileged voyeurism; and
3. Specific *relational context issues* such as parent–child relationship; victim/liberator; viewing the survivor as hero; and attention and attitudes toward Jewish identity.

These themes are reported, described, illustrated, and discussed in detail in a series of articles elsewhere (Danieli, 1980, 1982a, 1984, 1988a, 1988c, 1994).

Whereas society has a moral obligation to share its members' pain, psychotherapists and researchers have, in addition, a professional, contractual obligation. When they fail to listen, explore, understand, and help, they too inflict the "trauma after the trauma" (Rappaport, 1968), or "the 'second injury' to victims" (Symonds, 1980) by maintaining and perpetuating the *conspiracy of silence.*

[1]Indeed, the phrase *conspiracy of silence* has been used to describe the typical interaction of Holocaust survivors and their children with psychotherapists when Holocaust experiences were mentioned or recounted (e.g., see Barocas & Barocas, 1979; Krystal & Niederland, 1968; Tanay, 1968), as it had been used to describe the pervasive interaction of survivors with society in general.

COUNTERTRANSFERENCE IN TRAINING PROFESSIONALS WORKING WITH TRAUMA

Traditional training generally has not prepared professionals to deal with massive real (adult) trauma and its long-term effects. The Group Project for Holocaust Survivors and Their Children has provided short- and long-term training seminars and individual supervision to professionals since 1975. In-house, on-the-job training/supervision has been offered by other agencies. The International Society for Traumatic Stress Studies, among its other activities, has begun to ameliorate this lack of training through its initial report on the Presidential Task Force on Curriculum, Education, and Training (see Danieli & Krystal, 1989). This report contains model curricula formulated by leading international specialists in the field and is composed of subcommittees representing different technical specialties or interests including psychiatry, psychology, social work, nursing, and creative arts therapy; clergy and media; organizations, institutions, and public health; paraprofessionals and other professionals; and undergraduate education. The need to cope with and work through countertransference difficulties was recognized as imperative and necessary to optimize training in this field by all expert groups.

As early as 1980 (Danieli, 1980), when I published the preliminary thematic overview of the above-mentioned study, I stated:

> While this cluster [of countertransference reactions] was reported by professionals working with Jewish Holocaust survivors and their offspring, I believe that other victim/survivor populations may be responded to similarly and may suffer . . . similar [consequences]. . . . It will be of interest and importance to investigate what components of this cluster may be shared by different victim/survivor populations, and what other components may [constitute] clusters specific to other populations. Defining the[se] reaction-clusters . . . will lead therapists and investigators to be better able to [recognize them so that they can monitor,] contain and use them preventively and therapeutically. (p. 366)

In 1981 I noted that these reactions "seem very similar to alexithymia, anhedonia, and their concomitants and components which, according to Krystal, characterize survivors" (Danieli, 1981c, p. 201). In 1989, in the context of training (Danieli, 1989b) I referred to these phenomena as the "vicarious victimization of the care-giver."

These insights and hypotheses about the ubiquity of countertransference reactions in other victim populations have now moved to the forefront of our concern in the preparation and training of professionals who work with victims and trauma survivors. Indeed, the ensuing literature reflects a growing realization among professionals working with other victims/survivors of the need to describe, understand, and organize different elements and aspects of the *conspiracy of silence*. Haley (1974), Blank (1985), and Parson (1988) reported, and Lindy (1987) has adapted and revised, the countertransference categories mentioned above to compare and contrast them with responses from therapists of Vietnam veterans with post-traumatic stress disorder (PTSD). Comas-Díaz and Padilla (1990) and Fischman (1991) discussed countertransference themes related to torture; Mollica (1988) and Kinzie (1989), to refugees; Chu (1988) and Kluft (1989) to multiple personality disorder; McCann and Pearlman (1990), who similarly named these phenomena "vicarious traumatization," to adult survivors; and Herman (1992) to adult survivors of childhood sexual abuse among others, to name but some.

Countertransference reactions are integral to our work, ubiquitous and expected. Our work calls on us to confront, with our patients and within ourselves, extraordinary human experiences. This confrontation is profoundly humbling in that at all times these experiences try our view of the world we live in and challenge the limits of our humanity.

In reality, countertransference reactions are the building blocks of the societal, as well as professional, *conspiracy of silence*. They inhibit professionals from studying, correctly diagnosing, and treating the effects of trauma. They also perpetuate the heretofore pervasive absence of traditional training necessary for professionals to cope with massive real (adult) trauma and its (long-term) effects.

Although information cannot undo unconscious reactions, knowledge about traumata in their historic context does provide the therapist with factual and, for example, gender, ethnic, racial, religious, cultural, political perspectives that help him or her know what to look for, what may be missing in the survivor's account of his or her experience(s), and what types of questions to ask. But countertransference reactions interfere with the process of acquiring knowledge about the trauma as well. As one seminar participant reported about attempting to read one of the homework books assigned for a seminar discussion,

> "I can read it only a little bit at a time. Otherwise my head tunes off. I can't pay attention. It was too painful for me. He [Des Pres, 1976] writes so vividly, the imagery, that I couldn't read some of it, I just had to skip over sections. I wasn't tuning out. I was like putting the book down and looking for a less intense part of the book to read. It must have been very hard to put something like this into words."

The ensuing seminar discussion, in part, explored the implications of these reactions to her ability to listen fully to her survivor patients.

In another training seminar, a therapist, herself a child survivor of the Nazi Holocaust, reported that, "It's sitting at my bed table and I keep not reading it. I have read some [of the] other books ... I mean, I keep touching it ... but I just could not get myself to read it." Asked about the possible reasons for her particular ambivalence about reading *Children of the Holocaust: Conversations with Sons and Daughters of Survivors* (Epstein, 1979), she replied,

> "Oh, well now that you mention it ... truly, it didn't hit me till now, but since you are specifying it, I think that it probably has to do with me and my own children ... the specificity of it. ... For myself, I have put a lot of energy into trying to integrate in some way or another, but I have not dealt with it in my own children. And since that is what the book is about I think that's why. ... But I must say, I was not aware of it at the time while I was not reading it. ... Your notion of the conspiracy of silence has certainly been true in my family. ... The family colluded, ... they bought it ... not without attempts on their part. I mean, I think that they would have been open to it. They ... offered themselves but ... you know, the message from me was, 'Stay out of it.' So ... each of my children dealt with it in their own way, like when my son went to Brandeis and took all the courses he could on the Holocaust and that's how he dealt with it. But not, not with me. ...
>
> "It is a dilemma and there is a conflict. ... It's better to go into the field having dealt with that issue, but I haven't, neither with my children nor with my husband. I decided not to talk before the children came. ... My husband was sort of a stranger in the sense that he was American ... from another world. ... So I think I had a horror all the time that if I told him he would make special allowance for me for being a victim, special excuses, or he would be specifically supportive in a manner that I didn't want. ..."

Asked to elucidate, she elaborated, "that if I get angry, whatever negatives may be about me like anger or rage or weaknesses, that he would ... attribute it to that experience ... so that if I would be crazy because of what happened he would be more tolerant of it, and I would again be put in an inferior position vis-à-vis him."

In relation to her children,

> "I had a very clear motivation, that if I would scream at them ... I must say that in retrospect I am not sorry about that because when ... we take each other on now it's a different context ... and ... I did tell them that I am involved in this and they expressed mighty surprise, but they are pleased. The other reason was that I said, 'Well, it's enough that one person in the family is branded in some ways, scarred.' ... I just didn't want to pass that on to them also ... I knew that they wouldn't be able to get around totally, but I thought, later, when they are stronger. I don't know. I didn't think ... I didn't sit down and figure it all out. ... I just somehow thought that to experience it so directly through me was just

asking too much. And I would rather they experience it secondhand or thirdhand or fourthhand, or you know, through classes or whatever. . . . And I am sure that probably the main reason which I have not dealt with it was my own acceptance or nonacceptance of it. I'm sure that. . . . So that's why I couldn't read the book."

In addition to information about the trauma terrain, familiarity with the growing body of literature on the (long-term) psychological sequelae of the traumata on its survivors and their offspring also helps prepare mental health professionals. Nonetheless, they should guard against the simple grouping of individuals as "survivors," who are expected to exhibit the same "survivor syndrome" (Krystal & Niederland, 1968), or PTSD, and the expectation that children of survivors will manifest a single trans-mitted "child-of-survivor syndrome" (e.g., Phillips, 1978).

Many of the countertransference phenomena examined in my study were found to be reactions to patients' Holocaust stories rather than to their behavior. The unusual uniformity of psychotherapists' reactions sug-gests that they are in response to the Holocaust—the one element that all the otherwise different patients have in common. Because the Holocaust seems to be the source of these reactions, I suggested that it is appropriate to name them *countertransference reactions to the Holocaust,* rather than to the patients themselves. I also believe that therapists' difficulties in treat-ing other victim/survivor populations may similarly have their roots in the nature of their victimization *(event countertransference).*

PROCESSING EVENT COUNTERTRANSFERENCE[2]

Regarding event countertransferences as dimensions of one's inner or *intrapsychic, conspiracy of silence* about the trauma allows us the possi-bility to explore and confront these reactions to the trauma events prior to and independent of the therapeutic encounter with the victim/survivor patient, in a variety of training and supervisory settings and by ourselves.[3] I will now present an exercise process to work through *event counter-transference*[4] that I developed over the last two decades, which has proven helpful in numerous workshops, training institutes, debriefing of "front

[2]Portions of the following elaborate upon Danieli (1994). © 1994 by Yael Dan-ieli.

[3]Although event countertransference and personal countertransference (i.e., re-actions to the patient's behaviors) are not mutually exclusive, for training purposes it is useful to differentiate the two.

[4]The word *event* was chosen to specify the source of these therapists' reactions, not to imply that it was just one event.

liners," short- and long-term seminars, and in consultative, short- and long-term supervisory relationships around the world. While it originally evolved, and is still done optimally, as a part of a group experience, it can also be done alone and may assist the clinician working privately. As one veteran traumatologist who does it regularly stated, "It is like taking an inner shower when I am stuck with . . . [a] patient."

Instructions for Participants

In a group setting, I ask participants to arrange the chairs in a circle. After everyone is seated, without any introductions, I say:
"The first phase of the process will be private, totally between you and yourself. Take a large piece of paper, a pen, or a pencil. Create space for yourself. [If in group setting:] Please don't talk with each other during this first phase. Choose the victimization/trauma experience most meaningful to you. [When I lead this exercise, I always begin with the Holocaust, and after completing the total process described below about the Holocaust, only then do I ask the participants to take another large piece of paper and to choose the victimization/trauma experience most meaningful to them.] Please let yourself focus in to it."

Imaging

"Draw everything and anything, any image that comes to mind when you think _____ [the experience you chose]. Take your time. We have a lot of time. Take all the time you need."

Word Association

"When you have completed this task, turn the page, and please, write down every word that comes to mind when you focus on this experience."

Added Reflection and Affective Associations

"When you finish this, draw a line underneath the words. Please, look through/reflect on the words you wrote. Is there is any affect or feeling words that you may have not included? Please add them now. . . . Roam freely around your mind and add any other word that comes to mind now."

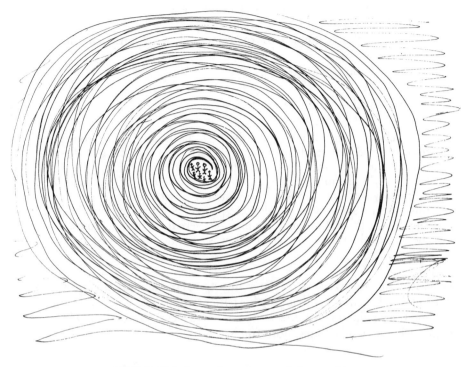

FIGURE 15.1. Image drawn by a workshop participant.

First Memory

"When was the very first time you ever heard of _____, the very first time?

How did you hear?
What was it like for you?
Whom did you hear it from? Or what did you hear it from?
Go back and explore that situation in your mind with as much detail as you can.
What was it like?
How old were you?
Where are you in the memory?
Are you in the kitchen, in the bedroom, living room, in class, in the movies, in the park? Are you watching TV?

Are you alone or with other people?—with your parents, family,
friends, strangers?
What are you feeling? Do you remember any particular physical
sensations?
What are you thinking?"

As one psychotherapist reported,

"As a child I remember very vividly, I had been scrounging around and
found an old carton of pictures. And discovered that my grandmother
had lost a sister and family. I felt terrible, having brought [this] to
everybody's memory. And I knew nothing about it at the time. And
everybody, of course, was crying and very upset when I brought down
this box and said, 'Who are all these people?' I was at my grandparents'
and I asked them. I assumed the pictures were from Europe. And I asked
them. And the result was everybody was crying. . . . I still feel guilty and
sad. . . ."

Presenting a case five sessions later into the seminar, this therapist recognized his difficulties with asking his patient questions. Working through
this memory helped place one source of his difficulty and enabled him to
explore his patient's issues more freely.

Choices and Beliefs

"Are you making any *choices* about life, about people, about yourself at
the time? Decisions like:

'Because this happened, therefore . . . ,' or
'This means that life is . . . that people are . . . that the world is. . . . '

"What are you telling yourself? Are you coming to any conclusions? This
is very important. Stay with that."

Continuity and Discontinuity of Self

"Think of yourself today. Look at that situation. Are you still holding
these choices? Do you still believe what you concluded then? Would you
say 'This is still me,' or 'This is not me anymore'? What is the difference?
What changed and why?"

Sharing with Others

"Have you *talked with other* people about it? Whom did you talk to, both in the past and now, if you did? What was their reaction? What was your reaction to their reaction?"

Secrets: Not Sharing with Others

"Is there anything about this that you haven't told anyone, that you decided that it is not to be talked about, that it is 'unspeakable'?

"Is there any area in it that you feel that is totally your *secret,* that you dealt with all alone and kept to yourself? If there is, please put it into words such as, 'I haven't shared it because . . . ,' or 'I am very hesitant to share it because. . . .'

"Please mention the particular people with whom you won't share it, and why."

Personal Knowledge of Survivors

[Moving to another aspect of the *interpersonal realm,*] "Do you personally know survivors of _____ or their family members—as friends, neighbors, or colleagues?"

Self Secrets

"There are secrets we keep from others to protect either ourselves or them, and then there are *self secrets.* Take your time. This is very important. Imagine the situation of the very first time you ever heard anything about it. Roam inside your mind. Is there anything about it that you have never talked to yourself about, a secret you have kept from yourself? An area that you have sort of pushed away and kept at arm's length from yourself? Or about which you say to yourself, 'I can't handle that'? Why is it the one thing that was too much for you? What haven't you put into words yet, that is still lurking in that corner of your mind you have not looked into yet?"

Personal Relationship to the Trauma

"What is your *personal relationship* to the trauma? Please, do write the answers, because even the way you write makes a difference. Did your place of birth figure in your relationship to the trauma? Does your age figure in your relationship to the trauma?"

Identity Dimensions

"What is your *religious, ethnic, cultural, political, class, racial,* and *gender* identity, and sexual orientation? Do these parts of your identity figure in the choices you made, influence your relationship to the experience? How? You can answer these one by one."

Professional Relationship to the Trauma

"Let us move to your *professional* self. What is your professional discipline? How long have you been working in it? What is your professional relationship to the _____? Within your professional practice, have you seen survivors of _____ or their children? How many?"

Therapeutic Orientation

"What therapeutic modality have you employed? Emergency/crisis intervention, short-term, long-term, individual, family, and/or group therapy? Has it been on an inpatient or outpatient basis? What modality have you found [or would you find] most useful, and why?"

Victim and Trauma Survivor Populations

"Is it the only victim/survivor population you have worked with professionally?"

Training in Trauma Work

"Have you ever been trained to work with victim/survivors of trauma?—in school, on the job? If you were, what have you found to be the crucial elements of your training without which you won't feel prepared to do the job?" One trauma therapist retorted, "Other than my personal experience I really had to go by the seat of my pants and not by what I was taught in school."

The sequence of the first phase of the processing of event counter-transference is from the immediate visual imagery through free associations to the more verbal–cognitive material. It then moves to articulate how the trauma fits within the therapist's experience, personal and interpersonal development, and the gender, racial, ethnic, religious, cultural, and political realms of her or his life. It begins with one's *private* world of trauma and proceeds through the context of one's interpersonal life to one's professional work. As one psychotherapist described it,

> "You reexperience the trauma through this. It takes you from the picture, being very concrete, . . . like the way the trauma occurs. You are very shocked and numb, shocked at recognizing your own reactions, the depth of them. And . . . then gradually words, and then not stopping there but go into feelings that you don't think of and don't have time to think of. And, like what happens in the retelling, putting things into words, from the impersonal to the inside. But then it pulls you out, to the professional. It lifts you back into reality so the therapist is not stuck in it."

Participants in group settings have frequently remarked on the feeling of intimacy that permeates the room even though the first phase of the process takes place in silence, perhaps reflecting the sense that it is opening ourselves to ourselves that allows for intimacy.

Although the material can be analyzed privately, the second phase of the process, the sharing and exploring phase, works best in a group setting, as is often the case with survivors and children of survivors of the Nazi Holocaust (Danieli, 1982b, 1988b, 1989a) and with other victims/survivors. As with victims and trauma survivors, therapists in a group are able to explore with each other and comprehend the consequences in their lives of the traumata they have experienced directly or indirectly, the conspiracy of silence that frequently follows them, and share their feelings and concerns. The group modality thus serves to counteract their own sense of isolation and alienation about working with trauma. As one psychotherapist described it,

> "You are invited for a Saturday night dinner or a picnic by very well-meaning people who want to connect you with other people whom they think you may like, and somebody introduces you as a person working with Holocaust survivors, and then you are expected to make small talk. It's like being in a crazy warp. And you are expected to entertain people with your work. You feel the same as you feel after death of a close person: Distance. As a result we ourselves devalue small talk because we feel distant, potentially reproaching banter and relief.
>
> "When I was deeply involved in interviewing for the book day and night, I remember feeling like I had a double life. When with friends

Saturday night I didn't dare to say anything. Carrying this burden, becoming deeper and deeper involved, do you have the right to disturb
other people? R. K. and M. T. [survivor friends] say that the survivor is
an irritant. When dealing with traumatized people you begin to think of
yourself as possibly an irritant to ordinary folk you interact with, family
and colleagues. I recall being referred to in my department as 'Holocaust
Lady,' and described as 'obsessed' and 'overreacting,' as if the material
emanates and, like the survivors, you are found to be so irritating that you
have to be put in a box, like a freak. It is victimization, not vicarious
victimization, of the caregiver. Really it is thanks to the International
Society for Traumatic Stress Studies that we all began to feel that there is
a place where we won't not be regarded as irritating, weird people."

A traumatologist who has worked with Vietnam veterans since the
early 1970s, similarly described being ostracized by his colleagues who,

". . . exempted from the war, . . . projected [their] strong anti-war senti-
ments towards the veterans themselves, making nasty remarks such as
'those guys shouldn't be allowed in here,' and by extension to me. Increasingly disturbed and moved by how the Vietnam war affected those
who fought it, . . . [and finding it] difficult to convey to others, who were
not interested, what I was learning and experiencing, I began to feel alone
and isolated . . . [until] . . . I felt more in common with Vietnam veterans
than with anyone else . . . offended by insensitive questions such as 'Are
they all screwed up?' and being protective of them. Through the grape-
vine I learned that my colleagues, called me the 'Vietnam vet' guy,
thought I was crazy and had some bizarre reason [for] what I was doing.
I thought to myself, 'Fuck them, fuck 'em all.'

"I existed in between different worlds. . . . There were years of loneliness, pain, searching, and self-questioning. However, one thing was
clear: I would never again be a traditional academic . . . or clinician. My
life had changed forever and there was no turning back. . . . Among the
things that made a difference was a growing affiliation with others doing
work with trauma survivors [which was] not only reassuring but validated
my commitment. . . . The network of colleagues around the country became a kind of family: trusted friends on whom I could call to sort out
my feelings and the impact of the work. . . . I now believe that everyone
involved in our field has to be profoundly affected by the work because
it impacts the soul of helpers in the same way that trauma scars the soul
of survivors."

Working privately with incest survivors, a psychotherapist stated:

"Individuals on their own have no place to go with it. I had such a lonely
feeling about this work and felt so shameful for having to do it. It was like
digging ditches. You don't tell anybody what you do. You don't tell them

how dirty your hands and your feelings got. It's a put-down, because I am associated with something so horrible and terrible, and being so helpless, that I became identified with the survivors."

After sharing with colleagues, however, the therapist said, "There was a different depth of feeling, attachment, and identity. Before there was no one. After that I felt different."

Elsewhere, in discussing the value of the group modalities for the victim/survivor patients, I suggest that groups have been particularly helpful in compensating for countertransference reactions. Whereas a therapist alone may feel unable to contain or provide a "holding environment" (Winnicott, 1965) for his or her patient's feelings, the group as a unit is able to. When any particularly intense interaction invoked by trauma memories proves too overwhelming to some people present, others invariably come forth with a variety of helpful "holding" reactions. Thus, the group functions as an ideal absorptive entity for abreaction and catharsis of emotions, especially negative ones, that are otherwise experienced as uncontainable (see Krystal, 1988). The group modality offers a multiplicity of options for expressing, naming, verbalizing, and modulating feelings. It provides a safe place for exploring fantasies, for imagining, "inviting," and taking on the roles and examining their significance in the identity of the participants. Finally, the group encourages and demonstrates mutual support and caring, which ultimately enhances self-care. These considerations apply to therapists working in groups as well.

This training process assumes that the most meaningful way to tap into event countertransferences is to let them emerge, in a systematic way, from the particularity of the therapist's experience. She or he is thus better able to recognize and become familiar with her or his reactions in order to monitor, and learn to understand and contain them, and to use them preventively and therapeutically. During the sharing phase, when participants describe the images they drew and the process of selecting them, they already put them into words. For example, the psychotherapist who drew the image in Figure 15.2 related,

"When you said draw a picture, I had the same reaction as always: that there was nothing that I could put on a piece of paper that could, for me, convey horror that is what I associate with, like this amorphous, just horribleness. Any of the scenes, whether it's the people on the lines to the gas chambers or the barbed wire, or the, you know, I wouldn't know where to start. Just the horror, that is what hits me. And there is nothing that I could pick out. Except that I . . . and then as I was sitting here, thinking, the thing that strikes me, of course, is . . . what I later wrote: the fates of death. It wasn't so much the death but the always-staring-into the

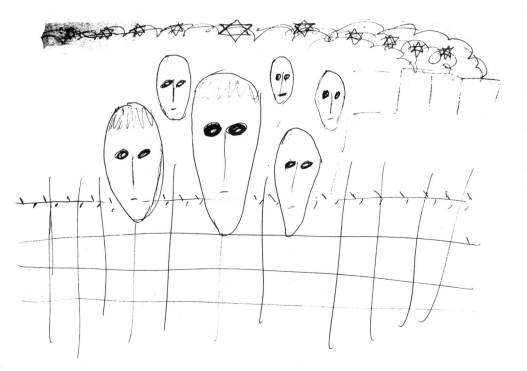

FIGURE 15.2. Image drawn by a workshop participant.

face of death, and always knowing: we're not now, but you are going to be there in the next two minutes. Never mind day, week, month."

Crying while writing, another therapist explained,

"It gets too close to . . . I am surprised . . . I cannot directly connect with the Holocaust without intense pain. . . . It's copeable with largely by avoidance. The Holocaust comes close to the ultimate of pain, beyond associations of, beyond endurance. The feeling of strengths are also there, but I am not connected with those. I feel most identified with the victimization and the overwhelming powerlessness against the horror."

Space does not permit describing the richness of what can be learned in ongoing, prolonged group supervision processes nor providing full narrative examples of the crystallization of countertransference reactions through repeated reviews; the interacting tapestries of, among others, event countertransference and person countertransference; the mutual impact of differing adaptational styles to the trauma (Danieli, 1981a) of therapists and patients; and the examination of mutual (counter)transferences among members played out in the group dynamics. One important instance of the latter is the attempted expulsion of the supervisor—the person leading the exercise process, who thus becomes the symbolic agent of the trauma—by/from the group for "victimizing" them and exposing their vulnerabilities by encouraging them to confront—(re)experience—the trauma.

The exercise incurs ambivalence as well. Claiming an inability to draw, and a preference to "only do the words part," is an obvious example of resistance. One psychotherapist attempting to do the exercise process alone stated,

> "Even for people who took a seminar it's very powerful and assumes a degree of training and sophistication. To do it in one clip is very traumatic. It forces you to meet, confront yourself, feelings and thoughts with regard to issues you would rather not deal with, that you usually won't do on your own. It's better to do it part by yourself and discuss it with another person, and then continue with the next part. You have to stop, because even though it's worthwhile, it is so difficult. It's easier and more productive to do it with somebody else because you have to convey a complete thought to another person. When writing it down you may fudge. It's individual. Some people perhaps can be very honest with themselves writing. But since it's such powerful and difficult material you need another person's support. If you fall, somebody will be there to catch you or stabilize you.
>
> "Even in a workshop you should be flexible and give people a choice—group, pairs, individual, and give them the opportunity to decide what is better for them even if they have to do it over ten times to meet everything. If you do it individually, do only as much as you can. Patients are entitled to human rather than ideal therapists. It is very powerful. I will do it when I am ready."

The exercise process does not aim to replace ongoing, analytical, supervisory countertransference work. It does, however, aim to provide a sorely needed focus on and an experiential multidimensional framework for the trauma aspects of the patient's and therapist's lives.

The process also helps build awareness of the caregiver's vulnerability to being vicariously victimized by repeated exposure to traumata and trauma stories and to the extent of the toll that countertransference reactions take on her or his intrapsychic, interpersonal, and family lives. One supervisee reported that "two people at the agency did a survivors' group and stopped after eight or nine sessions because they didn't want to come home every time and cry. It didn't get better with time. It got worse and worse. They couldn't handle it. They had nightmares. They were not in shape to get up and go to work."

The exercise process makes poignantly clear the paramount necessity of carefully nurturing, regulating, and ensuring the development of a self-protective, self-healing, and self-soothing way of being as a professional and a full human being. The importance of self-care and self-soothing is acknowledged in the exercise by building into the process instructional elements such as "take your time . . . take all the time you need," and by paying caring, respectful attention to every element explored.

The composition of the workshop or seminar group is unpredictable. One can be assured, however, that many of the psychotherapists present have themselves been, directly or indirectly, victims or trauma survivors. Their victimization either inspired and energized their choice of work/career or specialty, or interacts with their patients' traumata as part of their countertransference matrix. Invariable there will be both victims and perpetrators—such as a Cambodian boat girl and a Vietnam veteran turned psychotherapists, or survivors and children of survivors of the Nazi Holocaust and Germans—exploring together the legacy of their mutually shared history. Invariably, also, group members learn about cultures other than their own. They come to finish unfinished business with their patients and with themselves, to explore their wounds, clean the pus, and heal. They come to seek answers, to find forgiveness, compassion, and ultimately, understanding and camaraderie. They mobilize creative energy and allow themselves to transform as people, to be more authentic in their work and more actualized in their personal lives.

SOME PRINCIPLES OF SELF-HEALING

The following principles are designed to help professionals recognize, contain, and heal event countertransferences.

1. To recognize one's reactions:
   a. Develop awareness of somatic signals of distress—one's chart of warning signs of potential countertransference reactions, for example, sleeplessness, headaches, perspiration.
   b. Try to find words to accurately name and to articulate one's inner experiences and feelings. As Bettelheim (1984) commented, "what cannot be talked about can also not be put to rest; and if it is not, the wounds continue to fester from generation to generation" (p. 166).
2. To contain one's reactions:

    a. Identify one's personal level of comfort in order to build openness, tolerance, and readiness to hear *anything*.

    b. Knowing that every emotion has a beginning, a middle, and an end, learn to attenuate one's fear of being overwhelmed by its intensity by trying to feel its full life cycle without resorting to defensive countertransference reactions.

3. To heal and grow:

    a. Accept that nothing will ever be the same.

    b. When feeling wounded, take time, accurately diagnose, soothe and heal, so as to be "emotionally fit" again and able to continue to work.

    c. Seek consultation or further therapy for previously unexplored areas that are triggered by patients' stories.

    d. Acknowledge that any one of the affective reactions (e.g., grief, mourning, rage) may interact with old, un-worked-through experiences. Therapists will thus be able to use their professional work purposefully for their own growth. The child survivor, mother psychotherapist described earlier, through further integrating her insights and understanding, was able to turn her vulnerability into a source of sensitivity and strength and to use them not only for her patients, but also to enrich and deepen her relationships with her husband and children.

    e. Establish a network of people to create a holding environment (Winnicott, 1965) within which one can share one's trauma related work.

    f. Therapists should provide themselves with avocational avenues for creative and relaxing self-expression in order to regenerate energies.

Being kind to oneself and feeling free to have fun and joy is not a frivolity in this field but a necessity, without which one cannot fulfill one's professional obligations, one's professional contract.

CONCLUDING REMARKS

Countertransference reactions are integral to our work, ubiquitous and expected. Accordingly, this chapter reiterated the pivotal importance of working through countertransference difficulties in order to optimize and make meaningful the necessary, heretofore pervasively absent, training of professionals in the field of traumatic stress. Having previously introduced the concept of *event countertransference* to indicate that the source of these reactions is the nature of the patient's victimization or traumata (stories), the chapter presented an exercise tool for processing event countertransference, emphasizing the value of group modalities as a context for its sharing, experiential exploration, and working through. Following a brief description of some of the dimensions that emerge during training, supervisory workshops, and seminars, I presented some principles of self-care for the psychotherapists and others working with victims and trauma survivors.

The original conclusion of the quote with which I began this chapter was, "Unless humanity is willing to integrate this historical [fourth, *ethical*] narcissistic blow, the pessimistic prophecies stated by Freud (1930) in *Civilization and Its Discontents* may be fulfilled" (Danieli, 1984, pp. 31–32).

To make an analogy, I feel that unless our field is willing to integrate the professional, ethical narcissistic blow—the knowledge that we have participated in and perpetuated the conspiracy of silence by failing to listen, study, learn, explore, understand, train, and therefore help—victims and trauma survivors, their family members, the second generation, and possibly others to come will prove fully justified in feeling bitter and hopeless about receiving the right kind of help.

REFERENCES

Barocas, H. A., & Barocas, C. B. (1979). Wounds of the fathers: The next generation of Holocaust victims. *International Review of Psycho-Analysis, 6,* 1–10.
Bettelheim, B. (1984). Afterword. In C. Vegh, *I didn't say goodbye* (R. Schwartz, Trans., pp. 161–178). New York: E. P. Dutton.
Blank, A. S. (1985). Irrational reactions to post-traumatic stress disorder and Vietnam veterans. In S. M. Sonnenberg, A. S. Blank, & J. A. Talbott (Eds.), *The trauma of war: Stress and recovery in Vietnam veterans* (pp. 69–98). Washington DC: American Psychiatric Association Press.
Comas-Díaz, L., & Padilla, A. (1990). Countertransference in working with victims of political repression. *American Journal of Orthopsychiatry, 60,* 125–134.
Chu, J. A. (1988). Ten traps for therapists in the treatment of trauma survivors. *Dissociation, 1,* 24–32.
Danieli, Y. (1980). Countertransference in the treatment and study of Nazi Holocaust survivors and their children. *Victimology: An International Journal, 5*(2–4), 355–367.
Danieli, Y. (1981a). Differing adaptational styles in families of survivors of the Nazi Holocaust: Some implications for treatment. *Children Today, 10*(5), 6–10, 34–35.
Danieli, Y. (1981b). Families of survivors of the Nazi Holocaust: Some short- and long-term effects. In C. D. Spielberger, I. G. Sarason, & N. Milgram (Eds.),

Stress and anxiety (Vol. 8, pp. 405–421). New York: McGraw-Hill/Hemisphere.

Danieli, Y. (1981c). On the achievement of integration in aging survivors of the Nazi Holocaust. *Journal of Geriatric Psychiatry, 14*(2), 191–210.

Danieli, Y. (1982a). Therapists' difficulties in treating survivors of the Nazi Holocaust and their children (Doctoral dissertation, New York University, 1981). *University Microfilms International*, No. 949-904.

Danieli, Y. (1982b). *Group project for Holocaust survivors and their children* (Contract No. 092424762). Washington, DC: National Institute of Mental Health, Mental Health Services Branch.

Danieli, Y. (1984). Psychotherapists' participation in the conspiracy of silence about the Holocaust. *Psychoanalytic Psychology, 1*(1), 23–42.

Danieli, Y. (1985). The treatment and prevention of long-term effects and intergenerational transmission of victimization: A lesson from Holocaust survivors and their children. In C. R. Figley (Ed.), *Trauma and its wake* (pp. 295–313). New York: Brunner/Mazel.

Danieli, Y. (1988a). Treating survivors and children of survivors of the Nazi Holocaust. In F. M. Ochberg (Ed.), *Post-traumatic therapy and victims of violence* (pp. 278–294). New York: Brunner/Mazel.

Danieli, Y. (1988b). The use of mutual support approaches in the treatment of victims. In E. Chigier (Ed.), *Grief and bereavement in contemporary society: Vol. 3. Support systems* (pp. 116–123). London: Freund.

Danieli, Y. (1988c). Confronting the unimaginable: Psychotherapists' reactions to victims of the Nazi Holocaust. In J. P. Wilson, Z. Harel, & B. Kahana (Eds.), *Human adaptation to extreme stress* (pp. 219–237). New York: Plenum Press.

Danieli, Y. (1989a). Mourning in survivors and children of survivors of the Nazi Holocaust: The role of group and community modalities. In D. R. Dietrich & P. C. Shabad (Eds.), *The problem of loss and mourning: Psychoanalytic perspectives* (pp. 427–460). Madison: International Universities Press.

Danieli, Y. (1989b, August). *Countertransference and trauma: Vicarious victimization of the care giver.* Workshop presented at the Critical Incident Conference, Federal Bureau of Investigation, Behavioral Science Instruction and Research Unit Federal Bureau of Investigation Academy, Quantico, VA.

Danieli, Y. (1993). The diagnostic and therapeutic use of the multi-generational family tree in working with survivors and children of survivors of the Nazi Holocaust. In J. P. Wilson & B. Raphael (Eds.), *The international handbook of traumatic stress syndromes* (pp. 889–898). New York: Plenum Press.

Danieli, Y. (1994). Countertransference and trauma: Self healing and training issues. In M. B. Williams & J. F. Sommer, Jr. (Eds.), *Handbook of post-traumatic therapy.* Westport, CT: Greenwood/Praeger.

Danieli, Y., & Krystal, J. H. (1989). *The initial report of the Presidential Task Force on Curriculum, Education and Training of the Society for Traumatic Stress Studies.* Chicago: International Society for Traumatic Stress Studies.

Des Pres, T. (1976). *The survivor: An anatomy of life in the death camps.* New York: Oxford University Press.

Epstein, H. (1979). *Children of the Holocaust: Conversations with sons and daughters of survivors.* New York: G. P. Putnam.

Fischman, Y. (1991). Interacting with trauma: Clinician's responses to treating psychological aftereffects of political repression. *American Journal of Orthopsychiatry, 61,* 179–185.

Haley, S. A. (1974). When the patient reports atrocities: Specific treatment considerations in the Vietnam veteran. *Archives of General Psychiatry, 30,* 191–196.

Herman, J. L. (1992). *Trauma and recovery.* New York: Basic Books.

Kinzie, D. J. (1989). Therapeutic approaches to traumatized Cambodian refugees. *Journal of Traumatic Stress, 2*(1), 75–91.

Kluft, R. P. (1989). The rehabilitation of therapists overwhelmed by their work with MPD patients. *Dissociation, 2*(4), 243–249.

Krystal, H. (1988). *Integration and self-healing.* Hillsdale, NJ: Analytic Press.

Krystal, H., & Niederland, W. G. (1968). Clinical observations on the survivor syndrome. In H. Krystal (Ed.), *Massive psychic trauma* (pp. 327–348). New York: International Universities Press.

Lindy, J. D. (1987). *Vietnam: A casebook.* New York: Brunner/Mazel.

McCann, I. L., & Pearlman, L. A. (1990). Vicarious traumatization: A framework for understanding the psychological effects of working with victims. *Journal of Traumatic Stress, 3,* 131–149.

Mollica, R. F. (1988). The trauma story: The psychiatric care of refugee survivors of violence and torture. In F. M. Ochberg (Ed.), *Post-traumatic therapy and victims of violence* (pp. 295–314). New York: Brunner/Mazel.

Parson, E. R. (1988). The unconscious history of Vietnam in the group: An innovative multiphasic model for working through authority transferences in guilt-driven veterans. *International Journal of Group Psychotherapy, 38,* 275–301.

Phillips, R. D. (1978). Impact of Nazi Holocaust on children of survivors. *American Journal of Psychotherapy, 32,* 370–378.

Rappaport, E. A. (1968). Beyond traumatic neurosis: A psychoanalytic study of late reactions to the concentration camp trauma. *International Journal of Psycho-Analysis, 49,* 719–731.

Symonds, M. (1980). The "second injury" to victims. *Evaluation and Change* [Special Issue], 36–38.

Tanay, E. (1968). Initiation of psychotherapy with survivors of Nazi persecution. In H. Krystal (Ed.), *Massive psychic trauma* (pp. 219–233). New York: International Universities Press.

Winnicott, D. W. (1965). *The maturational processes and the facilitating environment.* London: Hogarth Press.

16

Beyond Empathy:
New Directions for the Future

JACOB D. LINDY
JOHN P. WILSON

Trauma strikes at the souls of those who survive extremely stressful life events. Individuals who become afflicted by post-traumatic stress disorder (PTSD) and associated states such as depression, anxiety, depersonalization, phobias, and alterations in the self often seek professional help. In the most severe cases, traumatic injury produces injury to the very core of ego processes and the degree of coherence of the inner self of the survivor. Specialists who work with survivors and victims of traumatic stress commonly have their emotions stirred close to their core as well, despite professional training and education. Empathic strain under these circumstances may well be a universal experience rather than the rare and often disdained exception characteristic of traditional literature on countertransference. It can be argued, however, that clinical work and research with severely traumatized persons is of a different nature than traditional psychotherapy or treatment approaches (Ochberg, 1988). If for no other reason, traumatized survivors have had a part of their humanness and individual identity severely scarred and, in many cases, permanently altered.

In the sanctuary of the therapist's office, a relationship can be created that allows for recovery, healing, and the integration of the traumatic life experience. We have suggested in this book that countertransference processes are an integral part of post-traumatic therapy. Among our goals in this volume has been to expand the understanding of countertransference for those working in the field of traumatic stress. In striving toward this goal, it soon became apparent that a conceptual paradigm was required to provide a structure to the broad range of countertransference phenomena reported by clinicians, researchers, emergency responders, consultants, supervisors, and others.

A CONCEPTUAL MODEL

In Part I, we elaborated a theoretical model that attempts to identify the core elements and dimensions of countertransferences and their relationship to PTSD. Our purpose in constructing a moderately complex paradigm that includes a large number of variables is to give wide berth to workers in the field so that they could describe and associate their particular clinical findings within a comprehensive whole. Through collaborative efforts with the contributors we have begun to discover a deeper underlying structure to countertransference processes and the various mechanisms that govern the specific configurations manifested by clinicians. The five core psychological dimensions that underlie Type I (avoidant) and Type II (overidentification) countertransference configurations include affect, defense, coping mode, role boundary impact, and intellectual rationalization. In a manner analogous to how amino acids combine to form nucleic acids and specific peptide chains (such as DNA), the five core dimensions can configure into specific subtypes of Type I and Type II countertransference processes. Thus, while it is apparent that there is a wide range of possibilities within Type I and Type II countertransference reactions (CTRs), these different configurations are indigenous to posttraumatic therapy, and therefore it is necessary to understand, manage, and utilize them as sources of clinical insight about the dynamics of the therapeutic relationship.

In the process of writing this book we worked in an active, collaborative way with the contributors, sharing ideas that evolved around the theoretical scaffold of the conceptual models. The ongoing and ever-changing process among us provided constant "feedback loops" such that, as the various authors used the conceptual model, they were better able to observe and structure some of their own field work, which was occurring even as the book was being written. Armed with the contributors' insights and discoveries, we were able to refine and elaborate our theoretical model to accommodate new information. It was a gratifying and creative process that extended well beyond the scope of a book of edited chapters.

Although it may seem like a truism, the dynamics of countertransference in work with PTSD are complex, intricate, and often enormously subtle in their manifestation. It proves to be a useful organizational tool simply to clarify that countertransference occurs in a context in which the specific trauma variables need to be acknowledged along with variables in the client, the therapist, and the institution. Laying out some of the predictable tension points that may cause ruptures in empathy and the stress recovery process also had merit. If nothing else, recognizing the ubiquity of countertransference in work with PTSD also serves a normalizing function by clarifying that such reactions are as expectable, if not predictable, as are the symptoms of stress response following trauma.

Transference and countertransference are "lock and key" phenomena; two halves of a complementary process in post-traumatic work. In this regard, aligning the many forms of empathic strain into Type I and Type II reactive processes provides therapists with reference points in their work. The four modes of empathic strain (withdrawal, enmeshment, repression, and disequilibrium) add depth and an inclusive context to the post-traumatic therapy literature.

The recognition that *trauma-specific transference* is common among victims of trauma enables a conceptual link to be made. Transference projects by a client and the clusters of affects thus mobilized in the therapist are associated with characteristic defenses and coping modes within a category of empathic strain as part of Type I and Type II CTRs. Viewed from this perspective, the particular ways in which the boundaries of the treatment are stretched seem typical of given post-traumatic situations. Thus, there are manifest predictable elements in the diagnosing of actual countertransference events. Further, the specific manifestation of countertransference within the treatment or research process characterizes both the conscious and unconscious ways in which the therapist is likely to play out some trauma role such as protector, rescuer, comforter, perpetrator, or significant figure involved in the traumatic event.

One of the purposes of delineating the contextual ideas in Part I of the book is to assist therapists and others and to transform the treatment, research, or work setting into a safer place, a new containing structure where the terrible affect associated with the trauma may surface and find resolution. As the client struggles to achieve integration and assimilation of trauma, the therapist strives to manage countertransference to illuminate as yet unmetabolized elements of the trauma experience.

The authors of chapters in this volume took on the task of conveying their ideas on countertransference and trauma within the context of their own and their study group's work. They needed to base these ideas on their own clinical experience in the absence of an agreed-upon format for the trauma field as a whole. Moreover, they agreed to try to illustrate their ideas with in-depth clinical material. Each author needed to overcome understandable resistances, personal and practical, in revealing the work of one's group, one's colleagues, one's students, and oneself. Respecting the privacy of the client and therapist sometimes conflicts with having sufficient openness to clarify one's ideas. Preserving anonymity in clinical vignettes that touch on such volatile experiences is also difficult. What emerged was an opening up of dramatic and revealing case material, which tended at first to raise more questions than it answered. During the course of the writing process, virtually all of the contributors experienced periods of vulnerability, uncertainty, and self-doubt about their efforts to explain adequately the phenomena of affective reactive processes in their clinical work. And yet, each author strove to present new insights and understanding related to the outcome of their work.

DISCOVERIES

As we continued to explore what clinicians were thinking and feeling as they had difficult and painful experiences with their trauma patients, we became aware that new theory and technique were being elaborated, which, if accurately communicated in this book, could increase the effectiveness of those of us who daily confront and try to help trauma survivors.

The following observations are of special note. First, clinicians empathizing with the trauma survivor may preconsciously elaborate their own fantasies of how the perpetrator might be avenged or the victim restored. Second, the clinician's access to these "intervention fantasies" is central to permitting similar or different ones to emerge from the otherwise silent trauma victim (Nader, Chapter 7). Third, based on our own experience, empathy is invariably askew as we try to follow the experience of our trauma patient. It is important to be aware that we often "miss a step" and to allow this faulty empathy to cue us about the possible interference of our own countertransference tendencies. In hermeneutic terms, the identification of such cues is part of "getting in step" with our trauma patient (McCann & Colletti, Chapter 4).

Therapists are not the only individuals who may become vicariously traumatized and consequently develop CTRs. Many helpers/rescuers at the scene of disasters are prone to similar responses, which are insufficiently understood (Raphael & Wilson, Chapter 13). The workplace is an area where concepts regarding countertransference can usually be applied as well (Dunning, Chapter 14). In this regard it may be important to rethink procedures of critical incident stress debriefing to take into account countertransference due to vicarious traumatization.

Society and the helping institutions within them are also prone to countertransference, some of which further poison the recovery environment and interfere with otherwise conscientious efforts to help. Among the Dutch, a dark side of Calvinist tradition seems to hold the trauma sufferer in contempt (Op den Velde et al., Chapter 12); a patriarchal and sexist society blatantly permits rape trauma survivors to be further damaged by the legal and medical procedures carried out on behalf of the greater society (Hartman & Jackson, Chapter 8); a racist and capitalist ethic turns a blind eye toward the trauma problems of children in inner cities of the United States (Parson, Chapter 6); even in systems designed to help trauma survivors, such as the U.S. Department of Veterans Affairs, there are profound needs to deny trauma (Maxwell & Sturm, Chapter 11).

The very context in which the trauma history is recorded offers an antidote to some of the damaging influences mentioned above. We all stand in judgment under a higher moral law regarding the actions of political states who torture their citizens; thus we introduce a powerful counterweight to society's tendency to extrude its tortured survivors (Agger & Jensen, Chapter 10). Yet clinicians, themselves wounded healers, who worked with survivors in countries that use torture as a political tool, risk avoiding the range of hostile countertransference that may also arise in this work.

Culture plays an important role in post-traumatic therapy. Sometimes, as we set up clinics for refugees, we are cast in healing roles that come from other traditions. Here the introspective work of the clinician helps to elaborate the contours of such figures as the "Asian wise man" (Kinzie, Chapter 9).

DIRECTIONS FOR THE FUTURE

Where do we go from here? Although we respect the diversity of factors leading to countertransference in work with trauma survivors, we believe that a more holistic approach may be taken regarding CTRs within the psychotherapy of PTSD. We believe the operational concepts presented here need to be refined and studied as an area of empirical research. This will help us distinguish more precisely which points are stumbling blocks for which groups of survivors and for which groups of therapists. Different schools of clinicians tend to deal with countertransference differently, but all acknowledge its presence and would profit from systematic study of its prevalence and impact.

Post-traumatic therapy education and training of trauma therapists and nonprofessional trauma caregivers continues to be a major task for the mental health professions. Danieli (Chapter 15) has demonstrated that training trauma therapists in countertransference should be first priority, so that therapists have the capacity to be effective in clinical roles. A literature of expectable responses and recommended approaches to getting derailed treatments back on track supervision and various forms of quality assurance in the area of trauma therapy. Other elements in the treatment situation with trauma survivors, such as transference, the working alliance, interpretations, and resistances, could be critically examined by authors working with different trauma groups.

CONCLUSION

The insights that have emerged from the contributors to this book have created a foundation for additional research, clinical training, and education about the role of countertransference in work with PTSD. There are many new challenges and directions yet to be explored. Illuminating the role of countertransference has made it possible to look beyond the role of empathy to the deeper dimensions of the healing process that enable survivors to overcome victimization. In the treatment process, the "dance of empathy" is always fragile, with many factors that can adversely effect the stress recovery process. We believe that through empathic "stretching," or the capacity to successfully manage and contain CTRs, a critical therapeutic structure can evolve as a safe sanctuary in which the work of recovery occurs. In the process, both the client and helper will experience pain, stress, and challenges to their capacity to function with integrity and meaning. For the traumatized client, the task of transforming trauma and restoring a sense of wholeness is an existential task that counterbalances despair and hope. For the clinician, the responsibility of caring counterbalances uncertainty and constancy in sustained empathic efforts. The understanding of the role of countertransference in the treatment process is an important tool in the self-care of the therapist and in the development of a genuine capacity to guide the recovery from traumatization. It is our belief that future research will reveal new insights on the critical role of countertransference in helping traumatized individuals to find their unique pathways of healing.

REFERENCE

Ochberg, F. (Ed.). (1988). *Post-traumatic therapy and victims of violence.* New York: Brunner/Mazel.

Index